Diagnosis and Management of
DERMATOLOGIC
DISORDERS
Made Easy®

Diagnosis and Management of DERMATOLOGIC DISORDERS Made Easy®

(Including STDs, Leprosy, HIV and AIDS)

SECOND EDITION

SK Punshi

MBBS (Indore) DDV (Mumbai)
FIMS FDS (London)
Senior Consultant in Skin Diseases
Rajkamal Chowk, Amravati
Maharashtra, India

Foreword
SJ Yawalkar

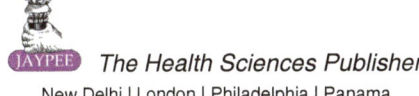

The Health Sciences Publisher
New Delhi | London | Philadelphia | Panama

Jaypee Brothers Medical Publishers (P) Ltd

Headquarters

Jaypee Brothers Medical Publishers (P) Ltd
4838/24, Ansari Road, Daryaganj
New Delhi 110 002, India
Phone: +91-11-43574357
Fax: +91-11-43574314
Email: jaypee@jaypeebrothers.com

Overseas Offices

J.P. Medical Ltd
83 Victoria Street, London
SW1H 0HW (UK)
Phone: +44 20 3170 8910
Fax: +44 (0)20 3008 6180
Email: info@jpmedpub.com

Jaypee Medical Inc
The Bourse
111 South Independence Mall East
Suite 835, Philadelphia, PA 19106, USA
Phone: +1 267-519-9789
Email: jpmed.us@gmail.com

Jaypee Brothers Medical Publishers (P) Ltd
Bhotahity, Kathmandu, Nepal
Phone: +977-9741283608
Email: kathmandu@jaypeebrothers.com

Jaypee-Highlights Medical Publishers Inc
City of Knowledge, Bld. 237, Clayton
Panama City, Panama
Phone: +1 507-301-0496
Fax: +1 507-301-0499
Email: cservice@jphmedical.com

Jaypee Brothers Medical Publishers (P) Ltd
17/1-B Babar Road, Block-B, Shaymali
Mohammadpur, Dhaka-1207
Bangladesh
Mobile: +08801912003485
Email: jaypeedhaka@gmail.com

Website: www.jaypeebrothers.com
Website: www.jaypeedigital.com

© 2015, Jaypee Brothers Medical Publishers

The views and opinions expressed in this book are solely those of the original contributor(s)/author(s) and do not necessarily represent those of editor(s) of the book.

All rights reserved. No part of this publication may be reproduced, stored or transmitted in any form or by any means, electronic, mechanical, photocopying, recording or otherwise, without the prior permission in writing of the publishers.

All brand names and product names used in this book are trade names, service marks, trademarks or registered trademarks of their respective owners. The publisher is not associated with any product or vendor mentioned in this book.

Medical knowledge and practice change constantly. This book is designed to provide accurate, authoritative information about the subject matter in question. However, readers are advised to check the most current information available on procedures included and check information from the manufacturer of each product to be administered, to verify the recommended dose, formula, method and duration of administration, adverse effects and contraindications. It is the responsibility of the practitioner to take all appropriate safety precautions. Neither the publisher nor the author(s)/editor(s) assume any liability for any injury and/or damage to persons or property arising from or related to use of material in this book.

This book is sold on the understanding that the publisher is not engaged in providing professional medical services. If such advice or services are required, the services of a competent medical professional should be sought.

Every effort has been made where necessary to contact holders of copyright to obtain permission to reproduce copyright material. If any have been inadvertently overlooked, the publisher will be pleased to make the necessary arrangements at the first opportunity.

Inquiries for bulk sales may be solicited at: jaypee@jaypeebrothers.com

Diagnosis and Management of Dermatologic Disorders Made Easy®

First Edition: 2010
Second Edition: **2015**

ISBN 978-93-5152-793-0

Dedicated to

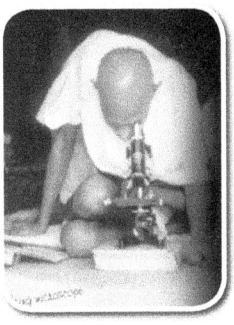

Father of the Nation—Mahatma Gandhi

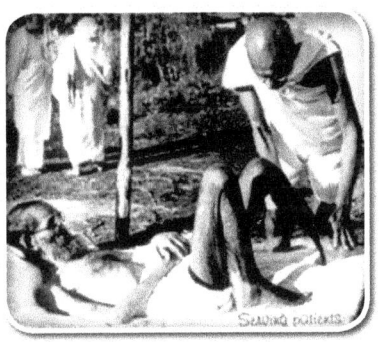

Mahatma Gandhi washing and dressing the leprosy ulcer of Acharya Parchure

"Leprosy work is not merely medical relief, it is transforming frustration in life into the joy of dedication, personal ambition into selfless service."

—*Rashtrapita Mahatma Gandhi*

Foreword

Skin is a living barrier between ourselves and the outside world. This largest organ of the human body, comprising of 15% of the total body weight, forms an effective barrier against invasion of the body by microorganisms and protects against loss of water. Part of our first line defence system is the non-specific mechanical barrier provided by the skin.

Skin diseases today constitute about 10 to 15% of the general practitioner's workload. The incidence of eczemas and allergic dermatoses is increasing every year, due to the ever-expanding range of cosmetics, detergents, dyes and chemicals.

The dermatologist is no more a "pimple and itch doctor" but is responsible for the diagnosis and treatment of serious diseases such as leprosy, skin cancers, exfoliative dermatitis and pemphigus. Due to recent impressive progress in this specialty, our understanding of skin diseases has considerably expanded. Dermatology, once a neglected subject, has now achieved the status it deserves. The old saying identifying dermatology with tons of Latin and ounces of vaseline is no more true. Corticosteroids have revolutionized the treatment of skin diseases. Therapy of cutaneous diseases may well be divided into: BC and AC (before corticosteroids and after corticosteroids).

Now, dermatologists have to cope up with the recent knowledge about genetic diseases, genes, RNA and DNA markers, etc. well and in the future the genetic dermatological diseases which may be cured can be prevented before birth. This monograph includes concise and clinically relevant information on commonly encountered skin diseases. There are quite a few books on dermatology but like paintings by different artists, each is different from the others. I am of the conviction that this book with typical photographs should be of immense use for general practitioners and dermatologists who do like to accept responsibility of the patient's skin condition once the consultant has given his opinion. I am sure that this interesting book will stimulate further reading on skin diseases and no doubt it would be a welcome addition to the current literature on dermatology.

SJ Yawalkar MD DVD
Dermatologist
International Clinical Research
Ciba-Geigy Ltd, Basel, Switzerland
Formerly, Director, Skin Department
GT Search Hospital
Grant Medical College
Mumbai, Maharashtra, India

Preface to the Second Edition

Since publication of the first edition in 2010 and pharmaceutical edition 2014, there have bean persisting demands for the revised edition in the previous years. There have been considerable advances in the field of dermatological therapy beside the understanding of the subject has been revolutionized.

My personal opinion is that emphasis should be made on clinical practice of the subject rather than on long winded hypothesis and jungle of terminology.

This book incorporates and encompasses the advances in the subject. The text has been modernized, expanded, revised and made up-to-date.

The dermatitis eczema, pyoderma, psoriasis, tuberculosis, vitiligo, melasma, and antiaging are completely revised and necessary additions have been made. New flowcharts and new clinical photographs have been added.

The book contains subject matter in a comprehensive manner with emphasis on clinical and etiological diagnosis, prognosis and treatment in all practical details as would be required by both basic doctor and specialist in this day-to-day practice.

I hope the second edition of *Diagnosis and Management of Dermatologic Disorders Made Easy* will help students and medical practioners to understand the vast subject of skin diseases and therapy and render service to the patients at large.

The father of nation Mahatma Gandhi gave stress to the eradication of leprosy and he washed the leprosy ulcers of Acharya Parchure.

Late prime minister Jawaharlal Nehru emphasized on the cure of vitiligo and leukoderma.

Prime minister Narendra Modi has given a slogan "Clean and Healthy India", the cleaning of the house and environment will prevent bacterial parasite infections like scabies, lice infestations, house mites, and dust that causes allergy, asthmas, itching and another skin diseases can be prevented by cleanliness. "Cleanliness is next to Godliness" is a common sense. I end with the following Vedic prayer:

"Oh God I don't want any kingdom nor desire to get a heaven,
I opt that my hands should cure and serve the poor and needy at large".

SK Punshi

Preface to the First Edition

*"I do not ask you either your opinion or
your religion but what is your sufferings."*
— **L Pasteur**

"For the uninitiated dermatology is difficult. Diagnosis seems impossible because different things look exactly the same and the similar things appear entirely different. Even when similar things turn out to be the same, there remains the problem of names," Mit Chell MD Practitioner 208, 597 (1972). Considering the above dictum, I have simplified the subject of dermatology for the students, general practitioners and dermatologists, especially working in rural and urban areas.

This book is more or less like a ready-reckoner and is meant for rapid reading.

I am not an expert diver, hence I could not dive deep into the bottom of vast and unfathomable ocean of dermatology hence could not bring out pearls. But I am confident I have collected a few pebbles while sitting and silently playing at the bank of river of dermatology.

In this book I have incorporated a few essays on most common topics which we see and confront in day-to-day practice hence I have not followed the standard textbook classification.

This book is concise, succinct, and aptly illustrated with clinical photographs. The treatment part is up-to-date.

I end these few words with them following Vedic prayer:
"Sarve Bhavantu Sukhinah
Sarve Santu Niramayah,
Sarve Bhadrani Pashyantu
Makashchid Dukh Bhag Bhavet"

Oh Lord! Keep all healthy and happy. Keep us all free from disease and decay, pain and sufferings. Please Lord, give us peace and bliss.

SK Punshi

Acknowledgments

I am thankful and highly indebted to the following for the publication of this book:
- Professor, Dr SJ Yawalkar, for writing the highly encouraging and thought provoking foreword for this book.
- Dr Rakesh, Rekha, Kavita and Poonam, for secretarial work and for arranging the photographs.
- Mr Rajesh P Salwe, Proprietor of Goldline Computers, Amravati, for computer manuscript work.
- I thank profusely my patients, who allowed me for the clinical photographs time to time for clinical research in the service of humanity at large.
- Lastly, I am grateful to Shri Jitendar P Vij (Group Chairman), Mr Ankit Vij (Group President) and Mr Tarun Duneja (Director-Publishing) of M/s Jaypee Brothers Medical Publishers (P) Ltd, New Delhi, India, for publishing this book in time and also for clear and meticulous presentation of the text and illustrations.

Contents

1. **GLOBAL PANORAMA OF DERMATOLOGY INCLUDING SCOPE OF SKIN DISEASES IN INDIA** — 1
   Introduction 1
   The Indian Scenario 2
   The World Statistics 2
   Scope of Dermatology 3
   Skin Conditions Caused by Parasites 4
   Stress and Skin 4

2. **STRUCTURE OF SKIN** — 9
   Layers of Epidermis 10
   Epidermal Cell Multiplication Cycle 11
   Important Cells of Epidermis 12
   Melanocytes and Biology of Melanin 12
   Epidermal Appendages 13
   Dermis 18
   Dermoepidermal Junction 19

3. **PHYSIOLOGY OF SKIN** — 20
   Immunological Function of Skin 22
   Embryology of Skin 22
   Allergy and Immunology 24

4. **DIAGNOSIS OF DERMATOLOGICAL DISEASES** — 27
   Symptoms 28
   Signs 30

5. CUTANEOUS INFESTATIONS: SCABIES AND PEDICULOSIS 52
Scabies 52
Pediculosis (Lice Infestation) 58
Human Demodex Mite: The Versatile Mite of
    Dermatological Importance 62

6. CUTANEOUS INFECTIONS WITH PYOGENIC BACTERIA 64
Impetigo (Impetigo Contagiosa) 64
Ecthyma 64
Folliculitis 65
Furuncle and Carbuncle 68
Carbuncle 69
Acute Paronychia 69
Periporitis (Multiple Sweat Gland Abscesses) 69
Erysipelas and Cellulitis: Pitted Keratolysis
    Therapy of Bacterial Infections 70

7. CUTANEOUS TUBERCULOSIS 73
Epidemiology 73
Etiology 74
Pathogenesis 75
Investigations 75
Diagnosis 75
Differential Diagnosis 76
Treatment 76
Clinical Features 76
Tuberculids 77

8. FUNGAL INFECTIONS (MYCOSIS) 79
Pityriasis Versicolor (Tinea Versicolor, Dermatomycosis,
    Furfuracea, Chromophytosis) 80
Candidiasis 81
Dermatophytosis 88
Deep Fungal Infections 102

Contents xvii

9. VIRAL INFECTIONS 114
Molluscum Contagiosum 115
Types of Viral Warts 116
Other Varieties of Warts 124
Varicella [Chickenpox, Primary Infection with Varicella Zoster Virus (VZVI)] 127
Herpes Zoster 127
Herpes Simplex 134
Herpes Labialis 135
Herpes Genitalis 136

10. ECZEMAS AND DERMATITIS 140
Etiologic Grouping of Eczemas 141
Etiology and Pathogenesis 144
Common Patterns of Eczema 147
Atopic Eczema 147
Contact Dermatitis 148
Atopic Dermatitis 148
Infantile Eczema (Eczema in Infants) 150
Seborrheic Dermatitis 162
Irritant Contact Dermatitis 167
Allergic Contact Dermatitis 169
Pompholyx 174
Lichen Simplex Chronicus 176
Nummular (Discoid) Eczema 177
Stasis Eczema (Gravitation Eczema) 178
Asteatotic Eczema 180
Diaper Dermatitis 180

11. DISORDERS OF SEBACEOUS AND SWEAT GLANDS 186
Acne Vulgaris 186
Acne Scarring 193

Rosacea (Acne Rosacea) 198
Perioral Dermatitis 198

12. PAPULOSQUAMOUS DISEASES   200
Psoriasis 200
Sympathetic Reception 225

13. DISORDERS OF PIGMENTATION   246
Albinism 247
Vitiligo 247
PUVA Therapy 262
Treatment 275

14. DRUG REACTIONS   293
Common Eruptions due to Drugs 293
Fixed Drug Eruption 295
Erythema Multiforme 296
Stevens-Johnson Syndrome 296
Toxic Epidermal Necrolysis 296
Miscellaneous Drug-induced Rashes 297

15. DISORDERS OF HAIR AND NAILS   304
Alopecia 304
Hypertrichosis 313
Nails 313

16. SKIN AND INTERNAL DISEASE   330
Skin Manifestations of
    Collagen Vascular Diseases 331
Lupus Erythematosus (LE) 331
Scleroderma 331
Skin Manifestations of Systemic Lupus
    Erythematosus (SLE) 332
Butterfly Rash 335

17. VESICOBULLOUS DISORDERS 337
Pemphigus 338
Dermoepidermal Bullae 344
Erythema Nodosum 348
Erythroderma (Exfoliative Dermatitis) 349
Nutritional Deficiencies 351

18. SKIN TUMORS 355
Cutaneous Neoplasms, Benign, Premalignant and Malignant Tumors of the Skin 355
Benign Neoplasms 357
Acanthosis Nigricans 357
Carotenemia 358
Cutaneous Hyperplasias 358
Nevi 359

19. MISCELLANEOUS DISORDERS 367
Subcutaneous Nodules 367
Vesicular Rash 373
Rash with Fever 374
Hirsutism 376
Prurigo Mitis 379
Aphthous Ulcer 379
Miliaria (Prickly Heat, Heat Rash) 380
Pruritus (Itching) 380
Urticaria, Angioedema 383
Skin Changes and Old Age 389
Hidradenitis Suppurativa 392

20. ICHTHYOSIS AND KERATODERMAS 400
Ichthyosis 400

21. LEPROSY (HANSEN'S DISEASE) 407
Mode of Transmission 407
Incubation Period 408

Prevalence 408
Classification of Leprosy Based on Clinical, Microbiologic, Pathologic and Immunologic Parameters 408

22. SEXUALLY TRANSMITTED DISEASES 423

Syphilis 426
Urethritis 431
Non-gonococcal Urethritis 433
Genital Ulcerative Disease (Including DD of Genital Ulcers) 434
Chancroid (Soft Chancre) 435
Filariasis 439
Lymphogranuloma Venereum (LGV) 439
Practical Management of STDs (Syndromic Management of STDs) 439

23. HIV AND AIDS 443

Human Immunodeficiency Virus 443
Immunopathogenesis of HIV Infection 444
Epidemiology and Transmission of HIV Infection 444
Natural History of HIV Infection 445
Clinical Features and Stages of HIV Infection 446

Bibliography 471
Further Reading 477
Index 481

CHAPTER 1

Global Panorama of Dermatology including Scope of Skin Diseases in India

INTRODUCTION

Dermatology is an essential part of general medicine and with clientele of family physician. Since the skin is not, by any means, foreign to the body which it covers. Diseases of the skin are a common occurrence. There are not many statistics to prove the exact frequency of skin diseases in this country, but commonly 20% of the skin diseases, a family physician and treating dermatologist encounters them in their day-to-day practice. A survey among school children in London revealed that skin diseases were responsible for an absentee rate of 23 per 100 children. Amongst the industrial workers covered by the Employees' State Insurance Scheme, there is a high rate of absenteeism due to skin diseases. While infections are more common in the tropics, chemical and psychogenic dermatoses are common in Western countries. There is no truth in the statement that skin diseases are to be found only in the tropics.

THE INDIAN SCENARIO

The skin diseases, which commonly found in tropical and developing countries like India, Pakistan, Bangladesh, Sri Lanka, Maldives are pyodermas, scabies, fungus infections, leprosy, STDs, HIV. The most commonly states in India affected by these diseases are Maharashtra, Tamil Nadu, Manipur, Central parts of Madhaya Pradesh and Chhatisgarh, Uttar Pradesh and Haryana.

THE WORLD STATISTICS

Most of the African countries still suffer from diseases occuring from malnutrition, avitaminosis, hypoproteinemia, leprosy, STDs, HIV, AIDS. The diseases in the developed and advanced countries are because of industrial pollution,

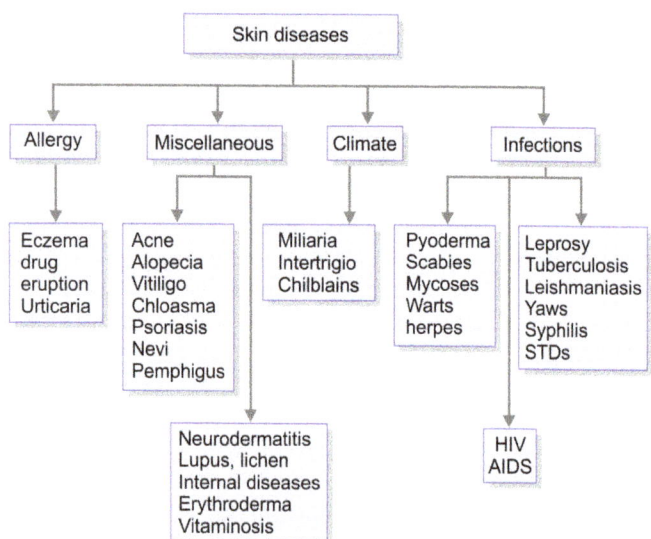

Flowchart 1.1: Skin diseases in India

chemical factories, rubber, nylon and synthetic dyes, etc. are the common causes of skin diseases. The modern stress and strain of human life are also contributing diseases like neurodermatitis, eczemas, vitiligo, etc.

The epidemiology of skin diseases, the etiology, prevalence of the skin diseases, effects of skin diseases on the life of human beings depend on the geographical, ecological, environmental, social factors above all the education, status and information of the masses.

SCOPE OF DERMATOLOGY

Skin reflects the internal disease process. It is more or less a glass and mirror of the body. There are various causative factors like physical, emotional, stress and strain and other

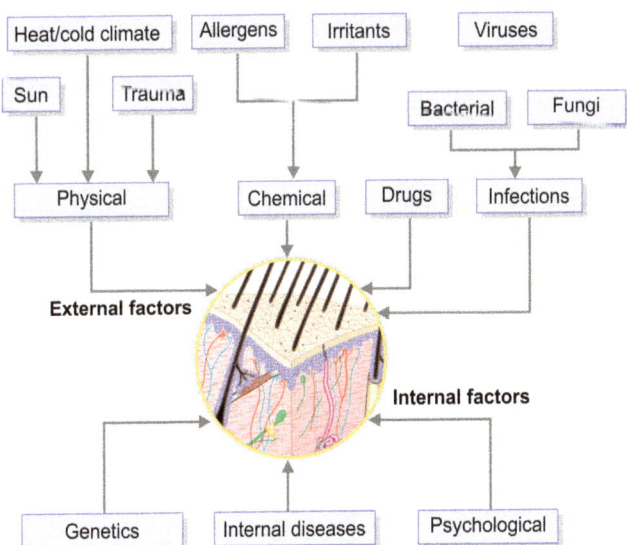

Flowchart 1.2: Etiology of skin diseases in general

known and unknown influences including genetics, genetic codes, RNA and DNA markers.

■ SKIN CONDITIONS CAUSED BY PARASITES

These infestations are caused by common insects. Mostly because of poverty, unhygienic conditions, crowded environments, poor nutrition and lack of education.

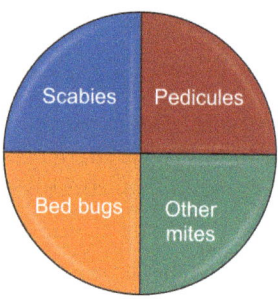

Fig. 1.1: Skin parasitosis

■ STRESS AND SKIN

Beauty is skin deep. It is a common saying. It is the largest organ of the body. It acts as a mantle or cover and protects from the external injuries. It is a important organ which creates unique shapes and hues in various individuals. If it is affected it will cause various reaction patterns.

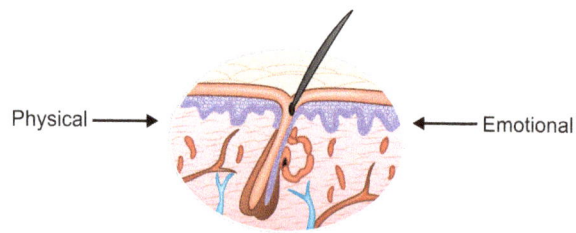

Fig. 1.2: Reaction patterns of skin

Skin disfigurement however may be a barrier to privileges and opportunities because of the profound social significance of appearance and the attitudes and prejudices of the society towards one whose appearance is atypical. Because of certain skin diseases, physically attractive people are believed to have more socially desirable traits than others.

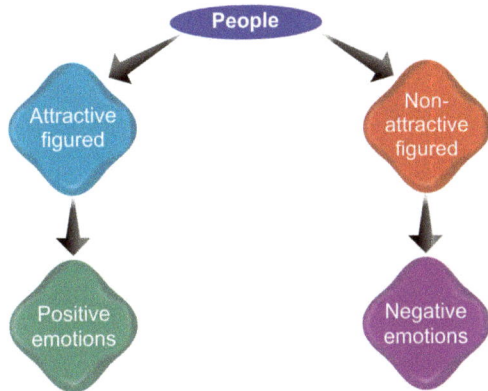

Fig. 1.3: Social attitude towards skin appearance

The outcome of the various response patterns may result into itching, pain, crawling, etc. The emotional responses may lead to disability and depression with negative thinking processes and causing into failures and disinterestedness in surroundings and in life.

The skin is affected by mind so called psyche. Also the human body is affected by emotions, stress and strain of life due to various factors, e.g. neurodermatitis, stress urticaria, etc.

The skin is the boundary between ourselves and the world around us. It is an important organ which acts as a mirror and window for the internal disease process which many times exhibits on the skin. This may produce not only psychological but functional and sociological impact on the patient and in severe cases, it may produce dejection and death.

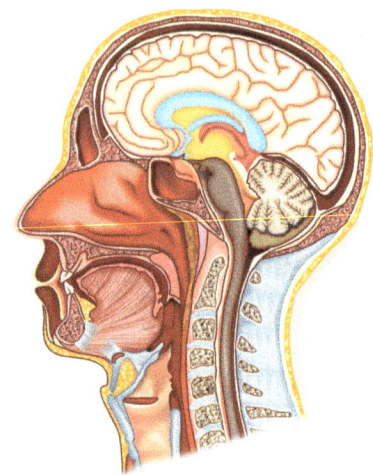

Fig. 1.4: Brain-mind-body axis

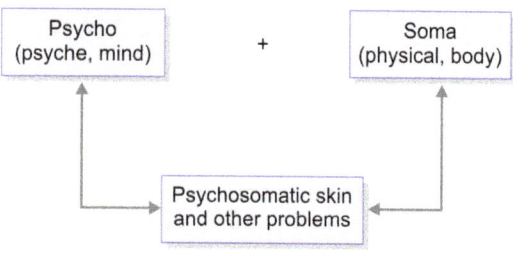

Fig. 1.5: Psychosoma

The course of the skin diseases is described and depicted as (1) Acute (2) Subacute (3) Chronic. Some of the disease are fatal, e.g. Penphigus, AIDS etc. The course and prognosis is depicted in the Figure 1.8.

Since time immemorial, over the course of evolution, nature prepared man to bear up to the various influences of his environment and to establish permanent contacts with changing environmental processes. During thousands

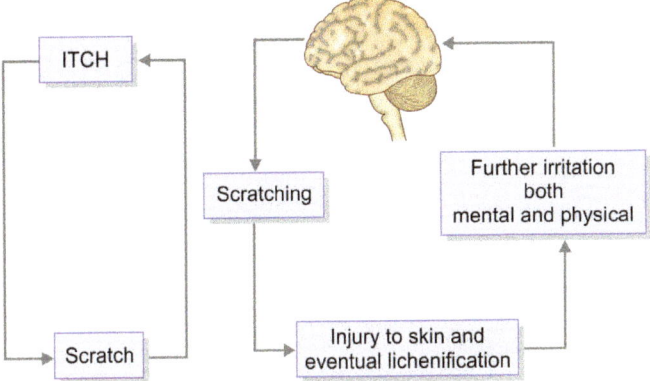

Fig. 1.6: Physiology of skin irritation

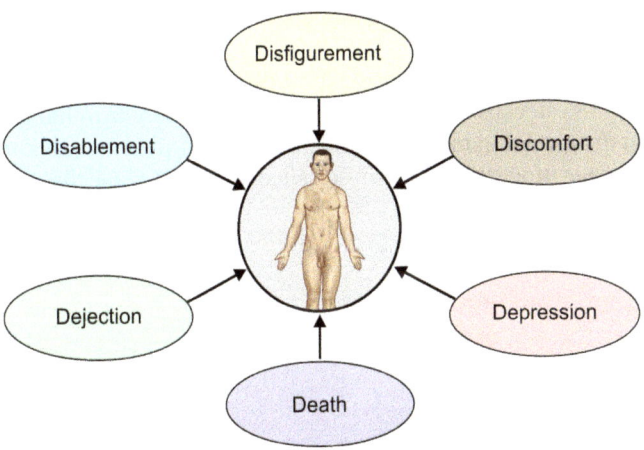

Fig. 1.7: Impact, perspective, course and outcome of skin disease

of years, biological rhythms developed in accordance with the activities of different functional systems of the body. Moreover, these rhythms changed parallel to changes in nature or environment.

Diagnosis and Management of Dermatologic Disorders

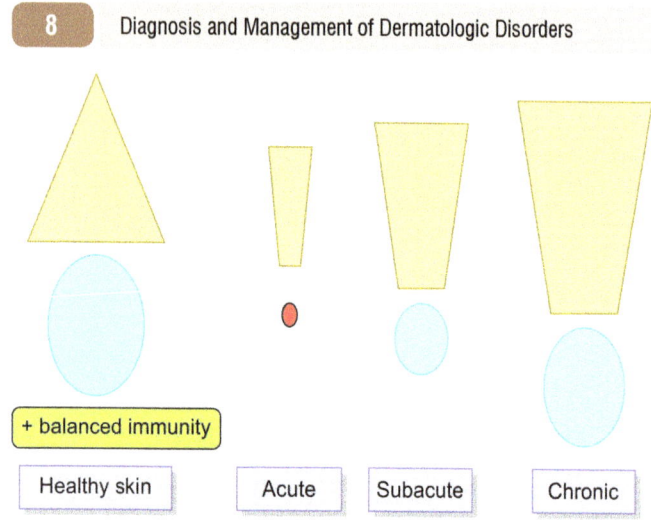

Fig. 1.8: The skin diseases

The skin is a mirror of the internal, systemic disease process. Because of the change of body immunity also changes in the local skin immunity will produce definite changes and disease process on the skin so called dermatological disease.

CHAPTER 2

Structure of Skin

Skin is the largest organ of the body. It is protective covering of the body. It, with all its specialized derivations, makes up what is called the integument (*Latin*: a covering) which covers the entire surface of the human body.

Skin consists of five parts (Fig. 2.1)

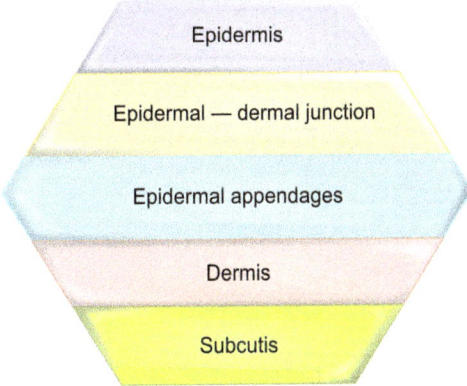

Fig. 2.1: Parts of skin

Diagnosis and Management of Dermatologic Disorders

The human skin shows wide regional variations in structure like scalp, face, ear lobes, back, palms and soles, etc. Thickness varies; the number of sebaceous glands, collagen fiber and vasculature differ in different parts of the integument.

LAYERS OF EPIDERMIS

Epidermis consists of:
- Stratum corneum (horny layer)
- Stratum lucidum
- Stratum granulosum (granular layer)
- Stratum malpighii (prickle cell layer)
- Stratum basale

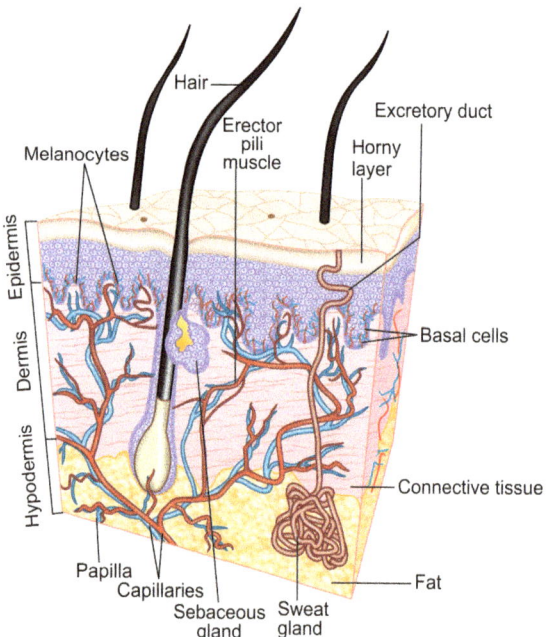

Fig. 2.2: Structure of skin

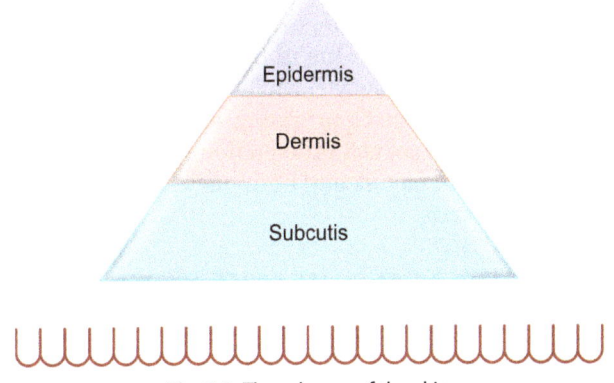

Fig. 2.3: Three layers of the skin

The epidermis is formed of nonvascular stratified epithelium. Its usual thickness is between 0.07 mm and 0.12 mm. But in certain parts like the soles of the feet and the palms of the hands, it is very thick, ranging from 0.8 mm to 1.4 mm. Squamous epithelium is 10–12 cells thick in the palms and soles and 3–4 cells over the eyelids and forearms. As viewed in three-dimensional manner the downward projections of epidermis are now referred to as rete ridges and not rete pegs. They are actually ridges of dermis.

The epidermis is mainly divisible into two main systems viz; keratinizing or malpighian system (keratinocytes) which forms the bulk and the pigmentary system (melanocytes) which produces the pigment. Melanin is transferred to the keratinocytes through the dendrites of melanocytes (cytocrine secretion).

EPIDERMAL CELL MULTIPLICATION CYCLE

The basal cell passes through a definite cycle as it multiplies. A newly formed cell is in the G_1 phase of the cell cycle. It synthesizes proteins, RNA and attains a definite size. It is then triggered to enter the S phase or the phase of DNA synthesis. The cell next enters the G_2 or postsynthetic phase and finally divides in the M phase. One of the daughter cells moves up to become a keratinocyte, while the other enters the G_1 phase (sometimes, the G_0 or resting stage). Various factors control the epidermal cell proliferation (epidermopoiesis). Cytokines, growth factors and hormones influence the rate of epidermopoiesis.

IMPORTANT CELLS OF EPIDERMIS

- Keratinocytes 85%
- Melanocytes
- Langerhans cells   } 15%
- Merkel cells

MELANOCYTES AND BIOLOGY OF MELANIN

Melanin pigmentation biosynthesis occurs under the influence of:
- Genetic factors
- Hormonal factors
- Ultraviolet radiation
- Other factors

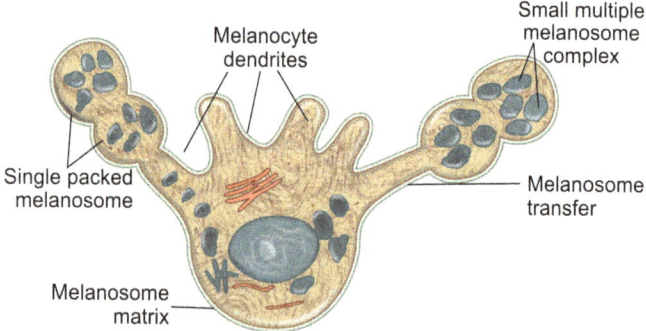

Fig. 2.4: Structure of melanocyte

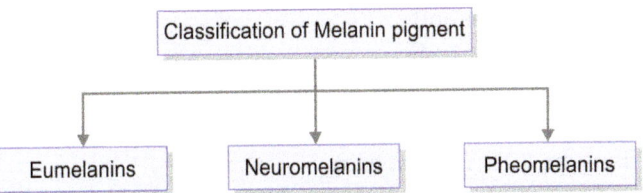

Fig. 2.5: Classification of melanin pigment

EPIDERMAL APPENDAGES

1. Hairs
2. Nails

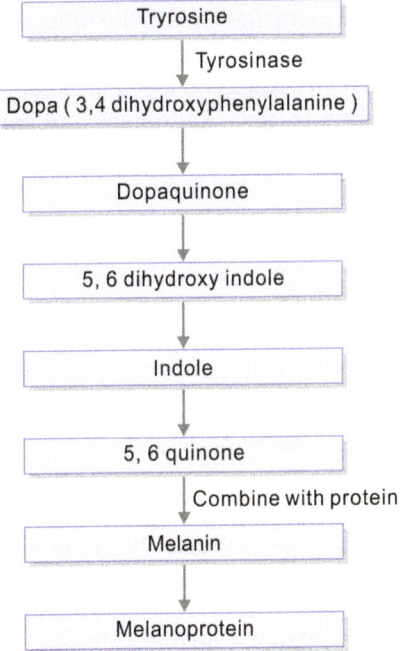

Fig. 2.6: Pathway of melanin pigment

3. Sweat glands and
4. Sebaceous glands

Hair

There are three types of hair:
1. Long, medullated, pigmented hair seen on the scalp.
2. Short, fine, nonmedullated and nonpigmented 'lanugo' hair seen in women, children, and on the faces and trunks of adults (vellus hair). Even in bald persons vellus hair may be present.
3. Thick bristles seen in the nose and ears.

Hair grows about 1–2 cm per month. The growth varies in different people, races and also on the different parts of the body.

Hair growth and development is under endocrine control. Fine balance of estrogens, androgens and gonadotropins determines the pattern in an individual.

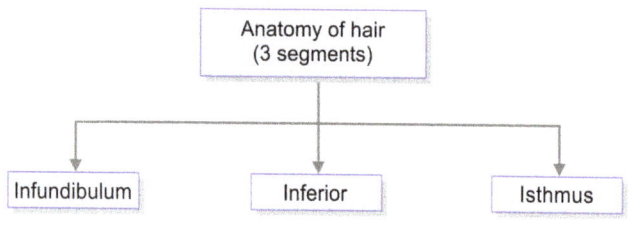

Fig. 2.7: Anatomy of hair

Life Cycle of Hair

The growth of the hair is cyclical. There are three phases in the life cycle of hair.

Anagen begins between the papillae and the undifferentiated cell. Mature anagens hair follicle consists of infundibulum. During catagen, entire inferior segment of

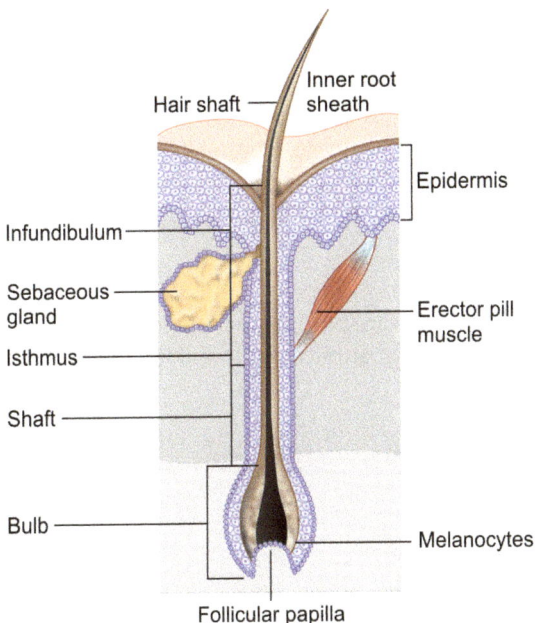

Fig. 2.8: Structure of hair

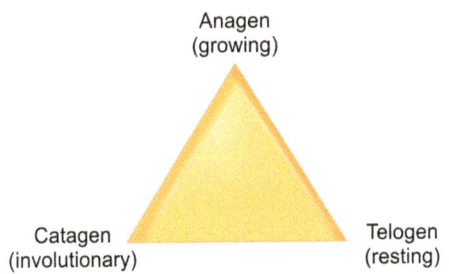

Fig. 2.9: Life cycle of hair

follicle shrivels upward as a thin cord of epithelial cells and is followed upward by the papillae. During telogen phase the hair melanocytes cease to synthesize melanin. This function of melanin formation begins against with anagen phase. Therefore, the root of the anagen hair is pigmented, whereas the tip of the telogen hair is unpigmented.

Arrector pili muscles are the small bundles of plain muscle fibers which extend from the connective tissue sheath of the hair follicles (below the level of the opening of the duct of the sebaceous gland) to the epidermodermal junction.

Nails

These are semi transparent, plate-like horny structures, covering the dorsal surfaces of the distal phalanges of the fingers and toes.

Structure of Nail

- Nail plate
- Nailbed
- Matrix
- Lateral nail-fold
- Lunula

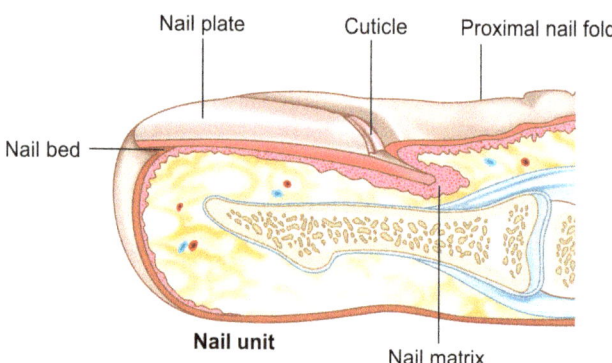

Fig. 2.10: Structure of nail

Functions of Nails

1. Protect terminal phalanges.
2. Cosmetic function.
3. Helps in appreciation of tactile stimuli.
4. Scratching of skin.
5. Helps in holding minute objects with finger tips.

Sweat Glands

There are three types:

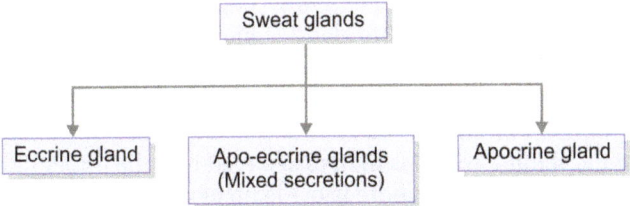

Fig. 2.11: Types of sweat glands

Eccrine Glands

They are the ordinary, small-sized sweat glands which are distributed all over the skin except on the beds of nails, margins of lips and the glans penis. Over 3 million sweat units are present and birth.

The glandular portion is a simple tube foled by a number of unequal twists into the shape of a ball.

Apocrine Glands

They occur in the axillae, areola and nipples of breasts, umbilicus, around the anus and the genitalia. Their glandular portion is very large and may measure 3-5 mm in diameter (the eccrine glands being only 0.3-0.4 mm in diameter). The myoepithelial cells are highly developed and more abundant in these glands. They are specialized sweat glands, and their secretion is odoriferous with a secondary sexual significance (pheromone).

Sebaceous Glands

They are scattered all over the intergument in association with the hair follicles. They are absent from the hairless portions of the body like the palms of the hands, the soles and sides of the feet. These glands, however, occur independently of hair follicules at certain places like the eyelids, margins of lips, external auditory meatus, nipples, anus and around the external genitalia, and at these sites the glands are more superficial. *Free* glands are found in the eyelids (Meibomian glands) mucos membranes (Fordyce spots), nipple, perianal region and genitalia. The gland is multilobed, being made up of lipid containing cells. The whole cell of the up of lipid containing cells. The whole cell of the sebeceous gland is secreted (this type of secretion is called holocine secretion) in the sebum, which is then discharged into the upper part of the hair follicle. Sebum is made up of a complex mixture of triglycerides, fatty wax esters, squalene and cholesterol.

DERMIS

This layer consists of bundles of collagen and elastic fibers arranged in a recticular fashion. It is profusely supplied with blood vessels. Superficially the dermis is condensed into a dense fibrous network—the basement membrane to which are attached the epidermal cells. Its deeper parts merge imperceptibly into the hypodermis. Beneath the basement membrane are distributed many blood vessels forming a capillary network which send up loops into the dermal papillae. These papillae are microscopic fiber—like processes projecting into the epidermis, which is moulded over and attached to them.

The connective tissue cells in the dermis are spindle—shaped and are more numerous in the superficial layers than in the deeper ones. Thickness of dermis is 1-3 mm.

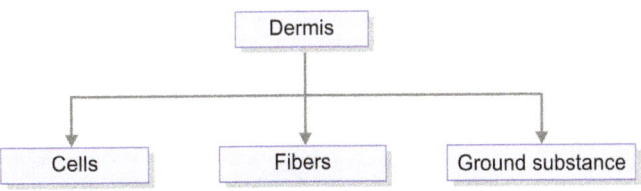

Fig. 2.12: Composition of dermis

Within the skin, the blood supply and drainage lie along well-determined pathways. There are rich capillary beds in the papillae and around the appendages and in subpapillary plexus; deep reticular plexus is much less rich. In the deeper layer of dermis, there is arteriovenous anastomosis surrounded by sphincter like group of smooth muscles under automatic control. Skin is richly innvervated by myelinated and nonmyelinated sensory fibers and via nonmyelinated autonomic fibers supplying blood vessels and appendages. Conspicuous nerve supply consists of plexuses in the papillae, Meissner's corpuscles, Pacinian corpuscles, Merkel's disks and nerve endings in the basal layer of the epidermis.

DERMOEPIDERMAL JUNCTION

Finger like projections extend upward from the papillary dermis and these are covered by epidermis so that the two interdigitate. To summarize, dermal tissue is composed of fibers
1. Collagen
2. Reticulum
3. Elastin
4. Ground substance
5. Cells
6. Blood vessels
7. Lymphatics
8. Nerves

and subcutis; it contains mainly fat and lower parts of eccrine and apocrine glands] hairs, nerves, lymphatics, vessels and cells, etc.

CHAPTER 3

Physiology of Skin

The skin perfoms a multitude of functions. These are:

(1) *Protective function:* As an organ of protection, the skin exhibits a wide range of modifications in the various species of animals. In human beings, the tough, horny, and keratinized waterproof epidermis, and appendages like hair and nails, provide sufficient strong barrier against injury.

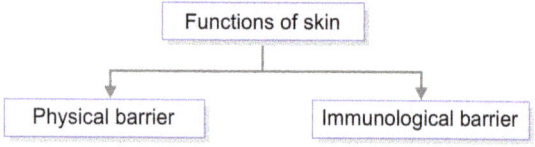

(2) *Sense organ:* The skin is richly supplied with nerves and various types of specialized sensory end-organs, which provide information regarding environmental changes.

(3) *Secretion and excretion:* The skin possesses various types of glands which pour secretions on the surface. Sweat in its composition consist of 1.2% solids (organic 0.4% and inorganic 0.8%) and 98.8% water. The important substances

excreted in it are: sodium chloride, sodium phosphate, sodium bicarbonate, keratin and a small amount of urea. Man perspires very little at low and moderate temperature, but his perspiration sharply increases at high temperature. The *sebaceous glands* of the skin secrete *sebum* which is composed of fatty acids, cholesterol, alcohols, etc. Excessive production of sebum is called seborrhea. Sebaceous glands undergo marked hypertrophy during puberty indicating hormonal control of these glands.

(4) *Body heat regulation:* The vital activity of warm blooded species like human beings is, in a large measure, independent of the temperature conditions of the external environments because of their constant internal temperature. *The skin plays the most important role in the regulation of heat loss.* It loses heat to the external environment in three ways: *by conduction,* by *radiation*. The heat loss through the skin is regulated by various physiological mechanisms which include (1) the reaction of the cutaneous vessels, (2) perspiration, and (3) the reaction of the smooth muscle fibers of the skin. *Hair also plays a major part in limiting the heat loss in animals.* Contraction of the arrector pili occurs at low temperatures.

(5) *Storage function of skin:* The dermis in conjunction with the hypodermis has a considerable capacity for string various materials, of these the best known are fat and blood.

(a) Fat is laid down in fat cells as a permanent store of subcutaneous adipose tissue. This provides the reserve stores of body energy. Incidentally, it also prevents heat loss, and is good shock absorber.

(b) Blood is stored in the rich subpapillary plexuses of the dermis. A rough estimate of its capacity in a normal adult comes to near about one liter. Whenever there is a greater requirement of blood by the muscles or other organs, blood is directed from this storehouse to those regions.

(c) The skin is also a good storehouse of ergosterol—the provitamin for vitamin D. This ergosterol is irradiated by the ultraviolet light of the sun and converted into vitamin D (calciferol).

(d) The other type of storage which occurs in the skin is what has been called by Cannon as *storage by inundation*. This, in fact, is the storage of extracellular fluid in the interstitial spaces.

(6) *Absorption:* It is almost an established fact that the uninjured skin is impermeable to watery solution of salts or other substances. Jons can, however, be made to permeate with the application of an electric current by a process known as *iontophoresis*.

(7) *Gaseous exchange through skin:* A small amount of gaseous exchange occurs through the skin. In man the amount of CO_2 exchanged through the skin is negligible compared to the amount exhaled from the lungs (near about 1/150–1/200 of that exhaled by the lungs). But in a thin skinned animal like the frog, the absorption of O_2 and the excretion of CO_2 through the skin may be sufficient for the proper oxygenation of its blood, so that it may continue to live even after the removal of its lungs.

IMMUNOLOGICAL FUNCTION OF SKIN

The skin immune system (SIS) is best considered as a functionally independent unit with components derived from the epidermis, dermis, blood vessels and lymphatics and acts as a immunological protective system or barrier.

EMBRYOLOGY OF SKIN

The whole of the skin, epidermis and dermis, is a unified integrated organ system, but it develops from two different primitive embryonic layers epidermis from the *ectoderm* and dermis from the *mesoderm*.

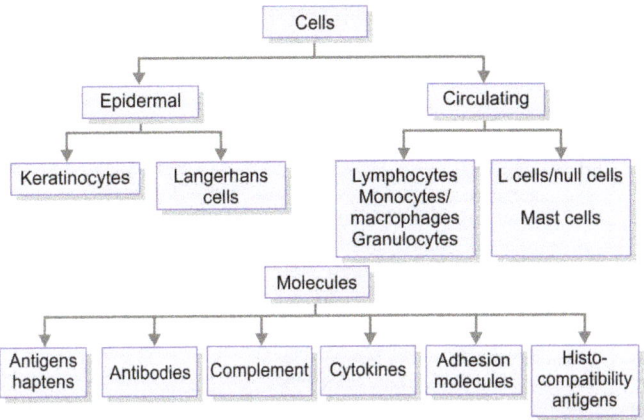

Fig. 3.1: Components of the skin immune system

SUMMARY

To summerise the functions of the skin
1. Barrier to the loss of water, electrolytes and macro molccules.
2. Regulation of body temperature.
3. Skin is sense organ for touch, temperature, pain and itch.
4. The skin surface has antibacterial and antifunal properties (normal flora and fauna).
5. Acid PH and negative electric charge on skin prevents bacteria, etc.
6. Vitamin D is produced on skin.
7. It is a secretary as well as excretary organ.
8. Skin regulates blood pressure.
9. Reservoir of electrolytes, water, vitamins, fats, carbohydrates, proteins, etc.
10. Immunological barrier.
11. It gives a clue to physician as indicator of internal disease process.

ALLERGY AND IMMUNOLOGY
Organs of the Immune System

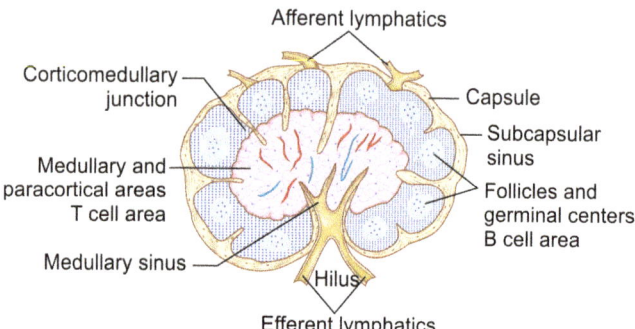

Fig. 3.2: Lymph node structure indicating primary T cell and B cell areas

Immune System Components

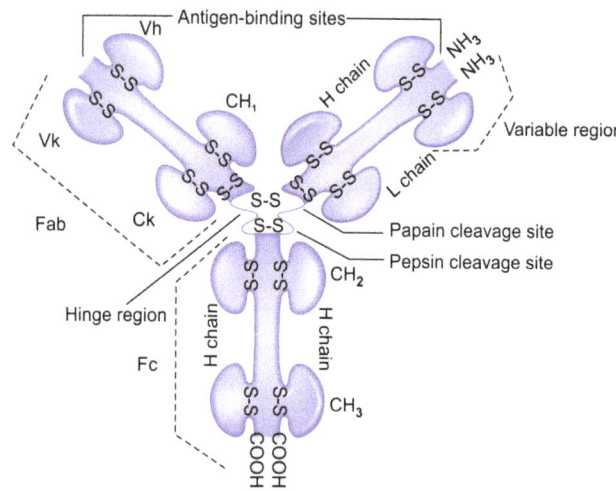

Fig. 3.3: Basic immunoglobulin structure with immunoglobulin subunits produced by enzyme

Antigen–Antibody Interactions Classification of Immunologic Reactions

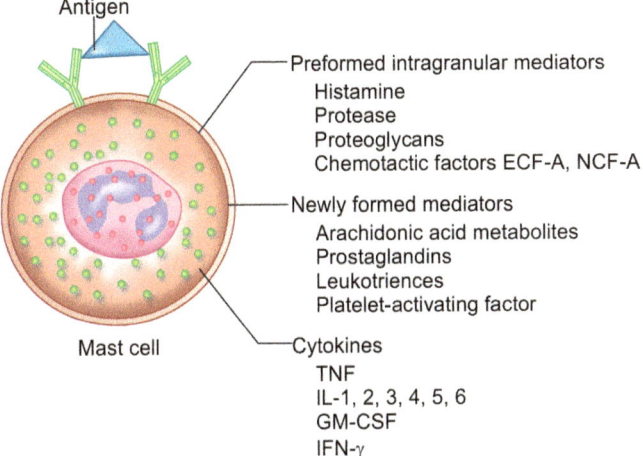

Fig. 3.4: Type 1: Anaphylactic of immediate hypersensitivity

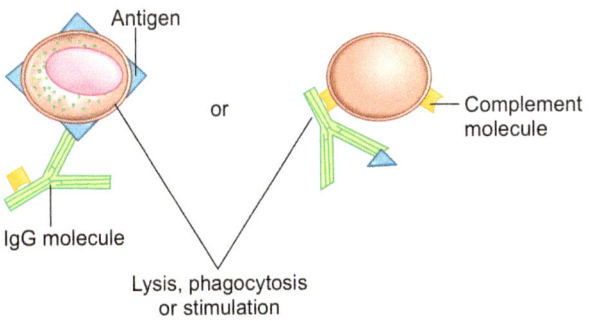

Fig. 3.5: Type 2: Cytotoxic reactions

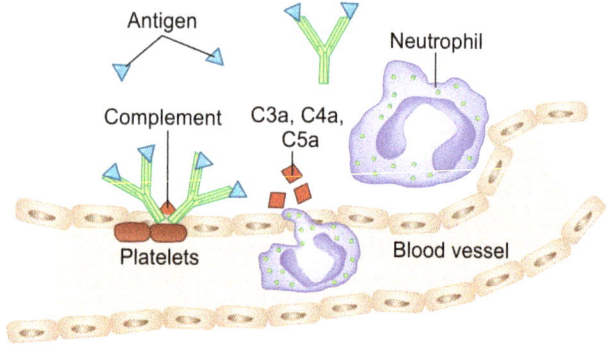

Fig. 3.6: Type 3: Immune complex-mediated reactions

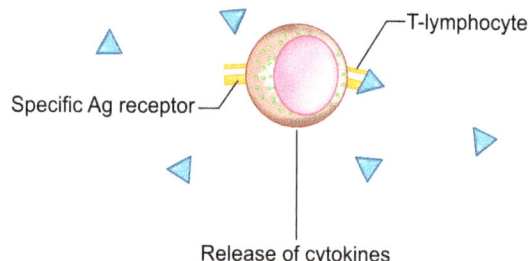

Fig. 3.7: Type 4: Delayed hypersensitivity

CHAPTER 4

Diagnosis of Dermatological Diseases

Three important steps in dermatological diagnosis are:
1. Morphological diagnosis based on morphological study, localization and distribution.
2. Clinical diagnosis—Etablishment of disease entity based on history and signs.
3. Etilogical diagnosis—establishment of cause or causes in the individual patient.

The ultimate aim of the treating physcian should be to establish the etiological diagnosis. Having established the diagnosis, information regarding activity, severity and acuity of the disease (prognostic criteria) be elicited and collected before treatment is prescribed.

The diagnosis of the skin diseases is started with the noting of clinical features, case statement and making general diagnosis which depends on the following factors:

History
a. Past history
b. Family history
c. Other history.

Social, occupational, travel and recreational history assist the physician in deducting a diagnosis.

Examination

Proper examination consists of:
1. Natural light
2. Examination of the whole body nakedly
3. Magnification
4. Looking for morphology of basic lesions which consists of
   (a) Shape
   (b) Distribution
   (c) Arrangement or configuration.

SYMPTOMS

The common symptoms of skin diseases are itching, pain and disturbed sensation in the nature of crawling, sense of heat, stinging, anesthesia or hyperesthesia. These subjective symptoms, as much as the apparent rash, are responsible for bringing the patient to the doctor for consultation.

1. *Itching (Pruritus).* It is an annoying complaint. Its intensity varies according to the disease and the sensitivity of the individual. It may be continuous or spasmodic, localized or generalized, accompanied or unaccompanied by a rash. The objective evidence of itching is scratch mark in the form of a linear excoriation. The common causes of itching are:

Scabies.	Urticaria.
Pediculoses.	Dermatitis herpetiformis.
Ringworm.	Neurodermatitis.
Eczema.	Insect bite.

Itching is typically absent in syphilitic rashes.

2. *Pain:* It may be localized to the skin, as in boils, abscesses, or radiate along a nerve, as in leprotic neuritis and herpes zoster.

3. *Crawling sensation (formication):* As if insects are crawling under the skin. It is a variety of itching e.g. acarophobia.

4. *Sense of heat:* In dermatological practice 'Heat in the blood' or Sense of Heat (in short, SOH) is not an uncommon complaint. It is seen as the first sign or symptom of drug eruption, in urticaria and allergy. Lay patients even call venereal diseases as Heat—'Garm' (Syphilis in Arabic means heat). Ayurveda, Hippocrates and Galen have laid stress on constitution, temperament and elementary qualities like heat, cold, dryness and moisture.

It is experienced as warm sensation to feeling of burning hot, warm to hot hands and feet, uncomfortable to burning sensation in the sun, and keeping feet and hands outside the covering while sleeping. Work done by Behl and Singh has convincingly proved that SOH is very significant in skin diseases especially of allergic origin. Almost every case of urticaria, drug rash and disseminated eczema is preceded or accompanied by SOH. This is more in cholinergic, physical urticarias. SOH, as a matter of fact, is a more useful guide than leukocyte count or allergy tests in urticaria and endogenous eczema. Further, according to our experience, persons with SOH are more prone to skin disease. May be change in eating and living habits (*Sattvic* vegetarian diet, no spices, chillies, tea, alcohol etc.) help to reduce the SOH and hence the predisposition to allergic dermatoses.

5. *Stinging sensation* is characteristic of stinging of insect bites.

6. *Hyperesthesia* signifies increased sensitivity, e.g. post-herpetic neuralgia.

7. *Anesthesia* signifies loss of sensations. It is noticed in leprosy, syringomyelia etc. The patient may notice the anesthesia himself, but usually it is found on physical examination. The sensations tested, pertaining to skin diseases are pain sensation (pin prick), touch and temperature (hot and cold).

SIGNS

Objective signs are more important in cutaneous diseases than subjective ones since cutaneous lesions are at once noticeable. Quite a few skin diseases are symptomless. Clinical lesions are basically, of two types:
1. Primary
2. Secondary

In case-taking, primary lesions are the most important. The differential diagnosis centers mostly around them. The clinician must look for the primary lesion in the most recently developed eruption or at the periphery of the rash. The history and observation of an intelligent patient will be helpful. With the passage of time, primary lesions either involute or transform or get modified into secondary lesions.

Primary Lesions

1. *Macule:* A macule is a small-sized, not raised, circumscribed lesion with alteration in color.

There are two types of macules:
(a) Erythematous
(b) Pigmentary

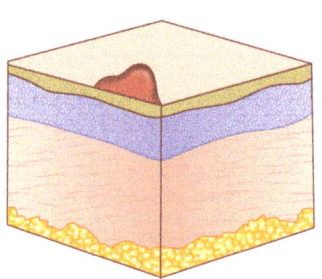

Fig. 4.1: Macule <1 cm

When of large size, this alteration in color is called a patch or a plaque or sheet of erythema or pigmentation.

A macule must be palpated for infiltration or induration which is typical of granulomatous diseases and reticuloses. Further, erythematous macules must be differentiated from purpuric macules. In the former, erythema disappears under pressure, while in the latter, the redness is brighter, and does not fade under pressure. Pigmentary macules are further differentiated into *hyperpigmented, hypopigmented, or depigmented types.*

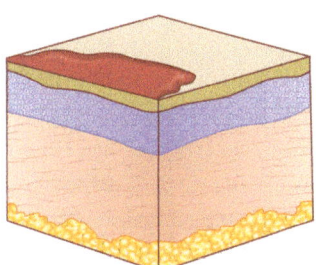

Fig. 4.2: Patch >1 cm

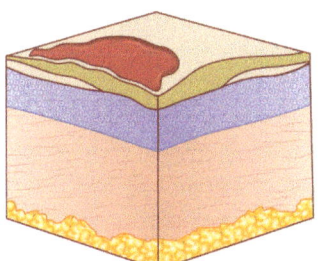

Fig. 4.3: Plaque >1 cm

The common causes of macular eruptions are:

Erythematous Macules
- Dermatitis
- Exanthemata
- Drug eruption
- Macular syphilide
- Erythema multiforme
- Tinea circinata
- Psoriasis
- Pityriasis rosea
- Leprosy

Heperpigmentary Macules
- Chloasma
- Fixed drug eruption
- Melanodermas
- Addison's disease
- Freckles
- Nevi
- Lentigines

Hypopigmentation
- Leprosy
- Tinea versicolor
- Pityriasis alba

Depigmentation
- Leukoderma
- Vitiligo

2. *Papule:* It is a solid, raised lesion about the size of a split pea or smaller. A similar lesion, but larger in size, is called, a *nodule* (as big as a hazel nut, or smaller), or *tumor* (bigger than a hazel nut). A papule may be a static lesion or a transition to other lesions; hence in practice, a dermatologist may come across *papulovesicular, papulopustular* and *erythematopapular lesions.*

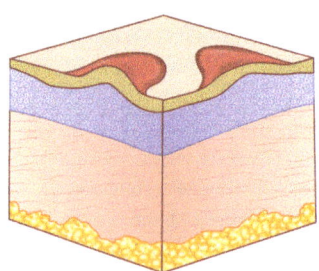

Fig. 4.4: Papule <1 cm

When dealing with papules, the points to be studied are: their size, shape, color; whether they be discrete or grouped; whether they be follicular or interfollicular; inflammatory or non-inflammatory in nature. Further, an attempt should be made to distinguish epidermic from dermic and mixed papules. An epidermic papule is usually superficial, dry, solid and flesh-colored; and dermic papule is deeper, elastic and raddish. The common causes of papules are:

- Warts
- Epidermal and dermal nevi
- Drug eruptions
- Syphilis
- Chickenpox and smallpox
- Psoriasis
- Lichen planus
- Lichen scrofulosorum
- Lichen spinulosus
- Eczema and eczematides
- Acne vulgaris
- Rosacea
- Prickly heat
- Tumors

Papules in Lines
- Warts
- Insect bites
- Psoriasis
- Lichen planus

Examples of Nodules
- Nevi
- Neurofibromatosis
- Skin cancer
- Dermal leishmaniasis
- Leprosy
- Syphilis
- Tuberculosis cutis
- Sarcoid
- Erythema nodosum
- Xanthomatosis
- Mycosis fungoides

Examples of Tumors
- Epithelioma
- Lymphosarcoma
- Mycosis fungoides
- Gumma
- Keloid
- Xanthoma
- Nevi
- Lipomas
- Neurofibromas
- Secondary carcinomatosis
- Sarcoid

3. *Vesicle:* It is a circumscribed, serum or plasma-containing elevation of the integument. When ruptured, the contents ooze out. The size of a vesicle varies from the size of a pin-

head to that of a small pea. A similar lesion, but larger in size, is called a *bulla*. The following characters of vesicles must be studied: their shape, size is there uniformity or irregularity of shape or size? Are they tense or flaccid, grouped or discrete? What is the mode of evolution? As a rule, vesicles are transitory and of short duration; they either rupture and ooze, or their contents coagulate to form crusts, or enlarge to form bullae, or transform into pustules, or their roofs get rubbed off to leave behind a moist, raw surface. On the palms of the hands, they are situated rather deeply, hence, their contents are discharged with difficulty. On the mucous membranes, their roofs get rubbed off very easily producing erosions. The common causes of vesicles are as follows:

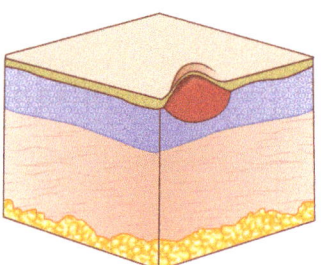

Fig. 4.5: Vesicle <1 cm

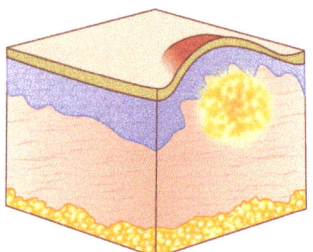

Fig. 4.6: Nodule >1 cm

Eczema, cheiropompholyx
Herpes simplex
Impetigo
Herpes zoster
Miliaria crystallina and rubra
Scabies
Smallpox
Chickenpox
Dermatitis herpetiformis
Tinea
Drug eruptions
Insect bites

The common causes of bullae are:

Impetigo contagiosa
Erythema multiforme
Pemphigus
Dermatitis herpetiformis
Insect bites
Epidermolysis bullosa
Hydroa aestivale
Drug eruptions

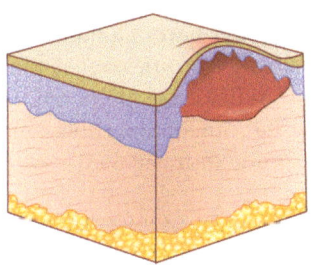

Fig. 4.7: Bulla >1 cm

4. *Wheal:* It is a flat, evanescent swelling of the skin caused by the local dilatation of blood vessels and increased permeability resulting in localized edema. The temporary, evanescent nature of a wheal and its duration (from a few hours to a maximum of 24 hours or so) is characteristic; it helps distinguish a wheal from a persistent granulomatous lesion. Wheals disappear without leaving any trace of stains, scars or atrophy. A wheal is usually pale in the center and red at the periphery, but it may be uniformly whitish or reddish. Common examples of wheals are as follows:

Urticaria
Insect bites
Trauma
Urticaria pigmentosa

Occasionally, a weal may be surmounted by a vesicle, e.g. papular urticaria of childhood, or accompanied by bulla formation, e.g. urticaria bullosa.

5. *Pustule:* It differs from a vesicle or a bulla in the nature of its contents. It is a purulent, fluid-containg elevation. It may arise as such, or it may be a transformation from a papule, or more so, a vesicle. The following characters should be studied: the size, shape, number. Is the pustule discrete or confluent, epidermal or follicular, superficial or deep?

An example of a superficial, epidermal pustule is impetigo, and of a deep, epidermal pustule is ecthyma. When a pustule is in the upper part of a hair follicle, it is called *folliculitis*. When it is in the deeper part of a hair follicle and involves the root of the hair which comes out as the core, it is called *furunculosis* (boil). When a conglomeration of boils forms a deep, dermic abscess with multiple holes on the skin through which pus is discharged, it is called a *carbuncle*. Pustules terminate by rupture, or desiccate to form irregular yellow crusts. Common examples of pustules are as follows:

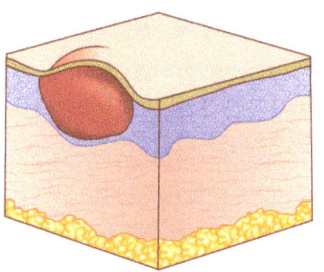

Fig. 4.8: Pustule <1 cm

Impetigo
Sycosis barbae
Carbuncle
Drug eruptions (iodides and bromides)
Acne vulgaris
Bacteroides
Furunculosis
Scabies
Anthrax
Tuberculides
Smallpox and chickenpox

Secondary Lesions

1. *Scale or Squama.* It is a dry exfoliation of the skin due to increased or abnormal formation of stratum corneum (hyper- or parakeratosis). It results from erythema or inflammation of the skin or increased dryness. Study the following characters: the color, shape; whether the scale is dry or greasy; whether it is thin or thick, loose or adherent, whether powdery or squamous etc.

In certain cutaneous diseases they are very characteristic, hence, of diagnostic value, e.g. the silvery layer-upon-layer scales of psoriasis, the greasy scales of seborrheic dermatitis, the cigarette-paper-like centripetal scaling of pityriasis rosea, the furfuraceous (powdery) scaling of pityriasis versicolor and the adhesive scale, with its nutmeg-like under-surface of lupus erythematosus. In other disorders, the diagnosis is

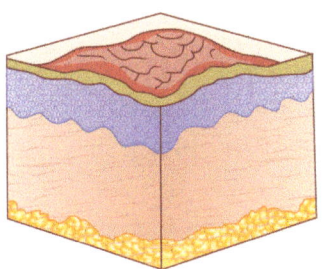

Fig. 4.9: Scale

based upon the primary lesion to which the secondary feature of scaling has been added. The important causes of scaling are as follows:

Dermatitis and eczema	Seborrheic dermatitis
Psoriasis	Pityriasis versicolor
Exfoliative dermatitis	Tinea corporis
Pityriasis rubra pilaris	Drug eruptions
Tinea capitis	Ichthyosis
Syphilis	Lichen planus
Lupus erythematosus	Malnutrition—pellagra
Exanthemata—following scarlet fever	Pityriasis rose

2. *Crust or scab:* It represents a dried-up mass of oozing and other products of inflammatory tissues particularly epithelial debris. Scabs form on vesicles, pustules, bullae, ulcers, erosions and excoriations. The color, thickness, adhesiveness, consistency and odour of a crust should be studied, also its underlying surface, visible only after the crust has been removed.

These characters of the crust, its underlying surface and the primary lesion which the crust has supplemented, are all helpful in the making of an accurate diagnosis. The common causes of crusts are as follows:

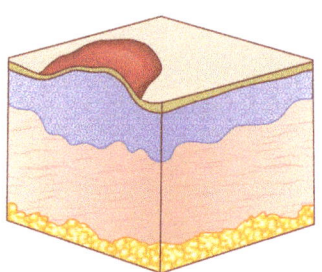

Fig. 4.10: Crust

Impetigo contagiosa, ecthyma
Sycosis

Seborrheic dermatitis
Pemphigus
Eczema and dermatitis

Exanthemata—chickenpox and smallpox
Herpes zoster

Ulcers
Kaposi's varicelliform eruption
Drugs—iodides, bromides and heavy metals
Syphilis—rupial and noduloulcerative
Scratch marks (blood crusts).

3. *Excoriations:* They are superficial, linear lesions characterized by the removal of the epidermis by scratching or by abrasion. An excoriation may be superficial or deep. It gets covered by a crust—simple, blood or impetiginous.

It is produced by trauma; an excoriation is an evidence of pruritus; a search should be made for its cause.

4. *Fissure:* It is a linear crack in the integrity of the skin reaching down to the papillary layer of the dermis, or deeper. It has length but unlike an ulcer, no breadth. A fissure is usually accompanied by pain which interferes with the use of the affected part. Because of the loss in integrity, there is risk of secondary infection. Common examples of fissures are as follows:

Chapping of hands as in extreme dryness
Chronic eczema of the palms and soles
Menopausal keratoderma
Syphilitic fissures
Fissure in ano
Angular stomatitis.

5. *Erosion:* Breach in skin continuity due to loss of part of whole of epidermis and without any dermal damage.

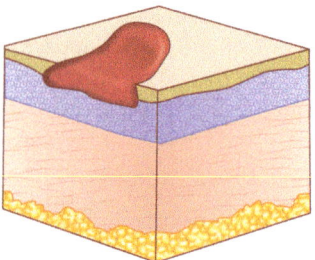

Fig. 4.11: Erosion

6. *Ulcer:* It is a circumscribed lesion starting from a break in the skin, reaching upto the level of the dermis. It has definite length, also breadth as opposed to a fissure. A clinician should study its size, contour, depth, edge, covering crust, contents, odour and the surrounding area of skin. The common causes of ulcers are as follows:

Traumatic	Actinomycosis
Pyogenic	Neoplastic ulcers
Tuberculosis	Varicose ulcer
Syphilis	Trophic ulcers
Dermal leishmaniasis	Peripheral vascular disorders
Leprosy	Metabolic disorders
Tropical ulcer	Syringomyelia and tabes
Veldt sore	Frost-bite.

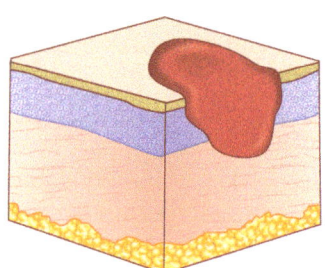

Fig. 4.12: Ulcer

Causes of Ulcers in the Mouth

Stomatitis	Tuberculosis
Dental irritation	Syphilis
Pemphigus	Epithelioma

7. *Scar:* It represents a healed destructive lesion of the dermis and deeper parts. Whenever any inflammatory or traumatic lesion destroys the basal layer of the epidermis and the underlying corium, a scar is formed. Superficial epidermal lesions heal without scarring; these are important points to be remembered in surgery and in the treatment of cutaneous lesions. A patient can be forewarned about whether or not a scar will be produced—a question asked by most patients with problems on the exposed parts of their bodies. In people with dark skins—Indians and Negroes—scars have a tendency to be keloidal. So, due precautions should be taken in surgery and in the treatment of burns. Certain scars are very characteristic, viz. the tissue-paper-like scars of lupus vulgaris, the wrinkled, chronic scars of leprosy, the depressed, pigmented scars of cutaneous leishmaniasis, pock marks of smallpox.

The clinician should study—the size, shape, color, texture, depression or elevation of the scar whether it is attached or free, whether there is any accompanying deformity and loss of sensations, hair, sebaceous or sweat secretion. The common causes of scars are as follows:

Traumatic
Ecthyma, acne necrotica and conglobata
Exanthemata—smallpox and chickenpox
Herpes zoster
Granulomata—tuberculosis, syphilis, leprosy, leishmaniasis, yaws and fungi
Varicose ulcer
Neoplasms.

Certain Dermatological Terms (Special Lesions)

Alopecia: It implies loss of hair resulting in a bald patch. Defluvium capillorum means fall or thinning of hair without areas of complete baldness. It must be remembered that hair occur in three states: Growing, stationary and falling. The last state comprises a very small percentage. For causes of baldness.

Atrophy: It means wasting away of the skin, which appears thin. There is loss of elasticity, wrinkling with diminished or complete loss of hair, sweat and sebum. All destructive disease processes of the corium with intact epidermis (i.e. without ulceration) leave behind atrophy. An atrophic patch may or may not be accompanied by scaling, pigmentation and telangiectasis.

Burrow: It is a straight or tortuous, slightly elevated, flesh-colored or slightly darker line found on the wrist, hand or genitalia in scabies. It represents the path or tunnel of the *Acarus scabiei* in the stratum corneum of the skin. At the deeper end of the burrow an acarus can be demostrated.

Cyst: It is a circumscribed collection of fluid or semi-solid substances in the skin surrounded by well-defined walls. Its size, shape, consistency, translucency, depth, and whether or not it is adherent to the skin and underlying structures, should be studied. The common cause of cutaneous cysts are as follows:

Sebaceous cyst	Milia
Implantation cyst	mucous cyst
Dermoid cyst	Benign cystic epithelioma
Pilonidal cyst	Hydrocystoma.

Comedone (blackhead): It represents a plug at the pilo-sebaceous opening. It consists of dried sebum and epithelial debris. To begin with, it is white. With the passage of time, the sulfur of sebum is converted into sulphide and the color becomes black. Comedones are usually found on the face, shoulders, sternal region and back in acne vulgaris and acneiform eruptions due to iodides and bromides. Tar, chlorine and oils, by contact, produce comedones on exposed parts like the face, arms and legs.

Circinata: It implies a circular lesion shaped like a coin or disk. If there is central clearing and spreading at the periphery, the lesions are called *annular*. Common examples are as follows:

Tinea circinata	Psoriasis
Impetigo	Infective eczema
Discoid dermatitis	Erythema multiforme
Lupus erythematosus	Granuloma annulare
Syphilides	Seborrhea corporis
Leprosy	Drug eruption
Lichen planus annularis	Pityriasis rosea.

Further special configurations may occur in different skin diseases viz. half circle (arciform), multiple circles joined together (polycyclic) or circular with central dots (iris). The latter is typically seen in erythema multiforme.

Erythema: It implies redness of the skin due to dilatation of blood vessels. It is a common early sign of most cutaneous diseases, but may be difficult to make out in dark people.

Erythroderma: It implies generalized redness and infiltration of the integument as is evident in pityriasis rubra pilaris, generalized dermatitis due to drugs and reticuloses. When accompanied by marked scaling and exfoliation of the skin, the term *exfoliative dermatitis* is employed. In reality, both terms mean more or less the same thing.

Erythematosquamous: It means a combination of erythema and scaling, e.g. psoriasis, tinea, syphilis, lichen planus, parapsoriasis, pityriasis rosea and exfoliative dermatitis.

Elephantiasis: It is a clinical term signifying elephant-like swelling due to extreme lymphedema and fibrous hypertrophy of a part of the body. The common causes are: filariasis, streptococcal lymphangitis, congenital lymphedema. The parts commonly affected are the feet, legs and the genitalia.

Granuloma: It is a chronic swelling usually in the form of a well-defined deep-seated, dermic nodule. Clinically it is marked by chronic induration and scarring; histologically, histiocyte infiltration in the corium is its special feature. They are very common in the tropics. Several causes of granulomas are as follows:

Infective
   Tuberculosis
   Syphilis, granuloma inguinale and lymphogranuloma inguinale
   Leprosy
   Yaws
   Leishmaniasis
   Septic
   Deep fungi like actinomycosis, etc.
   Sarcoid

Drugs
   Bromides
   Iodides

Neoplastic
   Epitheliomas
   Secondary metastases
   Reticuloses like mycosis fungoides, Hodgkin's disease, etc.

Keratosis: It is a circumscribed hyperplasia of the stratum corneum (horny layer) of the skin, e.g. senile keratosis, arsenical keratosis, seborrheic keratosis. Keratoses have a predisposition to malignancy. Follicular keratoses are seen in lichen spinulosus, keratosis follicularis, vitamin A, C or fatty acid deficiencies, pityriasis rubra pilaris, Darier's disease, lichen planopilaris, lichen scrofulosorum, etc.

Keratoderma: It signifies diffuse plaques of hyperplasia of the stratum corneum of the skin, particularly of the hands and feet, e.g. tylosis, congenital, arsenical, menopausal, chronic eczema, syphilis, psoriasis, avitaminosis, pityriasis rubra pilaris, etc.

Koebner phenomenon: It means linear lesions produced by scratching a primary lesion, which results in new lesions developing along the line of the scratch, e.g. lichen planus, warts and psoriasis.

Lichenoid: Violaceous or purplish, solid, firm papules, resembling lichen planus but not due to it. This term is loosely used till a proper diagnosis is established. Similarly terms like pemphigoid, leukodermoid and psoriasiform have been coined to describe cutaneous lesions morphologically.

Telangiectasia: It represents groups of fine, dilated capillaries. The common causes are: rosacea, spider nevus, alcoholism, liver disorder and X-ray burn.

Vegetations: They are cauliflower-like growths in moist areas like the ano-genital region, groins and axillae. If the stratum corneum is absent, vegetations look eroded—*erosive vegetations.* If the stratum corneum is hypertrophic, the vegetations are termed *verrucous vegetations.* The common causes are condylomata lata, pemphigus vegetans and pyoderma vegetans.

Zosteriform: Grouped lesions along the course of a nerve, usually unilateraly. Common example is herpes zoster. But zosteriform grouping may also be seen in nevi and vitiligo. Further zosteriform grouping should be distinguished from linear, retiform, herpetiform and corymbiform grouping.

Table 4.1: Shapes of papules and nodules

Shape	Example
Dome shaped	Molluscum contagiosum
Flat topped	Plane warts
Umblicated	Molluscum contagiosum
Acuminate	Genital warts
Verrucous	Verruca vulgaris
Pedunculated	Skin tags

Table 4.2: Shapes of skin lesions

Shape	Example
Nummular (Discoid)	Nummular dermatitis
Annular	Tinea corporis
Circinate	Herpes simplex
Arcuate (arciform)	Granuloma annulare
Gyrate	Some forms of tinea
Retiform (reticulate)	Macular amyloidosis

Table 4.3: Arrangement or configuration of the lesions

Arrangement	Example
Grouped	Herpes simplex
Linear	Linear epidermal nevus
Dermatomal	Herpes zoster
Serpiginous	Burrow
Arcuate	Granuloma annulare

Uncommon Configurations

1. Herpetiform
2. Aciform (arcuate)
3. Reticulate
4. Circinate
5. Polycyclic
6. Gyrate
7. Figurate
8. Geographic
9. Serpiginous
10. Cockade (concentric rings)
11. Corymbose
12. Whorled

Localization of Common Dermatoses

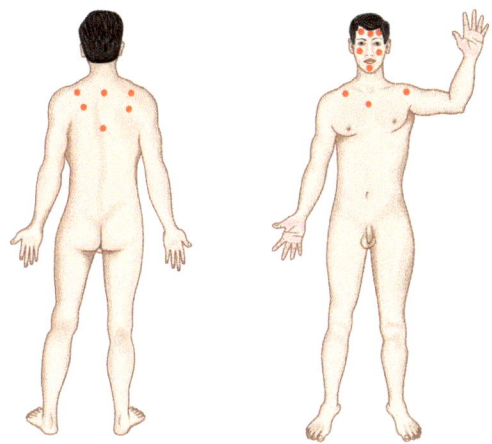

Fig. 4.13: Acne vulgaris

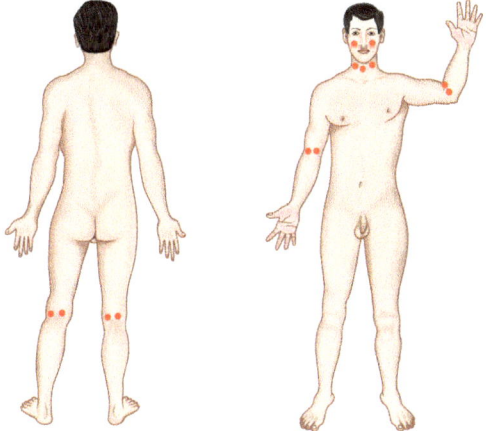

Fig. 4.14: Atopic dermatitis

48 Diagnosis and Management of Dermatologic Disorders

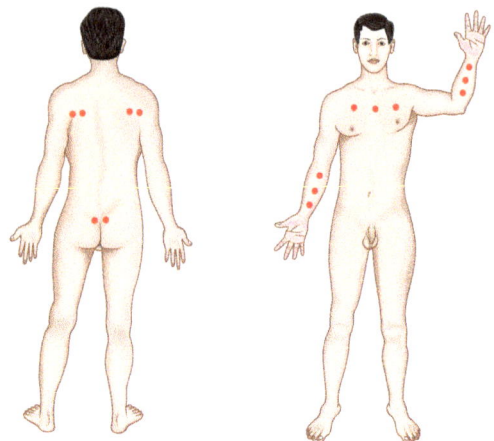

Fig. 4.15: Dermatitis herpetiforms

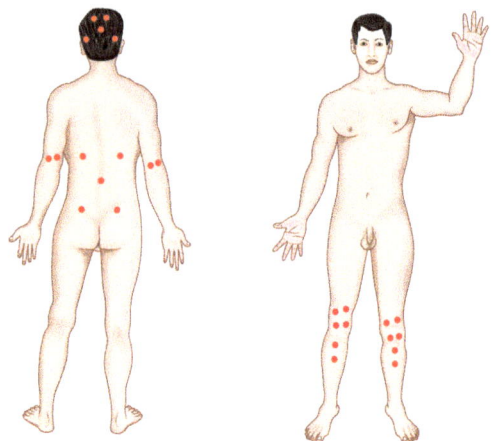

Fig. 4.16: Psoriasis

Diagnosis of Dermatological Diseases

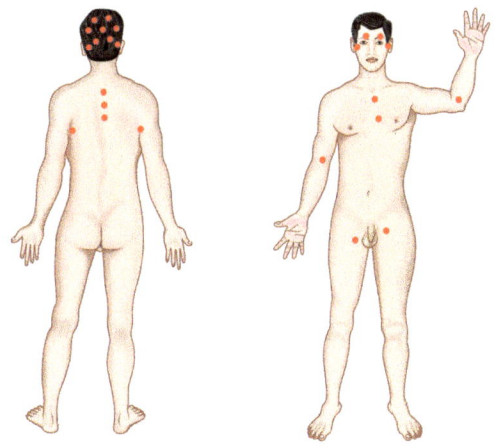

Fig. 4.17: Seborrheic dermatitis

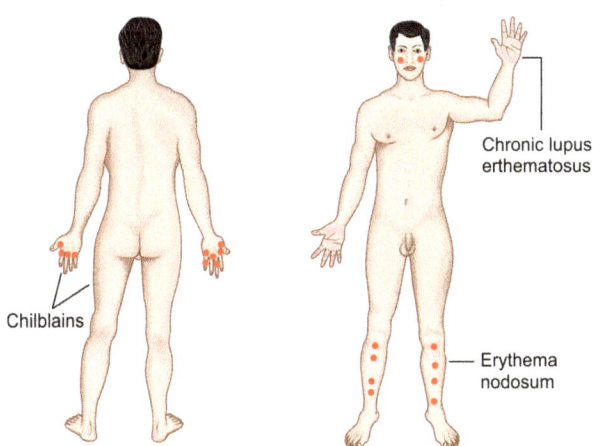

Fig. 4.18: Miscellaneous

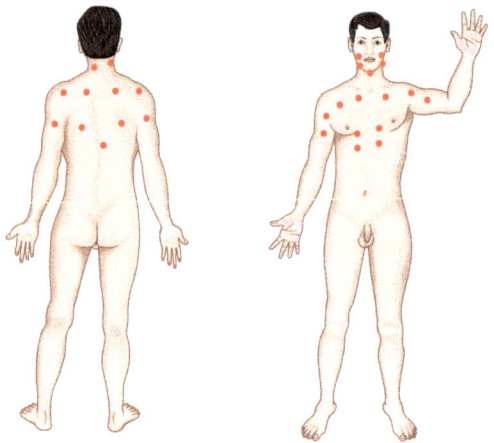

Fig. 4.19: Pityriasis versicolor

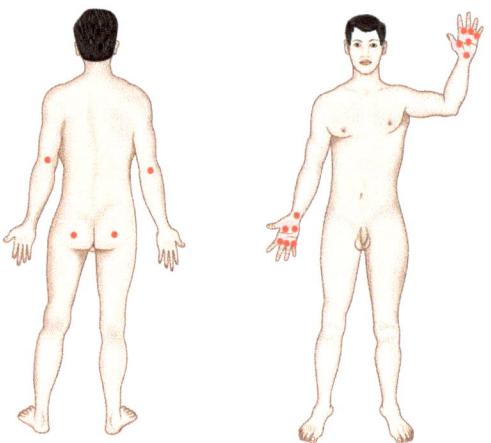

Fig. 4.20: Scabies

AIDS in Dermatological Diagnosis

Bacteriological studies
Smear
Culture
Sensitivity tests
Vaccine

Mycological studies
Fresh preparation
Staining
Culture

**Hematological
serological tests
for syphilis**
VDRL
HIV antibody detection test

Histological
Biopsy and cytological studies
IE cell
Tzanck test
Smear for cancer cells, etc.
Histochemistry
Immunofluorescence

Radiological

Dermatoscopy Epiluminescence microscopy, dermoscopy

Allergy tests
Patch tests
Intradermal or scratch tests
Basophil degranulation test

Biological tests
Tuberculin
Lepromin
Kveim test
Frei test

Wood's lamp examination
Blood—routine
Erythrocyte sedimentation rate
Cryoglobulin test
Chemistry—cholesterol
protein, vitamins, sugar, urea
copper, zinc, sodium, cortisol

Stool
urine
Routine
Porphyrin
17-ketosteroids

Biopsy Incision biopsy, punch biopsy.
Hair examinations and counts
Trichogram

CHAPTER 5

Cutaneous Infestations: Scabies and Pediculosis

SCABIES

Scabies is an infections communicable dermatosis caused by a parasite an octonarian—Sarcoptes scabiei var hominis de Geer, characterized by marked itching, burrows multiform lesions due to scratching distributed in typical locations.

Clinical Features

After 4-6 weeks of incubation period the patient develops intense nocturnal itching and burrows scratching produces other lesions like papules, papulovesicles, urticarial lesions.

These lesions may get infected and eczematized. The common locations are dorsal surface of interdigital webs of fingers. Medial aspects of wrists, exterior axillary folds, premaxillary area, genitalia, etc. The whole body may be

Cutaneous Infestations: Scabies and Pediculosis

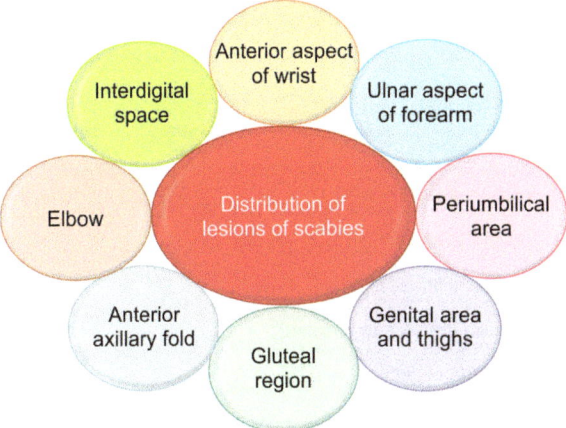

Fig. 5.1: Distributions of lesions of scabies

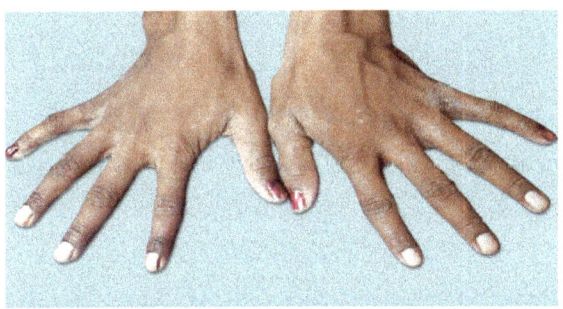

Fig. 5.2: Scabies-typical finger web spaces involvement with papular, vesicular and crusted lesions

affected. There may be some nodules due to hypersensitivity, The adult female mite or ova can be demonstrated under the microscope.

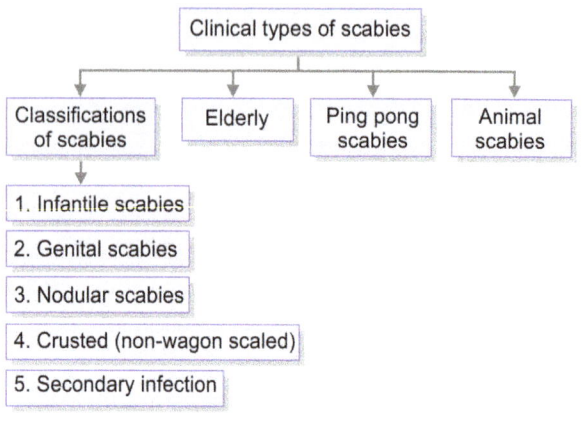

Fig. 5.3: Clinical types of scabies

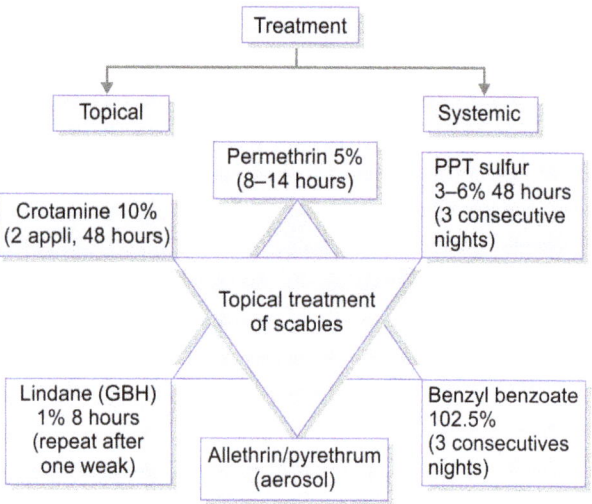

Fig. 5.4: Different method of treatment of scabies

Systemic
Ivermectin 200 μg/kg
Single dose, 56% cure/repeat 14 day later 96% cure.

Cutaneous Infestations: Scabies and Pediculosis

Keratotic scabies (Norwegian scabies) is a rare variant of scabies that affects immunosuppressed persons (lymphoma, HIV infections immunosuppressive therapy) or those who have lost the sensation of pruritus (leprosy) or are unable to take care of themselves (mental retardation, Down syndrome). Keratotic

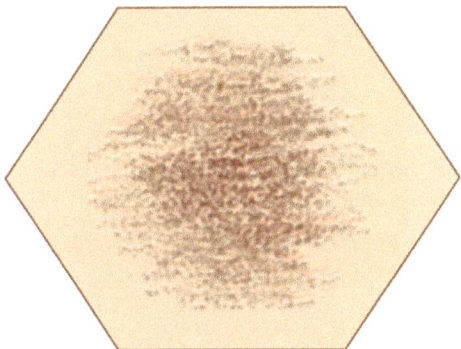

Fig. 5.5: Sarcoptes scabie var hominis Dee Geer

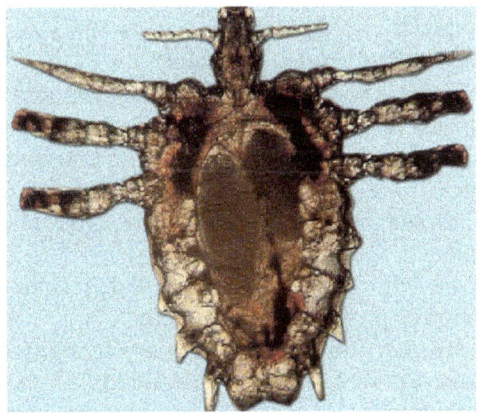

Fig. 5.6: Sarcoptes scabiei var hominis de Geer

and scaly erythematous plaques over trunk, extremities, scalp and face characterize this condition. These patients are highly infectious. Norwegian scabies responds to a topical keratolytic like 3% salicylic acid, in addition to repeated applications of an antiscabietic.

Supportive Treatment

1. Antihistaminics
2. Antibiotics: systemic, local
3. Emollients
4. Soaps?
5. Steroids: topical/systemic (eczematized scabies)
6. Keratolytics in crusted scabies.

Future trends: Local, ivermectin, tea, tree, oil, neem tree oil, etc.

Control Measures to Prevent Scabies

1. Treat all household members at the same time to avoid reinfestation.
2. All bed-lien (sheets, pillowcases, blankets) and clothing worn next to the skin (underwear, T-shirt, socks, pants) should be laundered in hot water).
3. If hot water is not available, places all linen and clothing into plastic bags and store it away for five or seven days. The mite does not survive beyond four days without skin contact.
4. Children may return to school the day after treatment is completed.
5. All those who have close contact with scabies patients may require prophylactic treatment.
6. Community education (i.e. early recognition and awareness of scabies) is recommended.
7. In widespread scabies epidemics, prophylactic treatment of the whole community may be optimal management.

Table 5.1: Treatment of scabies (summary)

	GBH	Permethrin	Benzyl benzoate	Sulfur	Crotamiton
Concentration (%)	1	5	25	5	10
No. of applications	1	1	3	3	3
Irritation	No	No	Yes	Yes	No
Relative Contraindications	Infants, Pregnancy	Nil	Children infected or eczematized scabies	infected or eczematized sc.	Nil
Efficacy	Good	Good	Good	Moderate	Moderate
Repeat after 10 days	Yes	Not Needed	Yes	Yes	Yes
Advantage	Effective and inexpensive	Ovicidal and effective as one application	Inexpensive	Inexpensive	Additional Antipruritic action
Disadvantage	Neurotoxicity in infants if overused	Expensive	Causes severe burning	stains, stinks and sticks	

The latest and most effective drug is Oral Ivermectin. 3 mg, 6 mg, 12 mg. Tablets are available which are effective in all types of scabies including Crusted Scabies and Norwegian Scabies.

PEDICULOSIS (LICE INFESTATION)

Pediculosis is an infestation of skin and hair caused by lice. This is an exceedingly common infection, particularly in the lower strata of the society in our country. The lice live on the blood sucked from the skin. The resulting excoriations and itchy dermatitis often get secondary infection. The pubic louse is the smallest while the body louse is the largest. The head louse is the most common.

Pediculosis Capitis

It is found chiefly among women and girls, especially at the nape of neck. Pruritus is annoying while excoriations and nits are disclosed, crawling lice may at times be seen. Secondary infection is usually present.

Treatment

1. 25% benzyl benzoate.
2. 1% gamma benzene hexachloride.

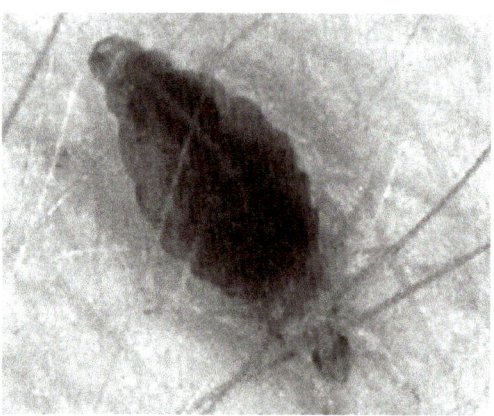

Fig. 5.7: Adult head louse

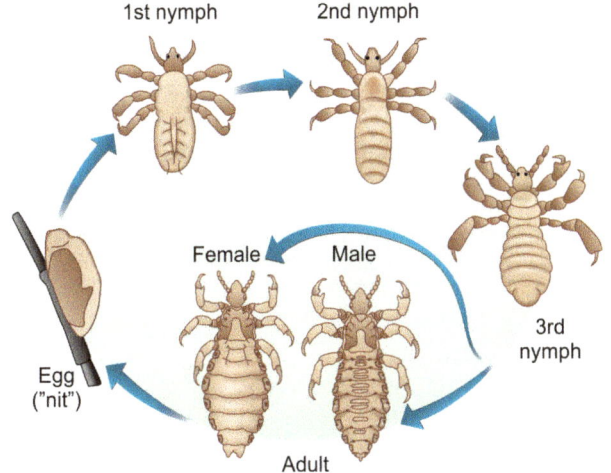

Fig. 5.8: Life cycle of head louse

Apply the solution on the scalp: Leave it for 24 hours. Then wash the scalp if required after 1 week, one more application may be used.
3. Permethrin.

Pediculosis Corporis

It is also termed as 'vagabond's disease'.

The causative lice live in the seams of human undergarments and are rarely found on the skin. Itching is intense. The finding of nit or lice on the clothes is diagnostic. Treatment is not of the skin but clothing should be boiled, dried in sun, Ironed and dusted with anti-infective agents.

Pediculosis Pubis

The infection is usually contracted as a result of sexual intercourse and is found commonly in the pubic area.

Treatment

The treatment in all cases consists of local application of 1% ointment of yellow oxide of mercury in vaseline base old treatment, and benzyl benzoate solution and crotamin lotion or ointment, and permethrin cream or soap.

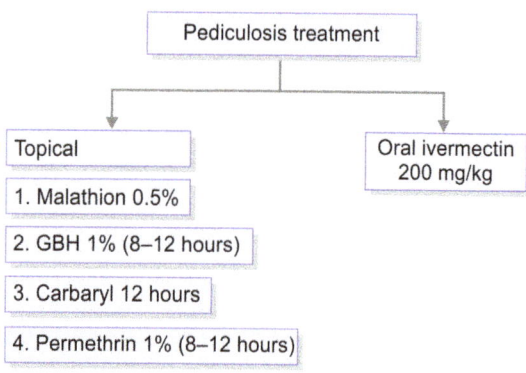

Fig. 5.9: Pediculosis (summary of treatment)

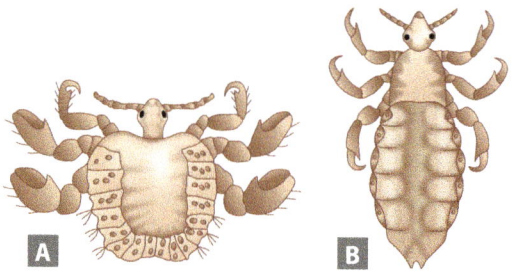

Figs 5.10A and B: Common types of louse: (A) Pubic louse; (B) Head louse

Cutaneous Infestations: Scabies and Pediculosis

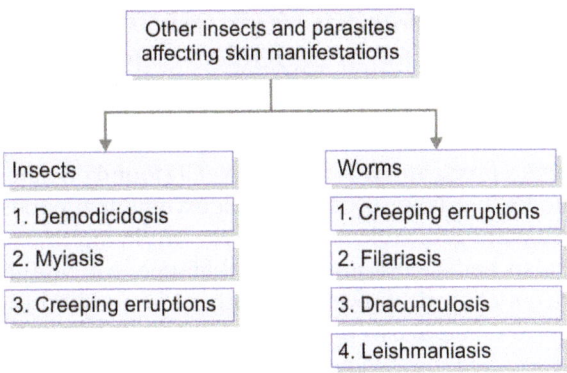

Fig. 5.11: Insects and parasites affecting skin manifestations

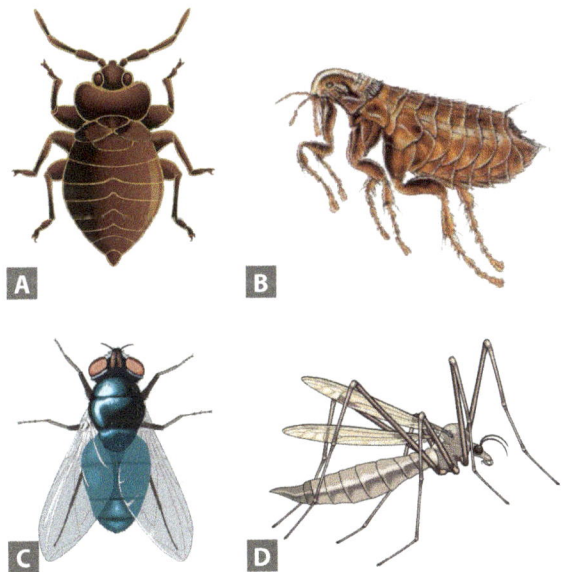

Figs 5.12A to D: Common types of insects: (A) Bed bug; (B) Human flea; (C) House fly; (D) Phiebotomus

HUMAN DEMODEX MITE: THE VERSATILE MITE OF DERMATOLOGICAL IMPORTANCE

Demodex mite is an obligate human ectoparasite found in or near the pilosebaceous units. *Demodex folliculorum* and *Demodex brevis* are two species typically found on humans. Demodex infestation usually remains asymptomatic and may have a pathogenic role only when present in high densities and also because of immune imbalance. All cutaneous diseases caused by *Demodex* mites are clubbed under the term demodicosis or demodicidosis, which can be an

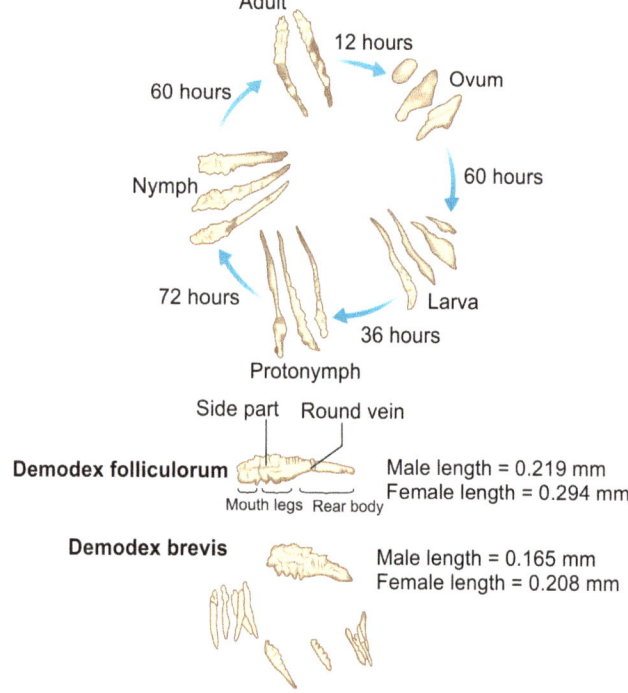

Fig. 5.13: Morphology and life cycle of the *Demodex* mite

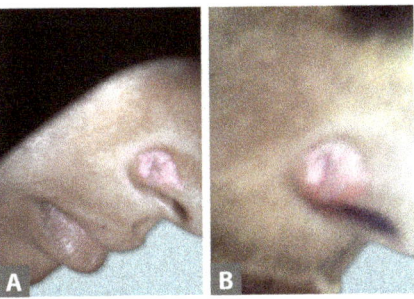

Figs 5.14A and B: Bacterial infection at the side of the nose

etiological factor of or resemble a variety of dermatoses. Therefore, a high index of clinical suspicion about the etiological role of *Demodex* in various dermatoses can help in early diagnosis and appropriate, timely, and cost effective management.

Human demodicosis is caused by the clinical manifestation of otherwise asymptomatic infestation of humans by two species of *Demodex mite*, i.e. *D. folliculorum* and *D. brevis*. The etiological role of this versatile mite should be kept in mind as human demodicosis can present as a variety of clinical manifestations mimicking many other dermatoses. This can help in early diagnosis and proper treatment, thereby saving time and at the same time being cost effective.

CHAPTER 6

Cutaneous Infections with Pyogenic Bacteria

IMPETIGO (IMPETIGO CONTAGIOSA)

This is a superficial bacterial infection caused by staphylococci or streptococci.

Impetigo is a superficial staphylococcal or streptococcal skin infection that presents in young children as erosions covered with thin honey colored crusts on face. Lesions begin as vesicles/pustules. Oral erythromycin or penicillin V is frequently necessary in addition to a topical antibiotic.

ECTHYMA

This deep bacterial infection, caused by streptococci, involves dermis.

Ecthyma is a deep streptococcal skin infection seen in older children or adolescents with poor hygiene as rounded ulcers covered with thick crusts over lower legs. Lesions heal with scarring after local cold compresses, topical antibiotics and oral erythromycin or penicillin V.

FOLLICULITIS

Although literally this term means inflammation of the follicle, it is generally used to denote follicular infection with pyogenic organisms. The most common causative agent is *Staphylococcus*, but occasionally, streptococci and gram-negative rodes *(E.coli, Klebsiella, Proteus, Pseudomonas)* are implicated.

Folliculitis is a staphylococcal infection of the hair follicle that affects adult males. Follicular pustules or papulopustules over beard region or anterior legs characterize the condition.

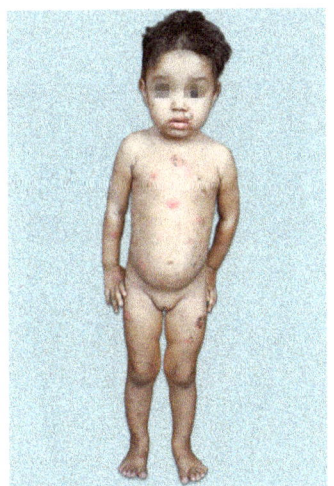

Fig. 6.1: Impetigo contagiosa—honey colored crusted lesions over the face, trunk, arms, hands, and legs

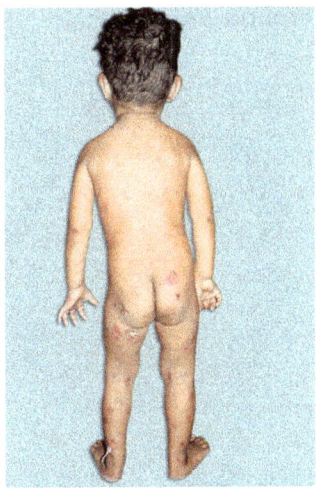

Fig. 6.2: Bullous impetigo—large pus filled blisters over the back side of the whole body

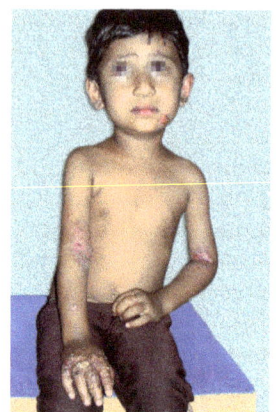
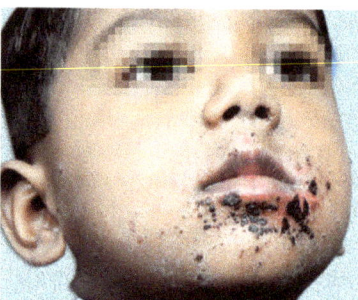

Fig. 6.3: Impetigo contagiosa—honey colored crusted lesions of the face, elbows, and hands

Fig. 6.4: Impetigo contagiosa—crusted lesions over the face of a child

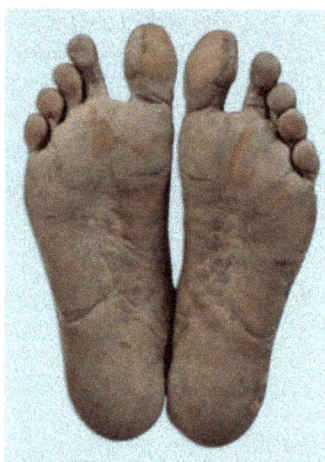
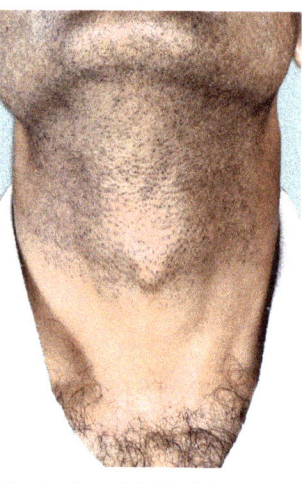

Fig. 6.5: Pitted keratolysis—soles demonstrating multiple pits

Fig. 6.6: Pseudofolliculitis—multiple follicular and perifollicular inflammatory papules

Cutaneous Infections with Pyogenic Bacteria

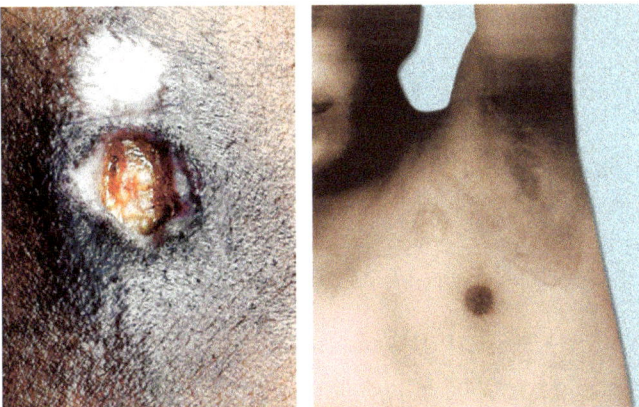

Fig. 6.7: Chronic legs ulcer going towards projections of a gangrene over the legs

Fig. 6.8: Erythrasma: noninflammatory brownish macule in axilla

Flowchart 6.1

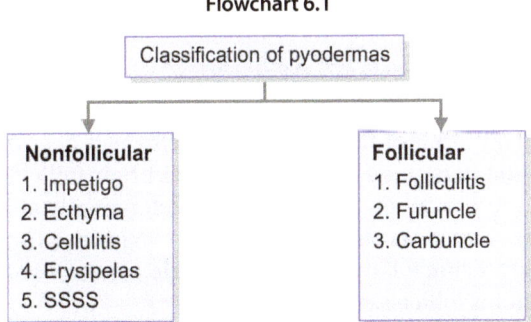

Classification of pyodermas

Nonfollicular
1. Impetigo
2. Ecthyma
3. Cellulitis
4. Erysipelas
5. SSSS

Follicular
1. Folliculitis
2. Furuncle
3. Carbuncle

Abbreviation: SSSS = Staphylococcal scalded skin syndrome

Extended application of a topical antibiotic is usually needed in addition to a short course of oral erythromycin or cloxacillin.

Flowchart 6.2: Etiological classification of pyodermas

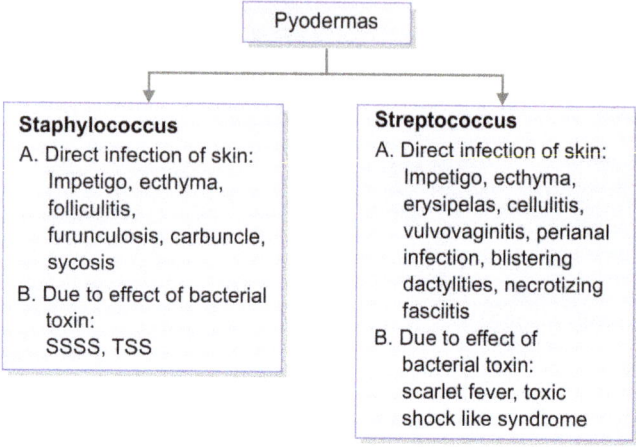

Abbreviations: SSSS = Staphylococcal scalded skin syndrome; TSS = Toxic shock syndrome

FURUNCLE AND CARBUNCLE

These two conditions, though clinically distinct, are essentially forms of deep folliculitis that involve, deep dermis and subcutaneous fat. Terminal (thick) hair follicles that extend to the subcutaneous fat are preferentially affected. *Staphylococcus* is the usual offender. Whereas furuncle involves a single hair follicle, carbuncle affects a group of contiguous follicles.

Furuncle is a deep *staphylococcal* infection of a terminal (thick) follicle/that reaches up to the fat. A painful, tender, erythematous nodule with central pointing is seen over either the axillae, buttocks or face. Abscess forms in a few days, bursts or needs drainage. Topical antibiotics are useful for a single lesion but oral cloxacillin or erythromycin are needed for multiple or recurrent lesions.

CARBUNCLE

Patient Profile

Most patients are adults with poorly controlled diabetes. Children are spared.

Carbuncle is a deep staphylococcal infection affecting a group of contiguous follicles that reach up to the subcutaneous fat. It typically affects diabetics. An extremely tender indurated erythematous plaque that, upon pressure, discharges pus through its sieve-like openings and later forms a deep ulcer over the nape of neck is characteristic. Desloughing, and later, grafting may be needed in addition to oral cloxacillin.

ACUTE PARONYCHIA

Paronychia is inflammation of the nail fold. Acute paronychia is caused by bacteria, mainly staphylococci, whereas chronic paronychia is usually intiated and perpetuated by *Candida albicans*.

Acute paronychia is a staphylococcal infection of lateral nail folds that is usually initiated by trauma. Tender erythema and swelling evolves into an abscess that is extremely painful. Oral cloxacillin and NSAIDs are needed in addition to incision and drainage for relief of pain.

PERIPORITIS (MULTIPLE SWEAT GLAND ABSCESSES)

Periporitis is a staphylococcal infection of facial skin of malnourished children. Lesions are nontender erythematous rounded papulonodules that may evolve into abscesses. Oral erythromycin or cloxacillin, improving hygiene and nutrition and drainage of large abscesses is needed.

ERYSIPELAS AND CELLULITIS: PITTED KERATOLYSIS THERAPY OF BACTERIAL INFECTIONS

Topical Antibiotics

Since these are easily administered, lack systemic side effects when applied over limited body regions and provide good concentration of the antibacterial in the skin, they are used in almost all pyogenic bacterial infections. Their only side effect, contact allergic dermatitis, is uncommon. It is preferable to use antibacterials that are not commonly used systemically since topical use promotes development of resistant strains in a community.

Neomycin 1% fusidic acid 1%, framycetin 1%, chlorhexidine 1%, sisomycin 1%, mupirocin 1%, nadoxin, betadin, metrogyl, gentamicin are some of the commonly employed preparations. A combination of neomycin (for gram negative bacteria), bacitracin (for gram-positive cocci) and polymyxin B (for *Pseudomonas*) is also available. Application to the skin lesions and perilesional skin 2–3 times a day gives good results. Topical antibiotics should preferably be continued for a week after all the lesions have healed, as this prevents reinfections and allows regrowth of protective normal flora.

Systemic Antibiotics

Indications for systemic treatment include extensive infections that recur or persist after adequate topical therapy. Associated regional lymphadenopathy and fever are other indications. Poor compliance for topical therapy, as in young children, is another situation for systemic therapy. In ordinary infections, 1–2 weeks of systemic therapy is sufficient. For recurrent infections, longer duration of therapy may be necessary.

Antibiotic sensitivity test should ideally be utilized for choosing the right agent. However, such testing is commonly reserved for recurrent, persistent or life threatening infections. Cloxacillin, erythromycin, cephalexin in doses of 250-500 mg qds are used for *staphylococcal* or *streptococcal* infections. Oral penicillin V 200-400 mg qds, inj. procaine penicillin (fortified or otherwise) 8 lac IU IM od after test dose are effective against most gram-positive cocci. Newer cephalosporins and macrolide antibiotics are also effective. Board spectrum antibiotics like ampicillin or amoxycillin with or without cloxacillin (250 mg each) are popular agents but are most useful for mixed and secondary bacterial infections. For unresponsive infections, a combination of ampicillin (250 mg) with clavulanic acid (125 mg), azithromycin, cephalosporins are recommended.

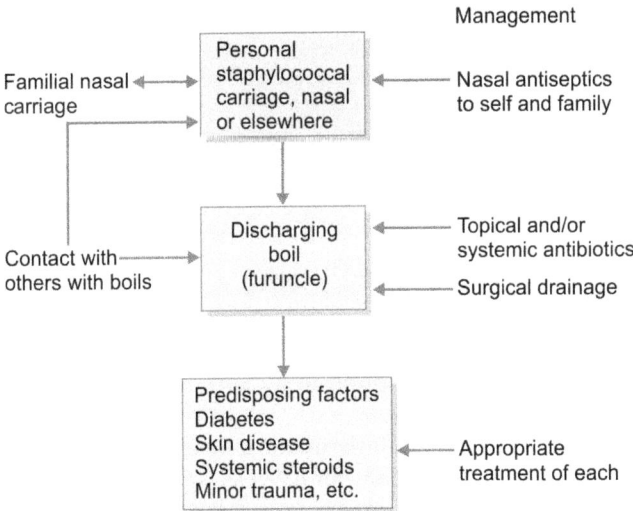

Fig. 6.9: Types of treatment of the family carriers

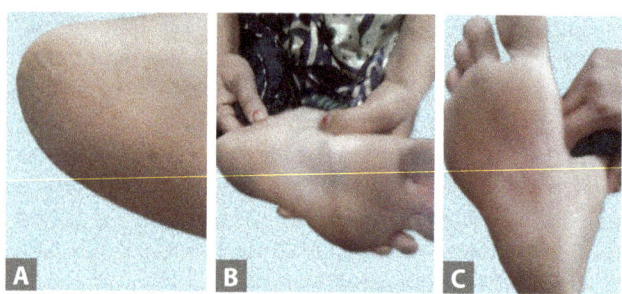

Figs 6.10A to C: Pitted keratolysis—soles demonstrating multiple pits

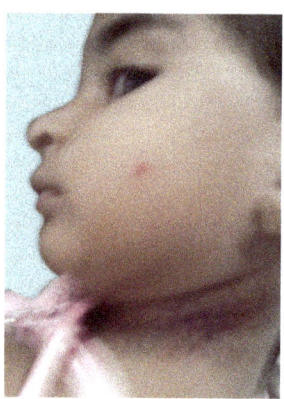

Fig. 6.11: Pyoderma

Summary of Treatment of Bacterial Infections

Acute episode will respond to an appropriate antibiotic; incision speeds healing.

In chronic furunculosis treat carrier sites, such as the nose and groin twice daily for 6 weeks with an appropriate topical antiseptic or antibiotic (e.g. chlorhexidine solution, mupirocin cream or clindamycin solution). Treat family carriers in the same way.

CHAPTER 7

Cutaneous Tuberculosis

EPIDEMIOLOGY

In India 2% (1950 and 1960). Then 0.1% by 1980s due to effective antitubercular drugs like streptomycin, isonex, pyrazinamide, kanomycin, etc.

Cutaneous tuberculosis may occur as a result of primary inoculation (tuberculous chancre), reinoculation (lupus vulgaris tuberculosis verrucosa cutis), contiguous spread (scrofuloderma) or uncommonly as autoinoculation (periorificial tuberculosis) or through hematogeneous spread (miliary tuberculosis). Prognosis is poor in the latter two. Diagnosis can be established by demonstration of bacilli and or a granuloma on biopsy. A four-drug regimen for two months followed by two drugs for four months is effective.

Cutaneous tuberculosis is a chronic granuloma of the skin due to *Mycobacterium tuberculosis*.

It is seen generally in the young age; most of the patients are in the first or second decades of life. The warty type is commonly seen in the bare-footed rural class of patients, is often due to an infection after a thorn prick, vaccination, piercing of the ear-lobules tattooing direct contact with an infected tuberculosis gland with sinus or sputum or auto infection from pulmonary or enteric lesions may lead to tuberculosis manifestations on the skin.

The manifestations of tuberculosis on skin can be broadly devided into localized and disseminate (tuberculids) groups.

Tuberculous chancre, lupus vulgaris, tuberculosis verrucosa cutis orificials are examples of the localized group.

ETIOLOGY

Cutaneous tuberculosis like tuberculosis elsewhere in the body, is caused by *Mycobacterium tuberculosis (M. tuberculosis)*. Sometimes cutaneous infection with atypical mycobacteria can also clinically resemble *M. tuberculosis* infection of the skin.

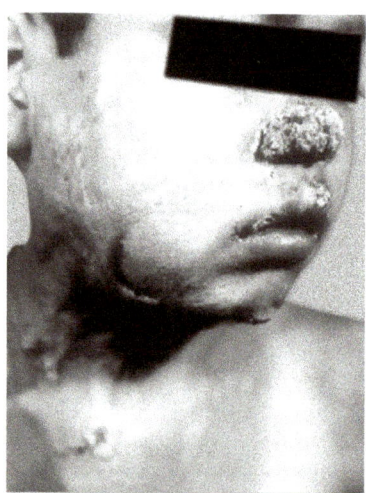

Fig. 7.1: Lupus vulgaris—verrucous plaque with active infiltrated border on the face of a child

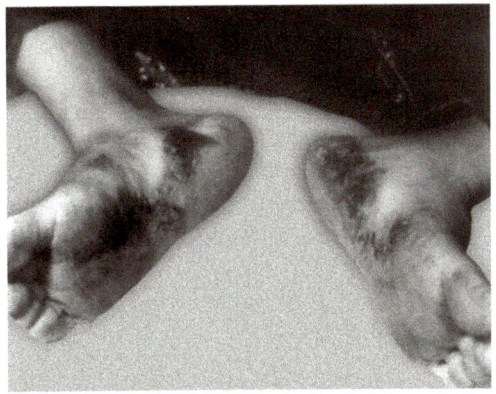

Fig. 7.2: Tuberculosis verrucose cuits—verrucous plaque with fissuring on the soles

PATHOGENESIS

The manifestations of *M. tuberculosis* infection in the skin depend on several factors:

Primary exposure or secondary exposure: Primary infection with tuberculosis occurs only rarely in the skin.

Immune status of the host.

Mode of entry of the organism.

Load of the bacteria.

INVESTIGATIONS

1. Histology
2. Culture
3. Chest X-ray

DIAGNOSIS

Chronicity of the lesions.
Characteristic morphology.

DIFFERENTIAL DIAGNOSIS

Discoid lupus erythematosus.

TREATMENT

Standard antituberculosis therapy with four drugs for two months followed by two drugs for four months is now recommended. All drugs are taken on an empty stomach once daily.

CLINICAL FEATURES

1. *Chancre:* It occurs chiefly on the face of children and is contacted usually through a kiss by lung tuberculosis patient.
2. *Lupus valgaris:* Although any part of the body may be affected, nose cheeks, neck and buttocks are the common sites the tuberculin test is a always positive. It has multiple forms:
   1. Lupus maculosus
   2. Lupus ulcerosus
   3. Lupus psoriaticus
   4. Lupus vulgaris verrulosus
   5. Lupus vulgaris mutilans.

   The lesions of lupus vulgaris are symptomless well-defind and indolent. Carcinoma may occur in 1–2% of the cases.
3. *Tuberculosis verrucosa cutis:* It is usually due to external inoculation. Hands and feet are common sites. Symptomless, indolent, warty, horny and papilliferous lesions are usually formed.
4. *Scrofuloderma:* This type is fairly common in our country. Neck and axillae are the common sites of prediction. The lymph nodes get swollen and adhere to the overlying skin on suppuration fistulae and sinuses are formed.

Table 7.1: Drug regimen for cutaneous tuberculosis

Phase	Duration	Drug	Dose	Side effects
Intensive	2 months	Isoniazid	5 mg/kg	Drug rash, pellagra-like rash, neuropathy, hepatic toxicity
		Rifampicin	10 mg/kg	Hepatic toxicity, discoloration of body secretions
		Ethambutol	15 mg/kg	Eye toxicity
		Pyrazinamide	30 mg/kg	Hepatitis, arthritis
Maintenance	4 months	Isoniazid	5 mg/kg	
		Rifampicin	10 mg/kg	

5. *Tuberculosis cutis orificiales:* It is commonly seen in perianal, genital and oral lesions due to spread from enteric, genitourinary, and pulmonary lesions.

TUBERCULIDS

These are due to hypersensitive reactions to tuberculosis. In these types the tuberculin reaction is strongly positive.

Treatment

Antituberculous therapy as for pulmonary tuberculosis is recommended. A common short duration regimen includes

Ethambutol	800 mg/day
Pyrazinamide	1500 mg/day
INH	300 mg/day
Rifampicin	450 mg/day

All for two months, and followed by the latter two drugs for a further period of 4 months.

```
┌─────────────────────────────────────────┐
│ Summary of therapy of cutaneous tuberculosis │
└─────────────────────────────────────────┘
                    │
         ┌──────────┴──────────┐
         ▼                     ▼
```

General measure
1. Notification
2. Identification and treatment of underlying tuberculosis focus
3. Coexistent infection, such as HIV
4. Anxillary measures

Specific chemotherapy
1. Phase I
2. Phase II

Polymerase chain reaction compared to other laboratory findings and to clinical evaluation in the diagnosis of cutaneous tuberculosis and atypical mycobacteria skin infection.

We have found that PCR was the best method in the diagnosis of CT and AMI. The positive tuberculin test and positive PCR analysis from samples with granulomatous tissue reaction were also very important for CT and atypical mycobacteria diagnosis. In our experience, tissue cultures have a poor yield, as well as AFB stain and BCG-IHC.

CHAPTER 8

Fungal Infections (Mycosis)

The various fungal infections which are commonly encountered commonly classified in Figure 8.1.

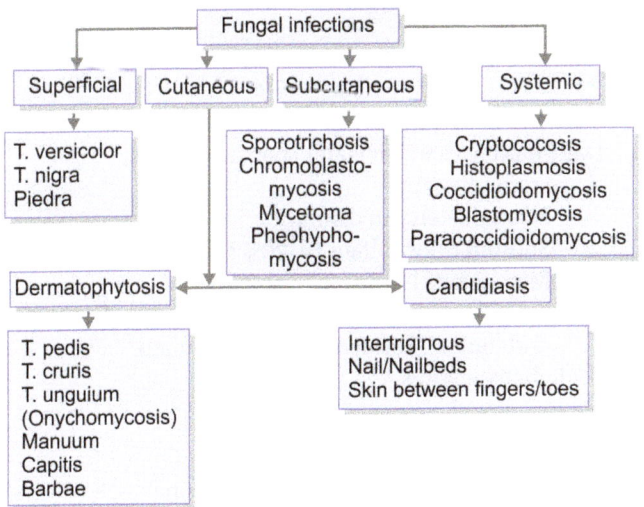

Fig. 8.1: Clinical classification of various fungal infections

PITYRIASIS VERSICOLOR (TINEA VERSICOLOR, DERMATOMYCOSIS, FURFURACEA, CHROMOPHYTOSIS)

Etiology

Caused by the fungus, *Pityrosporum orbiculare, p. ovale,* there are at least 7 species of lipophilic yeast—*Malassezia* on the human skin: *M. msympodialis* (most commonly found on the normal skin), *M. globosa* (most frequently associated with tinea versicolor), *M. restricta, M. dermatis, M. slooffiae, M. obtusa* and *M. furfuracea.* Pityriasis versicolor affects young adults. Hypopigmented macules and patches covered with fine, powdery scales, that are accentuated with stroking, typify this condition. Upper trunk, neck, axillae are usually involved. KOH mount demonstrates fungal spores and hyphae. Once daily topical use of 1% clotrimazole or 2% selenium sulfide for two weeks is curative. Oral ketoconazole or fluconazole are also useful.

Treatment

1. Undergarments should be boiled.
2. Daily bath with warm water soap are useful.
3. Local remedies are
   a. Selsun/selenium disulfide
   b. Sodium thiosuolfate 10–20% solution.
   c. Miconazole lotion.
   d. Tolnaftate lotion, fluconazole, ketoconazole, etc. oral and topical. Sertaconazole is assumed.
4. UV light exposures.

Diagnosis

Diagnosis of pityriasis versicolor is based on:

Hypopigmented perifollicular macules which become confluent. Lesions appear to be sitting on the skin.

Upper torso, neck candidal stomatitis (oral thrush, candidal glossitis).

Differential Diagnosis

Pityriasis versicolor should be differentiated from the following:

Vitiligo: The lesions of vitiligo are well-defined depigmented macules with no scaling while those of pityriasis versicolor are hypopigmented (sometimes hyperpigmented) with branny scales. The lesions of pityriasis versicolor are perifollicular; in vitiligo, hair may also be depigmented (leukotrichia) and on treatment perifollicular areas repigment first.

Leprosy: The hypopigmented lesions of leprosy show epidermal atrophy and sensory deficit and lack of the perifollicular character and the branny scaling of pityriasis versicolor.

Investigations

Potassium hydroxide mount is prepared from scrappings of the skin. It shows a mixture of short, branched hyphae and spores (spaghetti and meat ball appearance). Culture is of little help.

CANDIDIASIS

Candidal Intertrigo

Candidal intertrigo affects closely apposing and rubbing body folds that provide hot and humid environment for candida to grow. Obese, diabetic adults and chubby infants are frequent victims. Oozing erythematous erosions with marginal scales and satellite pustules are typical. Groins, axillae, inframammary and interdigital folds are involved. Smear shows budding yeasts. Topical 1% clotrimazole and correction of predisposing factors is curative. Oral fluconazole is useful in persistent or recurrent cases.

Clinical Manifestation

Candidal intertrigo manifests as:

A moist glazed area of erythema and maceration appears at sites of friction. The edges show soggy, frayed scaling, and satellite papulopustules.

Inframammary region, axillae and groins are favored sites; also in between fingers and toes.

Candidal Paronychia (Chronic Paronychia)

Candida thrives in the subcuticular space opened up due to damage to the cuticle by prolonged contact with soap and water. Pain,

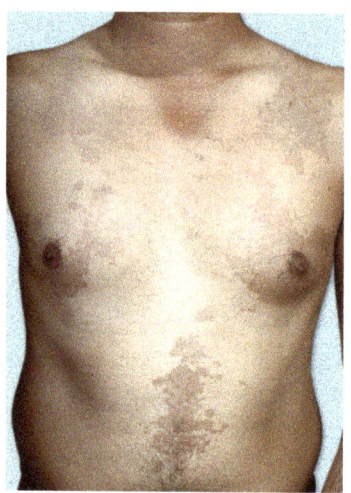

Fig. 8.2: Tinea versicolor—hypopigmented and hyperpigmented macules with fine scaling

Fungal Infections (Mycosis)

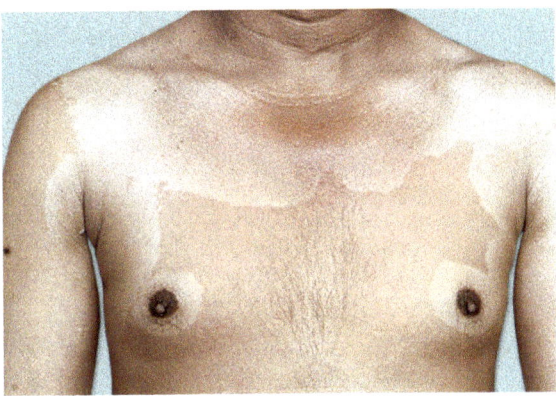

Fig. 8.3: Tinea versicolor—hypopigmented macules with fine powdery scales see the geometrical distributions on the chest

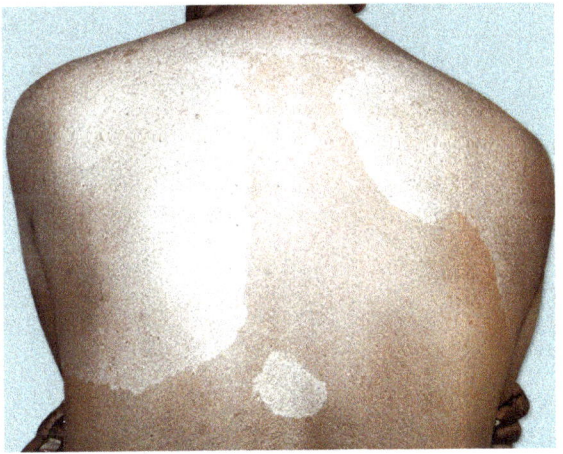

Fig. 8.4: Tinea versicolor—hypopigmented macules with fine powdery scales see the geometrical distributions on the back of the same patient

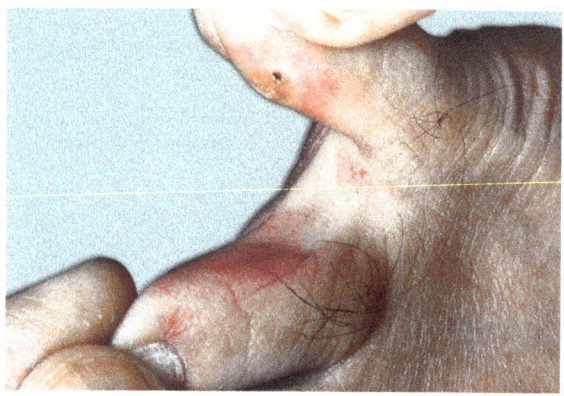

Fig. 8.5: Intertriginous candidiasis—toe cleft showing moist macerated lesion

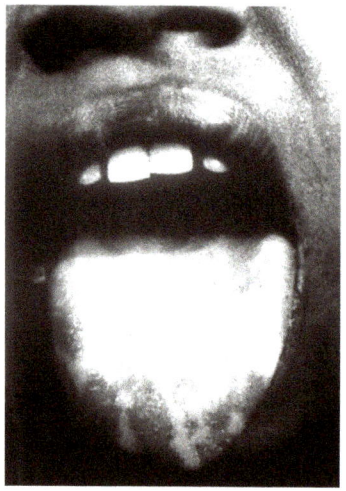

Fig. 8.6: Oral candidiasis with angular cheilitis

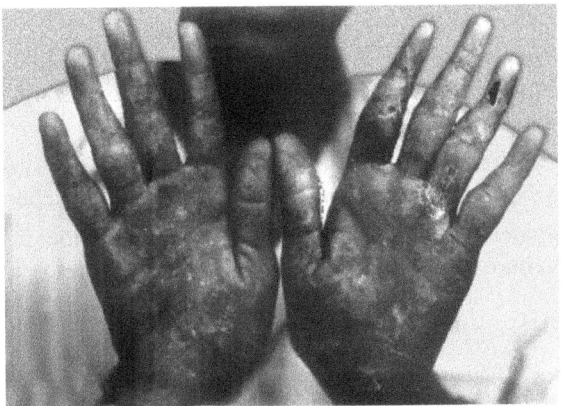

Fig. 8.7: Tinea manuum—scale lesions of both the palms

- Perleche (candidal angular stomatitis)
- Candidal vaginitis
- Candidal vulvovaginitis
- Perianal candidiasis
- Candidal balanoposthitis

Predisposing Factors

Wet work, poor peripheral circulation, diabetes and presence of vulval candidiasis are predisposing factors.

Clinical Manifestation

Inflammation of proximal nail folds which are red and rounded. Small beads of pus can be expressed from under the nail folds. Cuticles are lost. The adjoining nail plate becomes yellowish and shows ridging.

Genital Candidiasis

Predisposing factors: Predisposing factors include diabetes, antibiotic therapy, pregnancy and oral contraceptives. Conjugal spread is common.

Candidal vulvovaginitis: Most commonly presents as itching in the vulva along with presence of white curdy discharge.

Candidal balanoposthitis: Well-defined, erythematous lesions which may show tiny pustules on the glans and prepuce.

Oral Candidiasis

Several different forms are seen:

White adherent plaques which are difficult to remove; on removal, an erythematous base is revealed. Angular stomatitis usually in denture wearers.

Chronic Mucocutaneous Candidiasis

Predisposing factors: Several factors identified:

Genetic susceptibility, both an autosomal recessive and a dominant pattern recognized.

Candida endocrinopathy syndrome, characterized by hypoparathyroidism, Addison's disease and thymic tumors.

Manifestations: Persistent candidal infection in a number of sites.

Systemic Candidiasis

Seen against a background of severe illness, leukopenia and immunosuppression.

Investigations

A potassium hydroxide mount should be made and a culture from suspected lesion should be sent. Rule out diabetes in patients with recurrent problems.

Treatment

General Measures

Underlying predisposing factors should be sought and eliminated. Rule out diabetes mellitus.

Intertriginous areas should be kept dry. In paronychia, prolonged immersion in water is to be avoided.

Specific Treatment

Topical agents: Amphotericin, nystatin and imidazoles are effective.

Candidal intertrigo: Topical imidazoles (clotrimazole, miconazole, ketoconazole) are effective.

Candidal paronychia: Topical imidazole solutions. If acute paronychia is superimposed, then a course of antibiotic therapy may be necessary.

Oral candidiasis: Lotions and oral suspensions of imidazoles.

Genital candidiasis: Imidazole pessaries for vaginal infection.

Systemic Therapy

Systemic therapy is available in the form of ketoconazole, fluconazole and itraconazole. It is recommended in the following situations:

Candidal vulvovaginitis. Single dose fluconazole or itraconazole.

Recurrent oral candidiasis in immuno-compromised patients.

Chronic mucocutaneous candidiasis.

Synopsis of Candidiasis

Candidiasis is an opportunistic yeast infection caused by *Candida albicans* that thrives either in the warmth and moisture provided by body folds or when host immunity is compromised (diabetes mellitus, leukemia, steroid or immunosuppressive therapy). Erythema, tiny superficial pustules, erosions and a curdy white discharge that overlies them typify the disease. Oral thrush, vulvovaginitis, intertrigo, paronychia and balanoposthitis are some common syndromes of candidiasis. Correction of predisposing factors and topical antifungals (clotrimazole, nystatin) are effective. Oral fluconazole or ketoconazole are needed in unresponsive or immunocompromised patient cases.

DERMATOPHYTOSIS

The most common of all fungal infections, dermatophytosis is caused by dermatophytes, a group of fungi that survive by living on keratin. These may spread from human to human (anthropophilic, by sharing of clothes and personal articles), animal to human (zoophilic, by close contact

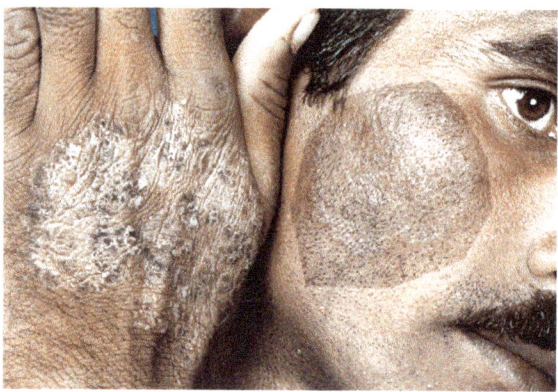

Fig. 8.8: Tinea faciei and tinea manuum dorsal aspect erythematous scale annular lesions over the face and hand—autospread

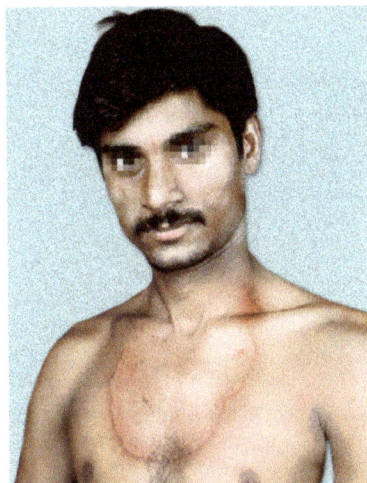

Fig. 8.9: Tinea corporis—typical annular erythematous ring like lesions on the chest spreading towards neck and face

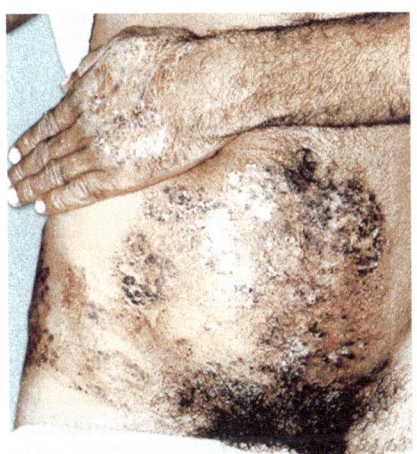

Fig. 8.10: Tinea corporis—circinate lesions with incomplete central with secondary bacterial infections on abdomen and hand—autospread

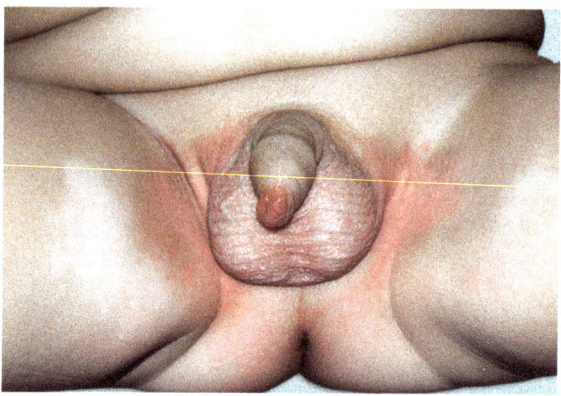

Fig. 8.11: Napkin candidiasis: acutely inflamed intertriginous areas with satellite vesiculopustules

with pets) and soil to human (geophilic, contact with soil). Microbiologically these fungi have been classified into three genera: *Trichophyton*, *Microsporum* and *Epidermophyton*.

Tinea Capitis

It is commonly known as ringworm of the scalp. It is highly contagious and appear in epidermis.

Etiology

Microsporum as *Trichophyton* genera may produce it.

Clinical Features

Clinical features vary according to the causative organisms. *M. audouinii* produces symptomless, grayish scaly patches of about 2" in diameter. In the affected areas the hair are broken, lustreless and fewer in number.

M. canis and *M. gypseum* tend to produce inflammatory lesions and lead to mild kerion formation. Kerion is due to strong local tissue reaction. Individual hair follicles how signs of marked inflammation leading to an acutely inflamed boggi granuloma. Secondary infection is often present and lesions contain pus.

Treatment

I. Isolate and treat
II. Get rid of infected hairs by epilation.

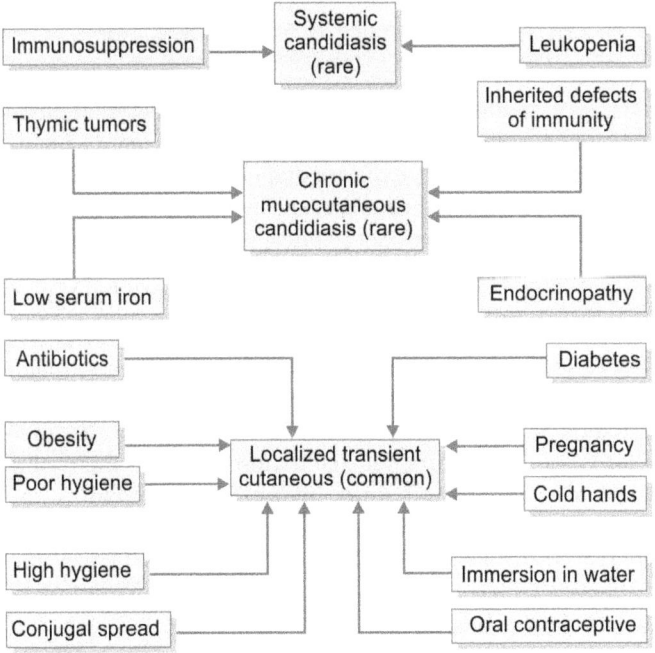

Fig. 8.12: Summary of contributors factors in the causation of candidiases

III. Secondary infection may be treated with sulfas, antibiotics.
IV. Kerion: should be treated with 25% hypertonic magnesium sulfate solution, 1:10,000 potassium permanganate solution compresses.
V. Local antifungal remedies.
VI. Grisovin 10 mg per pound body weight 8–12 weeks.

New topical remedies are buclosamide, chinoform, tolnaftate, and miconazole and clotrimazole and fluconazole preparations and the old local remedy is the whitefields ointments.

The Efficacy and Safety of Sertaconazole Cream (2%) in Diaper Dermatitis Candidiasis

Diaper dermatitis (DD) is an inflammatory irritating condition that is common in infants. Most cases are associated with the yeast colonization of *Candida* or diaper dermatitis candidiasis (DDC), and therefore, the signs and symptoms improve with antimycotic treatment. Sertaconazole is a broad-spectrum third-generation imidazole derivative that is effective and safe for the treatment for superficial mycoses, such as tineas, candidiasis, and pityriasis versicolor

Urine and feces: The interaction of urine and feces is a major contributing factor behind the development of diaper rash. Bacterial urease, an enzyme in the stool degrades the urea that is found in urine, releasing ammonia and increasing local pH. The warm, humid, high pH environment in the diaper provides the ideal setting microbial proliferation. The increased pH also activates the fecal enzymes, lipases and proteases which results in skin irritation and disruption of the epidermal barrier.

Activating factors
- Excess skin wetness
- Feces and fecal enzymes
- Interaction of feces and urine
- Increased pH leading to
  - Greater fecal enzyme activity
  - Increased skin permeability

Caretaker intervention
- Frequent diaper changes
- Lotion, ointment, cream
- Isolation of feces from urine away from baby's skin

Etiologic factors
- Fecal enzymes
- Skin friction
- Candida albicans (yeast infection)
- Unidentified chemical irritants

Fig. 8.13: Development of diaper rash

Tinea Barbae

Tinea barbae means the ringworm of the beard. It is also termed as "tinea sycosis" and is usually due to the endothrix or ectothrix trichophyton infection.

Clinical Features

1. Superficial dry scale lesions.
2. Sometimes deep boggy suppurative lesions.

Treatment

1. Beard should be clipped short.
2. Oxyquinoline ointment, tolnaftate ointment or lotion miconazole ointment are good.
3. Griseofulvin 1 g daily for 6–8 weeks.
4. Fluconazole.

Tinea Corporis

Tinea corporis means ringworm of the body. It has world wide distribution and may be due to the species of *Trichophyton*, *Epidermophyton*, and *Microsporum* genera.

Clinical Features

It consists of rings of branny, scaly itching lesions. The lesions may be circinate. Gyrate or concentric forms, the chest, abdomen back, axilla may be affected.

Treatment

1. Keep the undergarments, bedsheets, towels clean.
2. Locally—Miconazole ointment tolnaftate or whitefield ointment.
3. Griseofulvin 1 g/day 3-4 weeks or sometimes 6-16 weeks.
4. Fluconazole.

Tinea Cruris

It is ringworm of the genitocrural region. It is called as "dhobie itch". It is common in tropical countries, because of excessive perspiration, friction, shifting of acidic pH to Alkaline PH of the skin. Obese person, diabetes, chronic illness may predispose to the fungus infection.

Etiology

It is produced by Epidermophyton floccosum infection.

Clinical Features

I. The upper and medial parts of thighs, adjoining parts, ano-genital regions are particularly affected.
II. The lesions may be erythematosquamous, papulosquamous or erythematovesicular or pustular.
III. Margins are raised and active while center usually shows signs of healing.
IV. Itching is intense.
V. Secondary infection may supervene and recurrence are common.

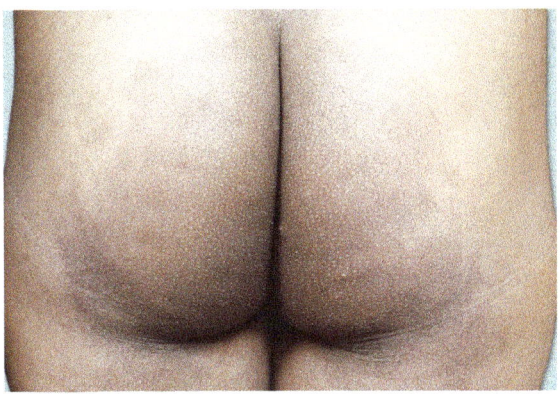

Fig. 8.14: Tinea cruris—marked hyperpigmentation with active border on the buttacks

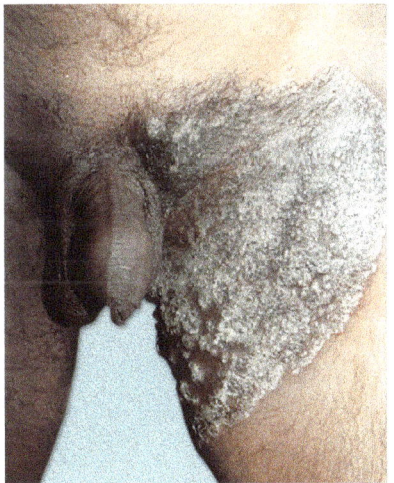

Fig. 8.15: Tinea cruris—marked hyperpigmentation with active border showing erythematous papules and secondary infections groin area

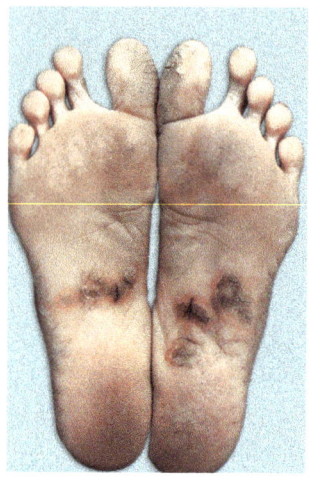

Fig. 8.16: Tinea pedis—scaly hyperkeratotic lesion on both the soles

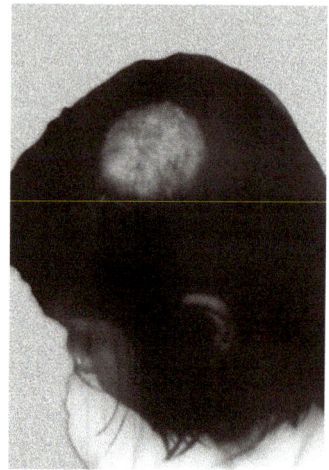

Fig. 8.17: Tinea capitis—boggy inflammatory swelling over the scalp "kerion type"

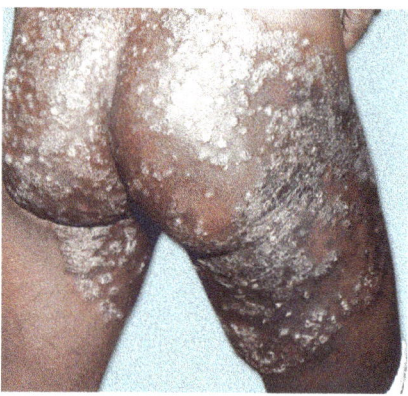

Fig. 8.18: Tinea cruris—marked hyperpigmentation with active border showing erythematous papules and secondary infections both buttocks areas

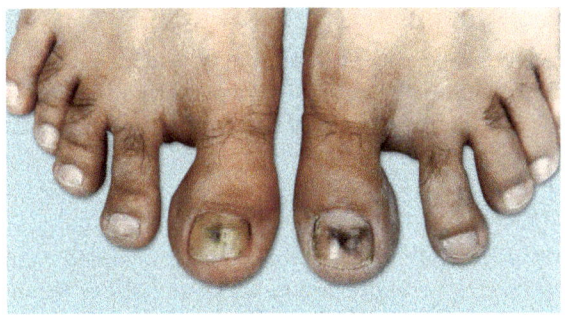

Fig. 8.19: Tinea unguium—thickening and dystrophy of involved nails of the toes both feet

Treatment

I. Keep the hygiene of the part.
II. Avoiding nylon or synthetic fiber underwears, etc.
III. Locally oxyquinotine ointment, chinoform ointment, toflnaftate, buclosamide, miconazole and clotrimazole ointment or solution.
IV. Orally griseofulvin 1 g/day 3–4 or 6 weeks, fluconazole, terbinafine.
V. Antihistamines, etc. for itching, etc. may be used.

Tinea Pedis and Tinea Manuum

Tinea pedis means ringworm of the feet while tinea manuum means fungus infection of the hands.

Etiology

Species of *Trichophyton* (*T. rubrum* and *T. gypseum*) and *Epidermophyton* genera are responsible. Tinea pedis is more common than Tinea manuum.

Clinical Features

There are three main presentation of this fungus infection (a) interdigital (b) vesicular (c) hyperkeratotic. Interdigital is the most important variety of tinea pedis. It is also called as athelets foot.

Treatment

Prophylactic: Walking bare foot should be avoided. Sandals, chappals may be worn. Nylon socks and shoes should be avoided. Hands and feet should be kept clean. Nails should be regularly clipped.

Curative
  I. Wash the affected areas with 1:10,000 of $KMNO_4$ solution

Local
  II. Whitefields ointment
  III. Castellani's paint
  IV. Buclosamide
  V. Tolnaftate
  VI. Miconazole
  VII. Clotrimazole
  VIII. Fluconazole

Oral
  IX. Griseofulvin 1 g/day 6 weeks.
  X. Superficial X-ray in resistent cases.

Tinea unguium: It is the fungal infection of the nails known as Onychomycosis, commonly caused by genus *Tichophyton* and *T. rubrum* is the common agent nails of the hands or feet may be affected together or seperately.

Clinical Features

Main types: (i) superficial (ii) Invasive, and (iii) hyperkeratotic.

The nail plates become opaque, discolored deformed, ridged and friable.

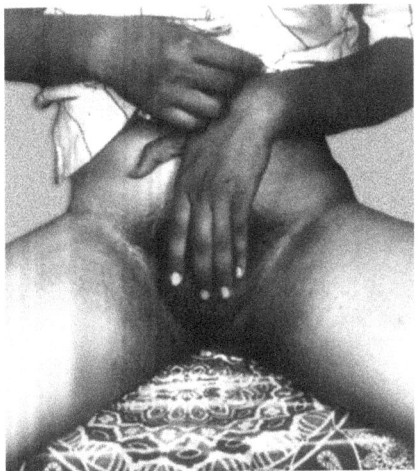

Fig. 8.20: Tinea cruris—marked hyperpigmentation with active border showing erythematous papules

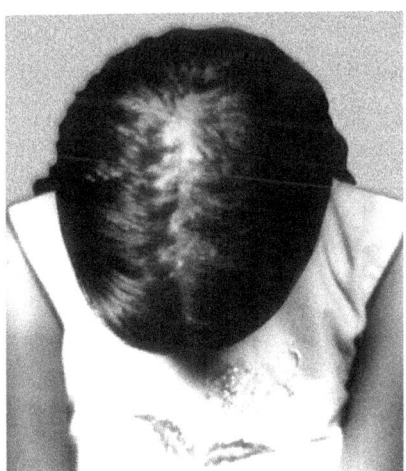

Fig. 8.21: Tinea capitis—partial loss of hair, remaining hair in the alopecia patch area are luster less "gray patch" type

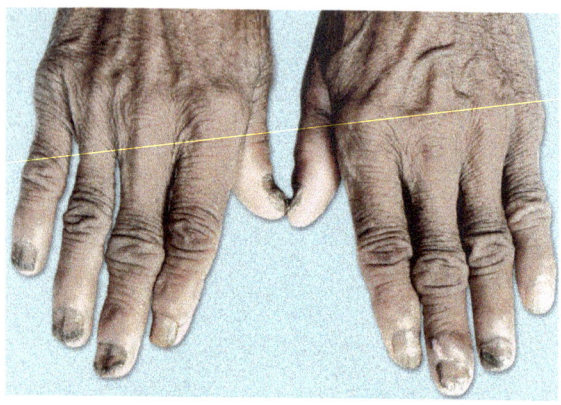

Fig. 8.22: Tinea unguium—thickening and dystrophy of involved nails

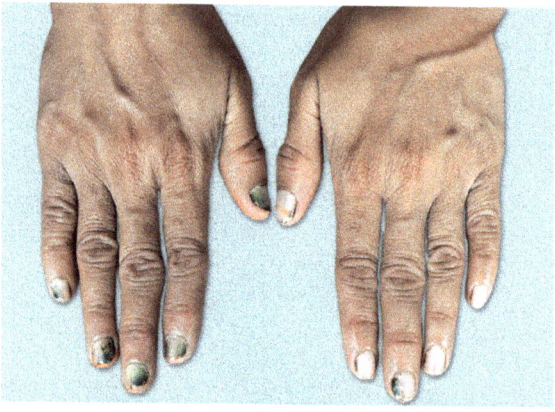

Fig. 8.23: Tinea unguium—thickening and dystrophy of involved nails

Fungal Infections (Mycosis)

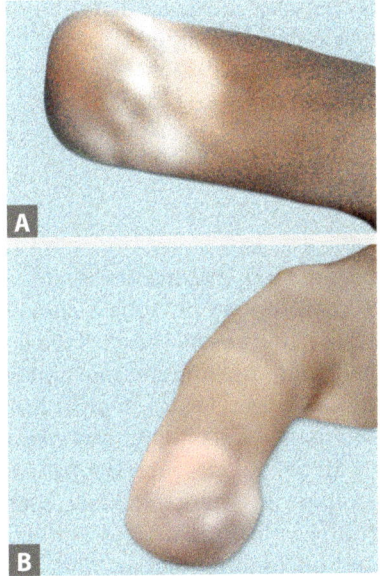

Figs 8.24A and B: Tinea unguium—thickeing and brittle nail with around secondary bacterial infection and whitlo

Treatment

1. Scrape the nails with some sharp edge of glass slide or knife blade.
2. Application of antifungal remedies like Whitefield's ointment, etc.
3. Griseofulvin 1–5 g/day for 6–9 months.
4. Surgical removal of nail.

Treatment

1. Undergarments should be boiled.
2. Daily bath with warm water soap are useful.

3. Local remedies are—
   a. Selsun/selenium disulfide
   b. Sodium thiosulfate 10–20% solution.
   c. Miconazole lotion.
   d. Tolnaftate lotion
4. UV light exposures.

Synopsis

Dermatophytes are fungi that live on keratin. According to the site of affection, dermatophytosis is classified into tinea capitis (scalp hair), tinea faciei (face), tinea cruris (groins), tinea corporis (trunk), tinea manuum (hand), tinea pedis (foot) and tinea unguium (nail). Typical lesion is a ring-shaped arrangement of erythematous papules, vesicles and pustules with central clearing. Hyphae and spores are seen when scaraping is mounted in KOH. Localized lesions respond to topical antifungals (clotrimazole) whereas widespread and unresponsive cases need griseofulvin 10 mg/kg/day for 4–6 weeks (corporis, cruris, manuum and capitis), 8 weeks (pedis) and 6 months to 2 years (unguium). Ketoconazole and fluconazole are newer drugs.

DEEP FUNGAL INFECTIONS

Mycetoma (Madura Foot)

Mycetoma is an uncommon subcutaneous infection caused by either Actinomycetes or true fungi that are introduced into the body by penetrating trauma. Multiple grouped nodules on foot that discharge pus and colonies of organisms (granules) are diagnostic. Causative organisms can be identified and cultured in the laboratory. Systemic antibiotic or antifungal therapy extended over many months may be successful.

Etiology

The causative organism of mycetoma varies from area to area but broadly two groups of organisms cause mycetoma:
  Actinomycetoma is caused by filamentous bacteria.
  Eumycetoma is caused by the fungi.

Table 8.1: Etiological organisms of mycetoma

Actinomycetoma	Eumycetoma
Nocardia brasiliensis	Madurella grisea
Streptomyces somaliensis	Madurella mycetomatis
	Petriellidium boydii

Clinical Features

Epidemiology: Although mycetomas are reported from all over the world, they are more commonly seen in tropical and sub-tropical regions where most people walk barefoot. The species causing mycetoma varies from country to country. Men are more commonly affected.

Morphology: Actinomycetoma and eumycetoma look alike clinically and begin as subcutaneous nodules which slowly eventuate into abscesses and draining sinuses. With further progress, the surrounding tissue becomes swollen and deformed by fibrosis. The discharge may be serosanguinous or seropurulent and contains granules. These granules are black in case of eumycetoma and white in case of actinomycetoma.

Site: Feet are the most favored site; infrequently, other sites of trauma like the hands may be involved.

Complications: Both are localized infections without systemic spread. Involvement of deeper tissues (bones of feet and hands) may cause deformities in long-standing cases.

Investigations

The following investigations need to be done to establish the diagnosis of mycetoma to identify the causative organism and to find the extent of local spread:

Histology: This helps to establish the diagnosis and may help to distinguish actinomycetoma and eumycetoma.

Examination of pus and granules: Examination of potassium hydroxide mount of the granules and culture of the granules help differentiate actinomycetoma and eumycetoma.

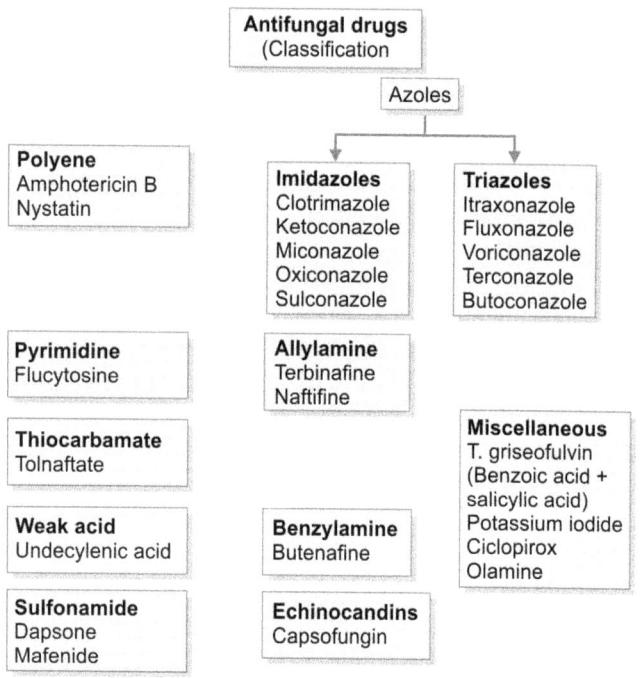

Fig. 8.25: Classification of antifungal drugs

Fungal Infections (Mycosis)

Table 3.2: Systemic antifungal agents

Drug	PV	Dosage/Schedule Dermatophytosis	Candidiasis	Side Effects	Precautions	Comment
Griseofulvin	NA	** 10 mg/kg × 4 week for corporis, × 6 week for manuum/capitis, × 8 weeks for pedis, 6 mth–1 year for finger nail, for toe nail–high failure rate	NA	Very uncommon headache, skin rashes	To be taken with food to improve absorption	Safe, inexpensive effective in dermatophytosis except toe nail
Ketoconazole	*200 mg CD 10 days	200 mg OD × 3–6 weeks for corp. × 6-8 weeks for cap/man/pedis × 6th for finger nail × 1 year for toe nail	200–400 mg. OD for 2 weeks.	Hepatotoxicity	To monitor hepatic transaminases	Expensive, hepatitis seen in 1:10000
Fluconazole	400 mg single dose	NA	**150 mg Single dose or 50–100 mg OD for 3–7 days or two weeks in immuno-suppressed	Gastritis, rarely, hepatitis	Take with food to avoid gastritis	Expensive but effective and safe in candidiasis
Itaconazole	*200 mg BD 5 days	*200 mg BD for 1 week, per month × 3 months for finger nails and × 4 months for toe nails 200 mg BD × 1 week for Tinea manuum/pedis/capitis	200 mg OD stat of for recurrent infections for 3 days. Not for oropharyngeal cand	rare, reversible hepatitis		Very expensive but effective and safe. Reduces treatment duration.
Terbinafine	NA	250 mg/day × 3 months for finger nail and × 6 months for toe nails	NA	Rare, hepatitis		Very expensive but effective in dermatophytosis. Reduces treatment duration.

Culture: To confirm the causative agent. X-ray of the affected part indicates the extent of involvement.

Treatment

Treatment depends on whether the mycetoma is actinomycotic or eumycotic.

Actinomycetoma: Responds to prolonged course (several months!) of combination of chemotherapeutic agents like:

Streptomycin + dapsone or cotrimoxazole.
Cotrimoxazole + amikacin.
Tetracyclines + streptomycin + rifampicin.
Penicillins + gentamycin + cotrimoxazole.
Eumycetoma: The following drugs can be used :
Ketoconazole.
Itraconazole.
Amphotericin B in resistant cases.

Surgical alternatives (deep debridement and even amputation) may need to be resorted to in case of recalcitrant cases.

Sporotrichosis

Causative agent *Sporothrix schenckii*.

Most frequently manifests as an asymptomatic nodule which eventually ulcerates. Over a period of time, a chain of asymptomatic nodules appear along the lymph vessel draining the area.

Potassium iodide solution or itraconazole are effective.

Other Deep Fungal Infections

Histoplasmosis: Associated with pulmonary infection especially in immunocompromised individuals.

Blastomycosis: Lesions are ulcerated nodules which have a spreading verrucous edge. The center shows scarring.

Treatment is with systemic amphotericin B or itraconazole.

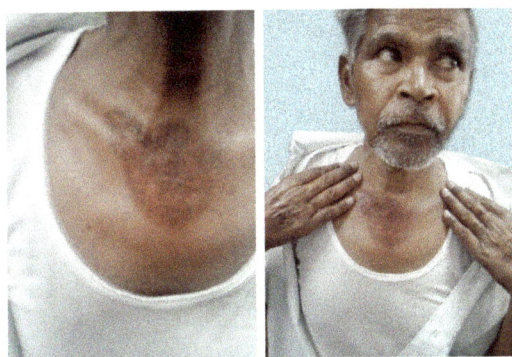

Fig. 8.26: Fungus infection

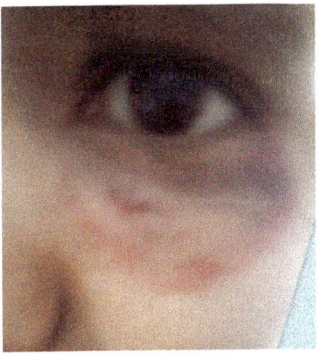

Fig. 8.27: Fungus infection of face

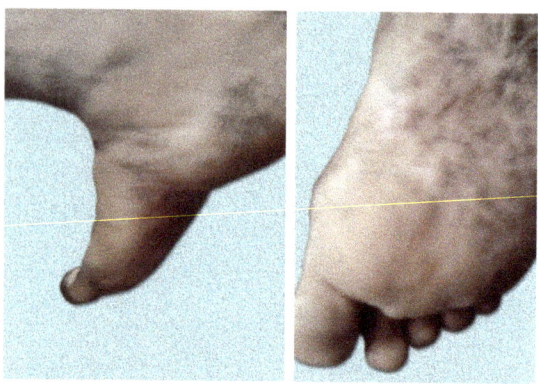

Fig. 8.28: Fungus infection of foot (different views)

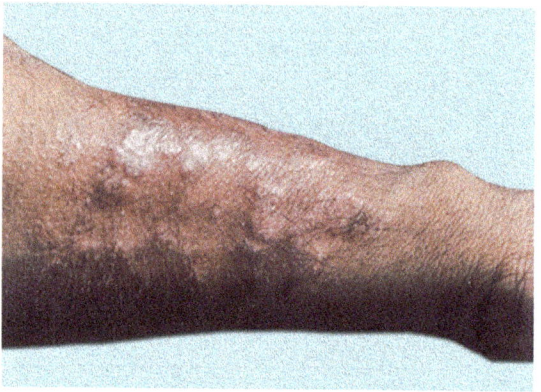

Fig. 8.29: Fungus infection on arm

Fungal Infections (Mycosis)

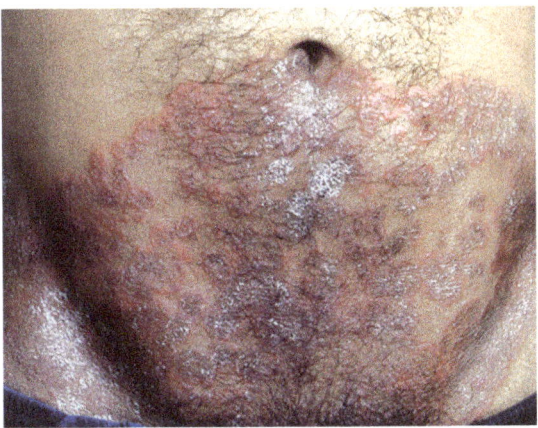

Fig. 8.30: Fungus Infection on abdomen and groin

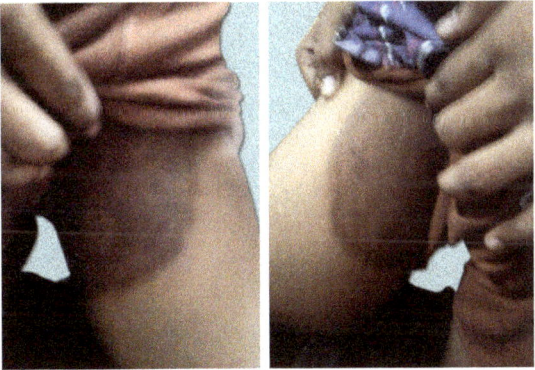

Fig. 8.31: Fungus infection of groin area

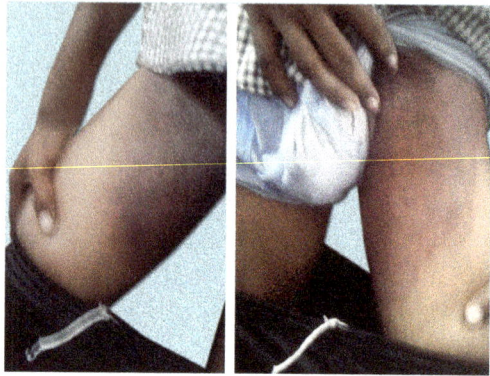

Fig. 8.32: Tinea cruris infection

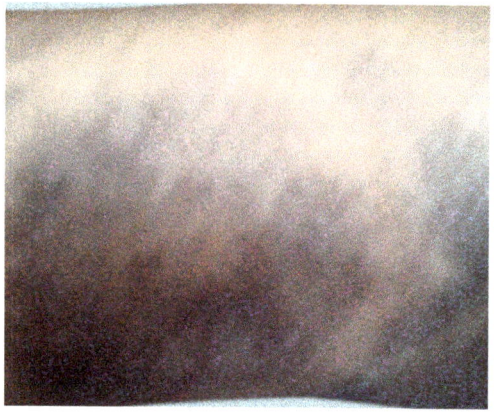

Fig. 8.33: Circular round itchy lesion superficial fungal infection

Fungal Infections (Mycosis)

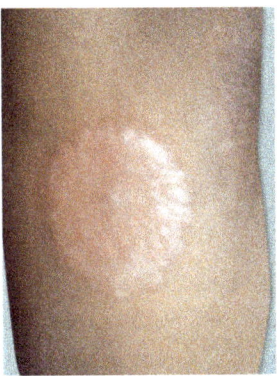

Fig. 8.34: Ringworm—classical ring of the superficial fungal infection

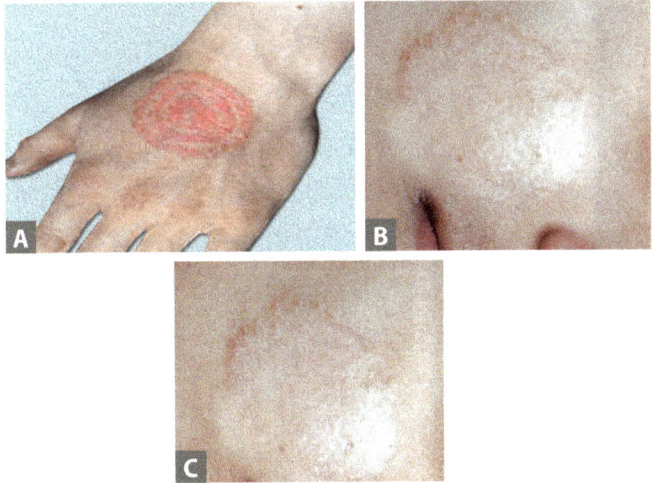

Fig. 8.35A and to C: Ringworm (fungal infection)

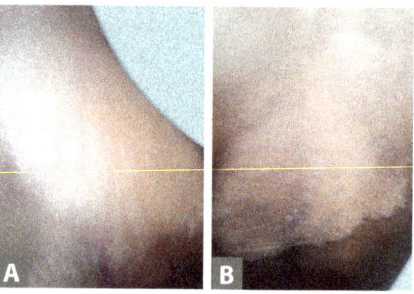

Figs 8.36A and B: Superficial fungal infection

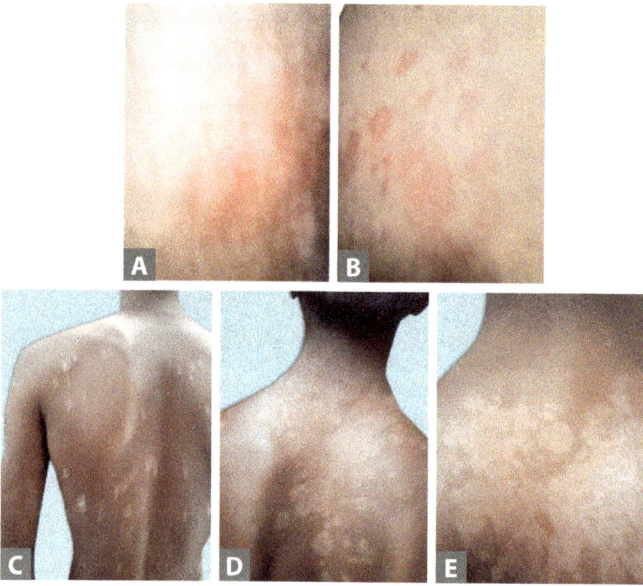

Figs 8.37A to E: Tinea versicolor

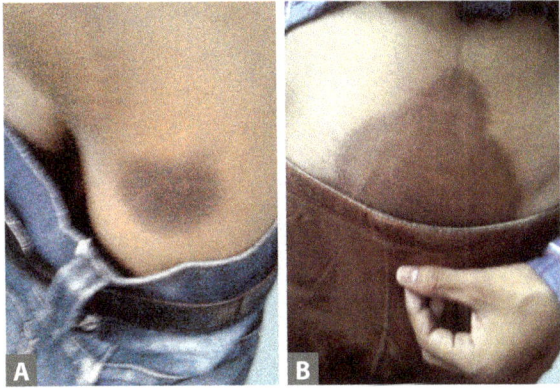

Figs 8.38A and B: Tinea cruris

Course

Lesions usually clear in about a years time without any sequelae, though some lesions may resolve with scarring.

Large solitary lesions may be indolent.

Extensive and difficult to treat lesions are seen in atopic patients and in those who are immunosuppressed.

CHAPTER 9

Viral Infections

The viral infections are divided into two groups local and systemic. Viral infections of skin are characterized by a definite morphology and distribution.

Flowchart 9.1: Classification of human viruses

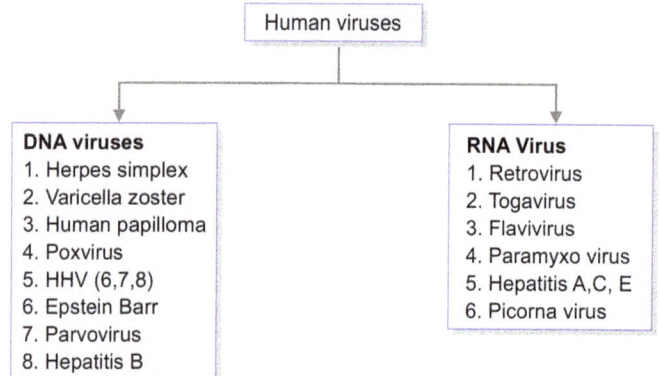

MOLLUSCUM CONTAGIOSUM

Etiology

Molluscum contagiosum, caused by a poxvirus, is transmitted amongst children through close contact and in adults through sexual contact. Its smooth, dome-shaped, pearly white, shiny papules with central umbilication are characteristics. Numerous extragenital mollusca in adults is a marker for HIV infection. Extraction, curettage and cautery are option for therapy.

It is a virus disease. The virus gets implated from a contact with infected individual.

Clinical Features

I. The disease is common with children.
II. Pearly white, smooth surfaced papules present on any part of the body.

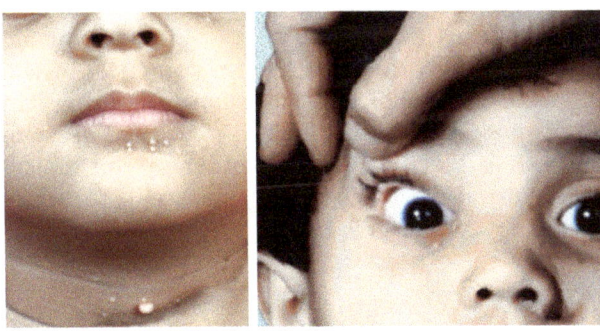

Fig. 9.1A: Molluscum contagiosum —over the face below the lips, chin, and neck of a male child

Fig. 9.1B: Molluscum contagiosum —lesions occurring over the face and on the above eyelid in a child

III. Bigger papules are umblicated in the center.
IV. If the papule is punctate white cheesy material comes out.

TYPES OF VIRAL WARTS

1. *Plane (flat):* These warts are common on hands and faces of children.

2. *Mosaic:* This wart is made of many single warts packed together in a plaque. Always hard to treat.

3. *Cauliflower:* Cauliflower and digitate patterns are most common in the beard and genital areas.

4. *Linear:* Warts may apperar in lines after the skin has been cut or scratched (the Koebner phenomenon).
(verruca vulgaris and verruca plana) or moist warts (condyloma acuminata).

Verruca Vulgaris (Common Warts)

Common warts (verruca vulgaris) are caused by human papilloma virus (HPV) that gets transmitted by contact or fomites amongst the young. Asymptomatic, grayish, rough, dry, sessile papules based on normal looking skin characteristics the disease. Hands, feet, face and neck are common sites. Electrocautery, cryotherapy and topical salicylic acid and imazaquin cream (Gracewell) are usually effective.

Clinical Features

Based on their features and location, warts are classifed into a variety of morphological variants:
- Verruca vulgaris
- Filiform warts

- Superficial mosaic—type of palmoplantar warts
- Deep hyperkeratotic palmoplantar warts
- Verruca plana
- Epidermodysplasia verruciformis
- Condyloma acuminata or anogenital warts.

Verruca Vulgaris (Common Warts)

Morphology: Common warts appear as single or multiple, circumscribed, firm, papules with verrueous, hyperkeratotic surface. Lesions are usually asymptomatic.

Sites: Common warts can occur anywhere on the body. They are most frequently seen on the hands but can also present on the face and genitals.

Filiform Warts (Digitate Warts)

Morphology: These appear as painless, thin, elongated, firm projections arising from a horny base.

Site: Filiform warts are most frequently seen in the beard region (spread by shaving) and on the scalp.

Superficial Plantar Warts (Mosaic Warts)

Morphology: These are hyperkeratotic plaques made up of multiple, small, warts which are tightly packed. They are usually not painful.

Sites: Mosaic warts occur on the soles and less often on the palms.

Deep Palmoplantar Warts (Myrmecia)

Morphology: These are painful, hyperkeratotic, deep-seated papules which protude only slightly from the skin surface and are surrounded by a horny collar. When this horny collar is removed using a scalpel, the wart proper becomes apparent as a soft granular brown papule. Further paring reveals oozing capillary loops. Although they may be multiple, deep plantar warts remain discrete.

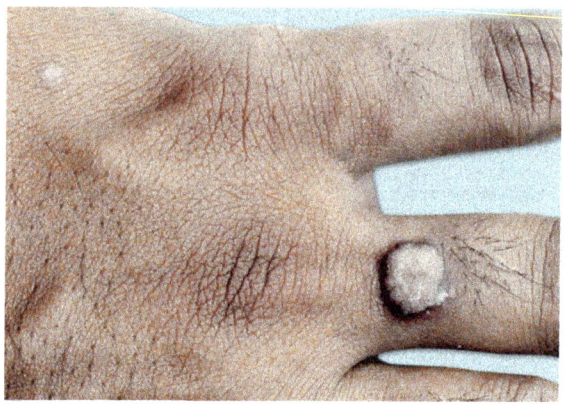

Fig. 9.2: Common warts—rough surfaced keratotic papules over the dorsa of hand

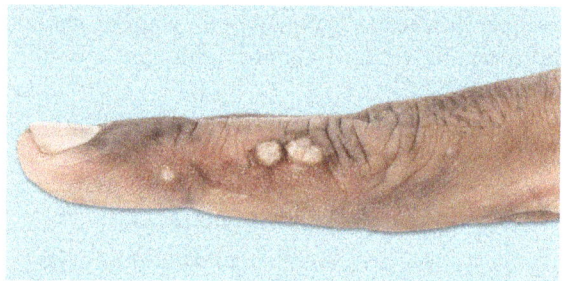

Fig. 9.3: Common warts—rough surfaced keratotic papules over the on the side of the finger multiple warts linear types

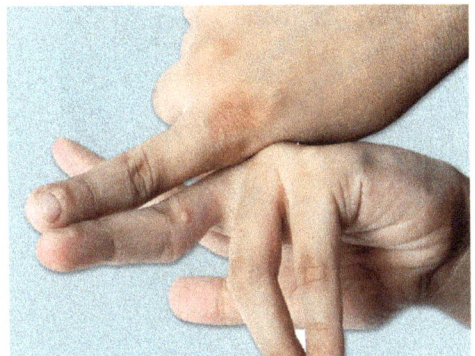

Fig. 9.4: Warts on the fingers and dorsum of the hands

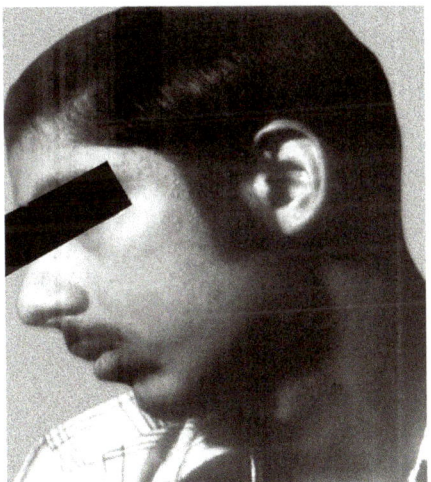

Fig. 9.5: Plane warts on the face and forehead

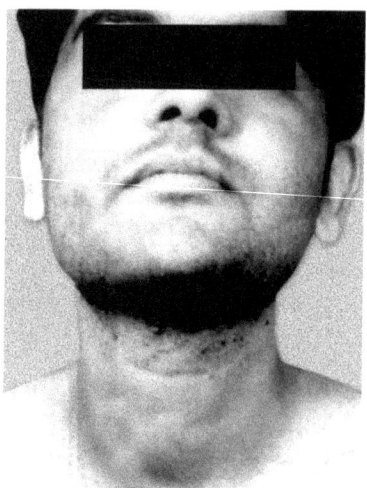

Fig. 9.6: Plane warts on the beard, neck, and chin area

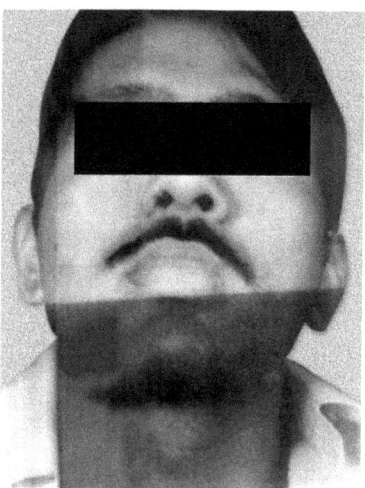

Fig. 9.7: Nasal warts. See inside right side of the nares

Site: Most frequently seen in the soles, deep plantar warts may also be seen on the palms and on sides of fingers.

Plane Warts (Verruca Plana)

Morphology: Plane warts appear as multiple, slightly elevated, flat, smooth papules. They are skin colored or have a brownish hue but may develop an erythematous halo.

Site: Seen on the face and on dorsal aspects of hands, the lesions may be arranged along a scratch mark (Koebner's phenomenon).

Epidermodysplasia Verruciformis

- Rare inherited disorder, characterized by an inefficient cell mediated immunity to certain types of human papilloma virus; this results in extensive infection. Development of Bowen's disease and invasive squamous cell carcinoma is common
- Two types of lesions are seen:
  (a) Plane wart-like lesions, many of which become confluent.
  (b) Pityriasis versicolor—like irregular, scaly macules.

Genital Warts

- Sexually transmitted disease
- Appear either as small flesh colored or as hyperpigmented papules or as cauliflower—like exophytic warts
- Seen most frequently on the glans, perianal region, vulva and cervix.

Course and Complications

In healthy individuals, the warts may resolve spontaneously as the host mounts as immune response to overcome the infection. Spontaneous regression clinically manifests as apperance of punctate areas of blackening (due to capillary thrombosis) in the warts and eventually. The wart resolves with no trace. Some warts like mosaic warts are, however, very recalcitrant. In the immunocompromised (patients on immunosuppressive therapy, those with lymphoreticular malignancy or those with HIV infection), the verrucae are persistent and extensive; some of these patients are also at risk of developing malignancies in the warts.

Diagnosis

Most warts are easily recognized because:
- They are characteristically warty papules with a rough, dry surface
  The morphology of the lesions, however, may be modified by site.
- Presence of Koebner's phenomenon, especially in plane warts
- Typical histology.

Differential Diagnosis

Most warts are easily recognized but the following conditions need to be differentiated:

These are smooth, dome shaped, pearly white papules with central umbilication, while warts have a verrucous, rough surface.

Corns

Corns occur as hyperkeratotic papules on points of pressure on the soles. The skin markings over the corn are not interrrupted. Paring of corn reveals a keratinous core; while in a wart, the core is made up of a leash of blood vessels.

Treatment

The treatment of viral warts depends on the site and type of lesion.

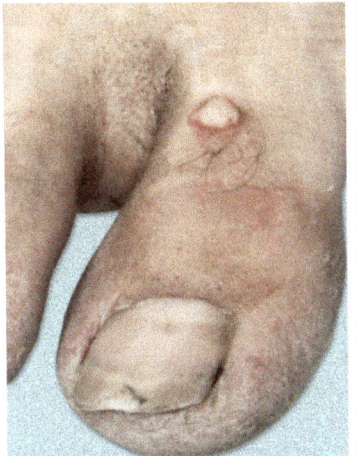 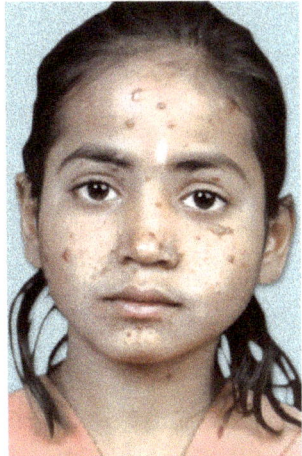

Fig. 9.8: Solitary wart on the toe

Fig. 9.9: Multiple warts on the face of a girl child

Removal of Warts

Several methods of destruction are available. It is not necessary to remove all the warts in a patient, since removal of some may stimulate the body's immunological response, resulting in the spontaneous resolution of remaining warts.

- *Mechanical removal:* Mechanical removal of warts using a curette followed by cauterization of the bleeding base using trichloroacetic acid or electric cautery
- *Electric cautery:* Small as well as slightly larger warts can be removed using an electric cautery. Electric cautery is the treatment of choice for filiform warts on the face
- *Cryotherapy:* Cryotherapy with carbon dioxide or liquid nitrogen is an effective procedure. A cotton-tipped applicator dipped in liquid nitrogen is applied firmly to the wart till a small halo of freezing appears on the adjoining normal skin. Blistering, often thought of as a

prerequisite for effective treatment, is not necessary. The same effect can be achieved with a carbon dioxide stick
- *Wart paints:* These remain the therapy of first choice, especially in children. Most wart paints contain salicylic acid (10-20%). The wart paint is applied daily after the warts have been softened by soaking in hot water about 10 minutes. The paint is apppplied so as to cover the wart but not the surrounding skin. Before the next application, the dead tissue and old paint are removed, the feet soaked in hot water and wart paint reapplied. Warts on the plantar surface should be covered with plaster. Wart paints are best avoided on face and on anogenital warts
- *Formalin soaks:* These are ideal for multiple small plantar warts. The feet are soaked in a 4% formalin solution for about 10 minutes. A few patients, however, develop allergic contact dermatitis to formalin
- *Cryotherapy:* This can be tried as for verruca vulgaris.

Plane Warts:
- Few lesions, when present, can be touched with 10% trichloroacetic acid or treated with careful freezing
- Multiple, extensive facial lesions can be treated with topical retinoic acid (0.05%).

OTHER VARIETIES OF WARTS

(1) Verrucae plana (plane warts, juvenile warts)
(2) Palmoplantar warts
(3) Condyloma acuminata.

Condyloma acuminata are caused by a human papilloma virus that is transmitted by sexual contact. Early lesions are pink conical papules. Pink, fleshy, pedunculated, cauliflower like growths are seen in advanced cases. Topical podophyllin (20%) is usually effective.

The latest treatment of all type of warts is by local application of imiquimod. Imiquimod is an immune response modifier. Chemically, imiquimodis 1-(2-methylpropyl)-1 H-imidazo [4,5-c] quinolin-4-amine. Imiquimod has a molecular formula of $C_{14}H_{16}N_4$ and a molecular weight of 240.3.

Imiquimod has no direct antiviral activity in cell culture. A study in patients with genital/perianal warts comparing imiquimod cream and vehicle shows that it induces mRNA encoding cytokines including interferon at the treatment site. In addition HPVL 1 mRNA and HPV DNA are significantly decreased following treatment. However, the clinical relevance of these findings is unknown.

Flowchart 9.2: Pathogenesis of HPV-associated anogenital warts

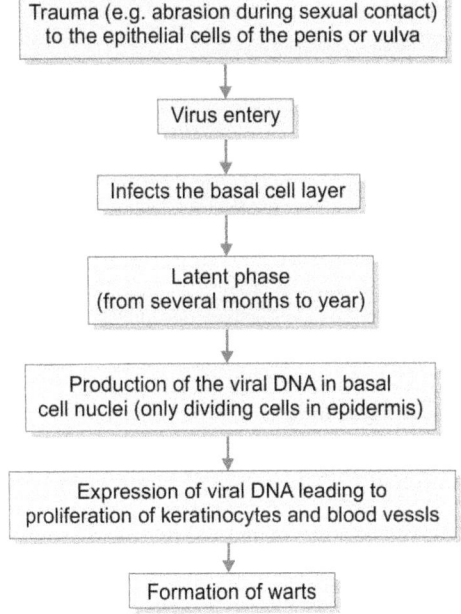

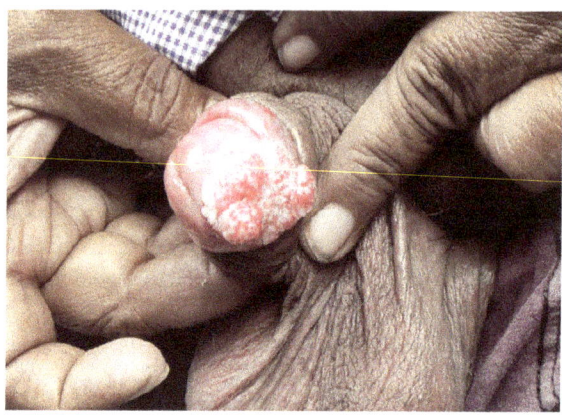

Fig. 9.10: Pathogenesis of HPV

Table 9.1: Different type of therapy agent and their mechanism of action

Therapy agent	Mechanism of action
Local excision	Surgical removal
Cryotherapy	Physically freeze/thaw to destroy tissue
CO$_2$ laser vaporization	Vaporization of tissue
Electrocautry	Physical destruction of tissue
Podophyllin	Antimitotic
Podophyllotoxin	Antimitotic
Trichloroacetic acid	Chemical destruction
Interferon	Antimitotic

Alternative Therapy
- Topical cantharidin
- Tretinoin (0.05–0.1%)
- Cidofovir (1–3%)
- Imiquimod (5%)
- 10% KOH application
- Silver nitrate

- 5-FU topically
- Trichloroacetic acid (30–100%) application.

VARICELLA (CHICKENPOX, PRIMARY INFECTION WITH VARICELLA ZOSTER VIRUS [VZVI])

Varicella (chickenpox) is a manifestation of initial infection with varicella zoster virus. It is common in children, who usually have a mild, self limiting disease. Clear colored fluid containing vesicles with surrounding erythema are characteristic. Papules, umbilicated vesicles and pustules also occur. Complications include bacterial infection, pneumonitis and encephalitis. Oral acyclovir is used in immunocompromized persons or for complications.

HERPES ZOSTER

Herpes Zoster (Reactivation or Secondary Attack of Infection)

After an attack of varicella, the virus of varicella remains dorments in the neurons of posterior root ganglia and becomes reactivated at times when body immunity is low. Therapy is symptomatic for this self-limiting disorder. Oral or topical acyclovir, used early may shorten the duration of disease but does not present recurrences. Oral acyclovir is useful in the immunoincompetent.

Advanced Antiviral Therapy Simplifying Herpes Management

Famciclovir

Indication	Immunocompetent	Immunocompromised
Herpes zoster	500 mg tid × 7 days	500 mg tid × 10 days

Genital Herpes

First episode of 250 mg extremely important to explain to the patient the causes that underlie initiation and perpetuation of the disease and advise here or him to take corrective measures. Measures specific for each variety of eczemas are discussed with their clinical features. Apart from this, the principles of managing eczema remain similar and they depend on the extent and chronicity of the condition. The more acute an eczema the more bland region innervated by that nerve segment.

Factors that precipitate an attack of herpes zoster include unusual stress, or an immunocompromized state like HIV disease or lymphoma, systemic administration of immuno suppressives or steroids or irritation of nerve roots due to

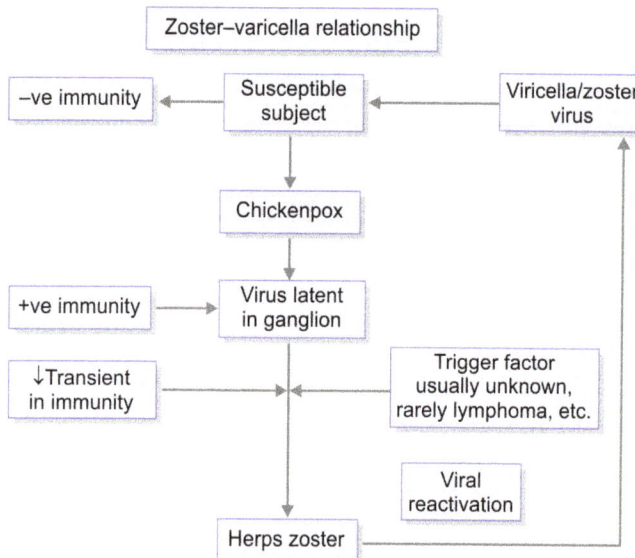

Flowchart 9.3: Zoster–varicella relationship

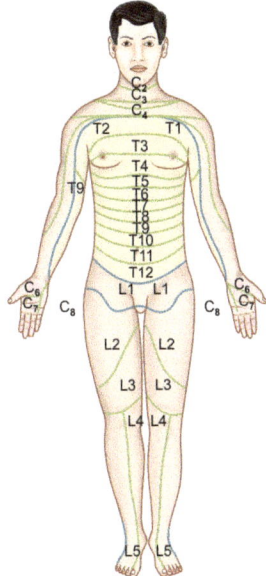

Fig. 9.11: Distribution of herpes lesions

trauma, surgery or tumors. Pattient remains infective till skin lesions get crusted. Since the virus of varicella and zoster are the same, a patient with herpes zoster can transmit the infection to a previously unexposed child causing varicella. However, since herpes zoster represents reactivation rather than reinfection, contact with a case of varicella cannot result in herpes zoster.

Patient Profile

Males and females are affected equally. Elderly individuals are common victims. However, it is not incommon in middle aged or even young adults. Young adults are affected more frequently in the HIV era. Zoster in a young adult male is considered a marker for HIV infection and it is necessary to screen such patients for HIV infection.

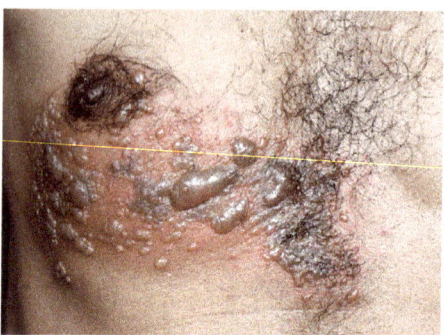

Fig. 9.12: Herpes zoster-grouped vesicles on erythematous patches in thoracic dermatome

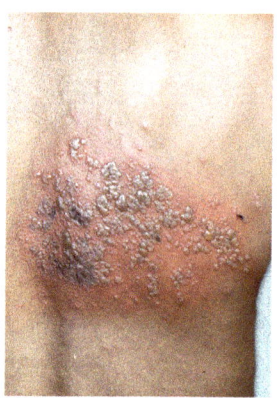

Fig. 9.13: Herpes zoster-grouped vesicles on erythematous patches in back dermatome

History

It is common for pain and hyperesthesia to precede the skin lesions in the affected segments. Hence, patients with zoster commonly present to specialists other than dermatologists with complaints of pain in extremities, chest, abdomen, back ear or tooth or headache. Pain may be severe or mild or even absent especially when zoster occurs in younger individuals. pain precedes skin lesions by a few days. Prodromal symptoms of fever and malaise are noted in occasional cases. Skin lesions appear in one to three crops over 3-4 days.

Morphology

Grouped tense vesicles containing clear fluid that have a base or a halo of erythema and edema are seen in the developed stage of the disease. Erythematous macules, papules and papulovesicles in grouped configuration constitiute the earlier lesions. In servere cases, such groups of vesicles are so closely placed as to become confluent. Individual vesicles may also coalesce forming bullae. Vesicular fluid may become hemorrhagic or turbid at times. In immunocompromized patients, the lesions may turn ulceratcive or gangrenous.

In a stereotypical case, lesions evolve over one week and than the center of the vesicles becomes dry and depressed leading to crust formation. Crusts fall off within 10-15 days leaving behind dyspigmentation. Scarring occurs only when the lesions develop secondary bacterial infection or are unusually severe.

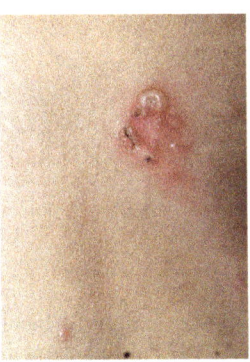

Fig. 9.14: Typical lesions of herpes zoster

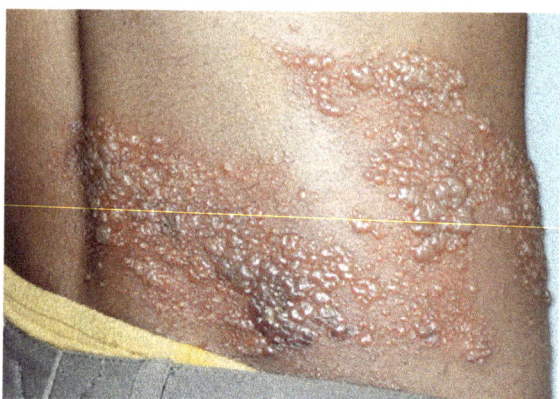

Fig. 9.15: Herpes zoster-grouped vesicles on erythematous patches in back dermatome, extensive lesions

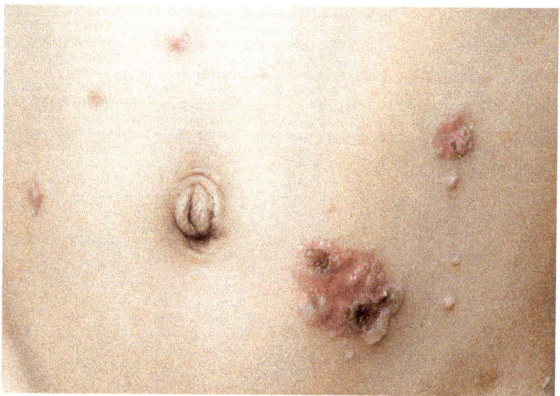

Fig. 9.16: Chickenpox—vesicular erupion over the abdomen

Distribution

Zoster involves one or two contiguous nerve segments. Hence, the lesions are arranged in a unilateral segmental distribution either across the trunk or along an extremity. A few lesions outside the involved segment do not signify dissemination. Commonly involved segments include divisions of trigeminal are segments supplying the trunk (T3 to L1).

Complications of Herpes Zoster

Common complications of zoster include secondary bacterial infection, scarring and postherpetic neuralgia. Postherpetic neuralgia is common in the elderly and may be prevented by early administation of a short course of systemic steroids. When severe, it may disturb sleep and needs to be treated with analgesics or antiepileptics.

Other complications may be related to the following:

Morphology
Bullous, confluent, hemorrhagic, ulcerative and gangrenous lesions in immunocompromized patients.

Distribution
Multisegmental zoster, disseminated zoster involving the skin.

Segment Affected
Ophthalmic: Keratoconjunctivitis, glaucoma extraocular muscle palsy, delayed cerebral angiitis leading to hemiplegia.
Facial: Facial palsy, deafness, vertigo (Ramsay Hunt syndrome).
Upper cervical: Unilateral paralysis of diaphragm.
Systemic: Myelitis, meningoencephalitis, radiculitis.

Therapy

Being a self-limiting viral infection, a typical case of zoster does does not warrant antiviral therapy. Systemic antiviral agents are usually reserved for patients with underlying immunodeficiency or case with unusually dense, deep or disseminated or painful lesions. Oral acyclovir 400 mg 5 times a day shortens the course of zoster and lead to faster heading of lesions in severe cases. It needs to be administered early

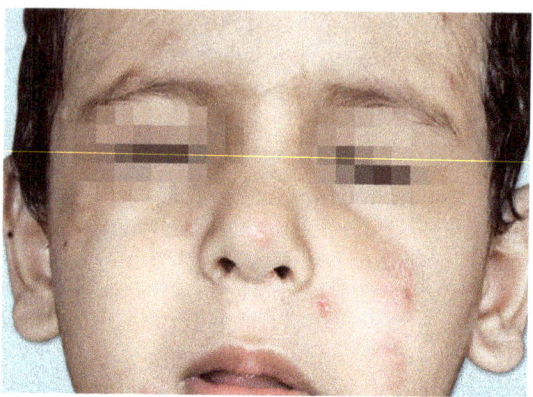

Fig. 9.17: Chickenpox—vesicular eruptions on the face

in the course of the disease (within 2-3 days of the eruption) to be of significant benefit to the patient.

Summary

Herpes zoster is due to reactivation of the dormant varicella-zoster virus under conditions of stress. Grouped vesicles on an erythematous, edematous base in a unilateral segmental pattern are typical. Branches of the trigeminal nerve are commonly affected. Ophthalmic branch involvement can lead to keratoconjuctivitis. Other complications are postherpetic neuralgia and, in immunocompromized persons, visceral dissemination. Oral or intravenous acyclovir is useful for such patients.

HERPES SIMPLEX

Herpes simplex virus I causes stomatitis and keratoconjunctivitis and HSV II causes genital infections that are trasmitted sexually. The virus has a tendency to remain

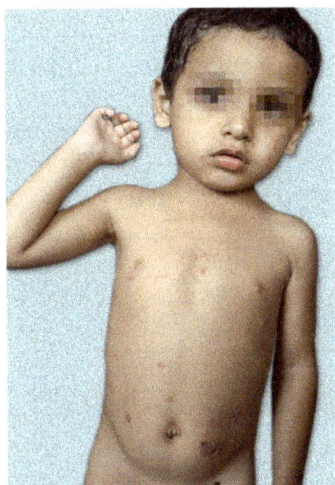

Fig. 9.18: Chickenpox lesions on the face, ears, neck, abdomen, arms and hands

dormant and cause recurrences at frequent intervals. Grouped vesicles on erythematous bases characterize the disease. Regional lymphadenopathy is common. Lesions last for about 1–2 weeks. Oral acyclovir does not prevent recurrences but hastens healing of lesions.

HERPES LABIALIS

Caused by HSVI, herpes labialis usually reperesents secondary attack following initial herpetic gingivostomatitis. Attacks are precipitated by fever, trauma or stress. Grouped vesicles on a base of erythema on or around the lips, including their mucosal aspects are characteristic. Regional lymphadenopathy is common in severe episodes. Therapy is symptomatic for. This self-limiting disorder. Topical acyclovir, used early, may shorten duration of disease.

HERPES GENITALIS

Caused by HSC II, a primary attack of herpes genitalis tends to be severe with regional lymphadenopathy. Secondary attacks are common and are precipitated by trauma of intercourse or stress. Grouped vesicles on a base of erythema on glans, prepuce or the shaft of penis.

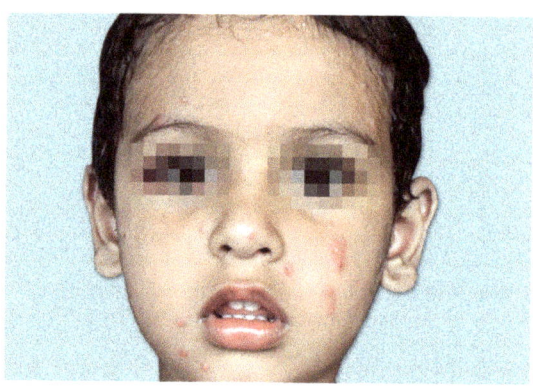

Fig. 9.19: Chickenpox lesions on the face, ears and below the eyes and nose

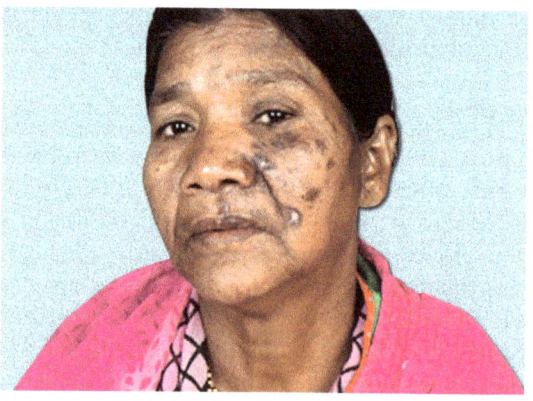

Fig. 9.20: Postherpetic scar on face

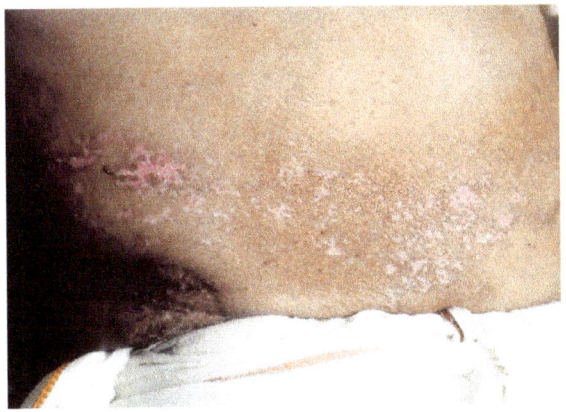

Fig. 9.21: Postherpetic scar on the thoracic dermatome

Table 9.2: Advanced antiviral therapy simplifying herpes management: Famciclovir

Indication	Immunocompetent	Immunocompromised
Herpes zoster	500 mg tid × 7 days	500 mg tid × 10 days
Genital Herpes First episode of genital herpes	500 mg tid × 7 days	500 mg bid × 7 days
Treatment of recurrent genital herpes	125 mg bid × 5 days	500 mg bid × 7 days
Suppresive treatment of recurrent patients, interrupt the genital herpes therapy at 6–12 months	250 mg bid × 1 year	500 mg bid for HIV

Table 9.3: Advanced antivital therapy simplifying herpes management: Valcivir

Indication	Valcivir
Herpes zoster	1 g 3 times daily for 7 days
Genital herpes	1 g twice daily for 10 days
Initial episode	500 mg twice daily for 3 days
Recurrent episode	1 g once a day in patients with normal immune function
Suppressive therapy (more than 9 episodes a year)	500 mg once a daily
Suppressive therapy (less than 9 episodes a year)	500 mg once a daily
Suppressive therapy HIV patients	500 mg once a daily for source partner
Reduction of transmission	2 g twice a day for one day taken
Herpes labialis 12 hours apart	

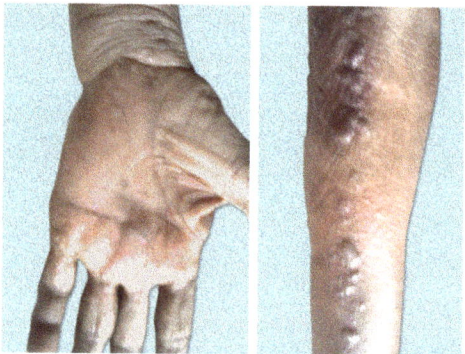

Fig. 9.22: Herpes zoster lesons—linear vesicular painful lesions on the course of the nerve root ulner nerve extending to arms and palm

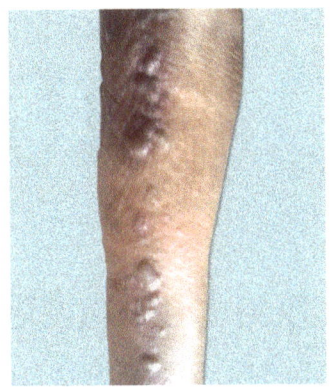

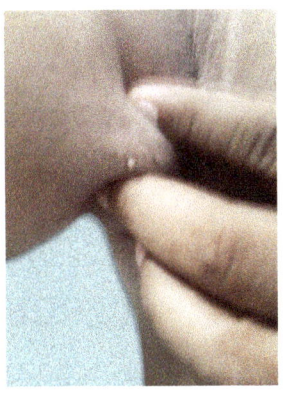

Fig. 9.23: Herpes zoster lesons—linear vesicular painful lesions on the course of the nurve root ulner nerve extending to palm

Fig. 9.24: Hanging warts

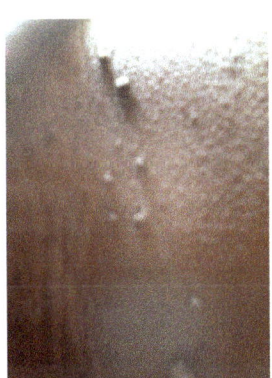

Fig. 9.25: Warts

Statins and the risk of herpes zoster: a population-based cohort study.

Statins are widely used lipid-lowering drugs with immunomodulatory properties that may favor reactivation of latent varicella-zoster virus infection.

CHAPTER 10

Eczemas and Dermatitis

DEFINITION

Eczema is an inflammatory condition of the skin that is characterized by erythema, edema, papulovesicles, oozing and crusting in the acute stages and lichenification in the chronic stages. 'Ekze' in Greak means "to boil over". All the eczemas are dermatitis but not all dermatitis are eczema. Eczema are group of etiologically unrelated conditions that have similar clinical morphology. They have been defined a pattern of skin inflammation that has characteristic morphologies in acute, subacute, and chronic phases, as shown in Table 10.1.

Table 10.1: Pattern of skin inflammation in acute, subacute, and chronic phases

Acute phase	Erythema, edema, vesiculation, oozing and crusting
Subacute phase	Hyperpigmentation, scaling, and crusting
Chronic phase	Lichenification (a combination of thickening, hyperpigmentation and prominent skin markings)

The term dermatitis is usually used synonymously with eczema. The word eczema should preferably not be used without a preceding qualifying term as in contact eczema or xerotic eczema. Histopathologically, this group on condition is typified by epidermal intercellular edema (spongiosis).

The natural history of eczema is diagrammatically represented in Figure 10.1.

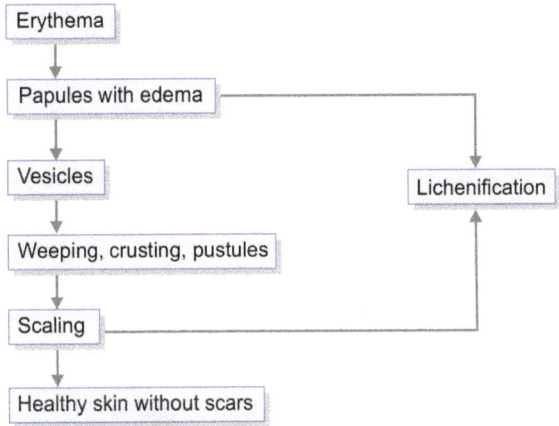

Fig. 10.1: Natural history of eczema

ETIOLOGIC GROUPING OF ECZEMAS

Exogenous eczemas: An external cause for the eczema is identifiable and when this is removed, eczema does not recur. Contact dermatitis is the prototype of exogenous eczemas.

Endogenous eczemas: An internal cause or an inherent property of the skin is responsible for the occurrence of eczema. Prime example is seborrheic dermatitis.

Combined eczemas: Some eczemas may have an exogenous as well as an endogenous component, e.g. xerotic eczema precipitated by cold and dry winter climate and excessive use of soap a multifactorial etiology.

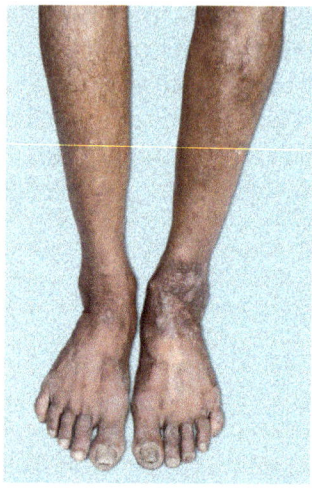
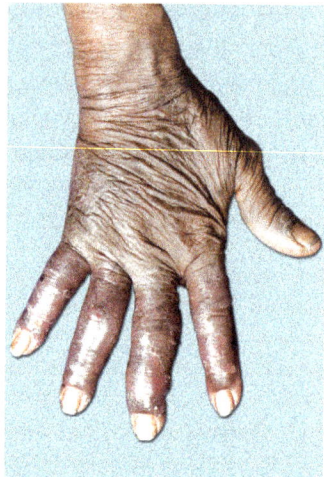

Fig. 10.2: Chronic Eczema of both feet and legs—lichen simplex chronicus

Fig. 10.3: Eczema on the hand—swelling and infection scaling and hyperpigmentation

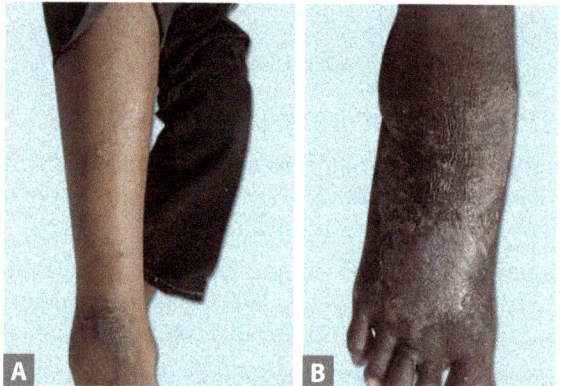

Figs 10.4A and B: A. Infected eczema, swelling and pus; (B) Chronic eczema and change of skin color

Eczemas and Dermatitis

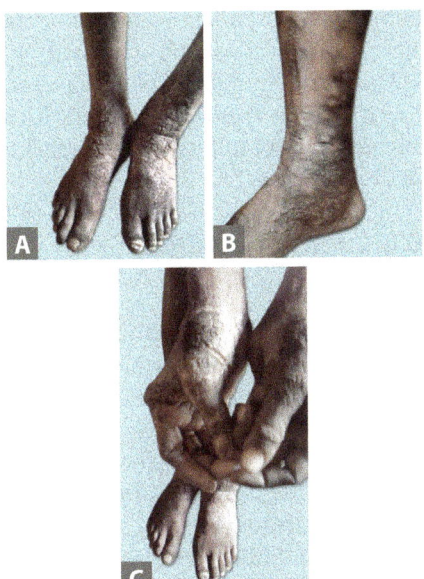

Figs 10.5A to C: Chronic eczema of both feet and legs—lichen simplex chronicus. There is infection and swelling of both the feet; there is crusting also

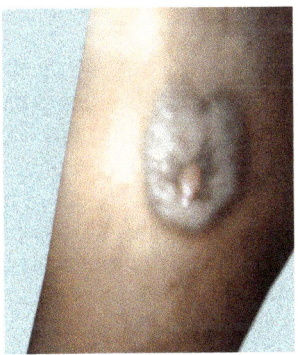

Fig. 10.6: Circular, round single lichenified, thickened, lesion of eczema on skin of the leg

Atopic dermatitis is an endogenous eczema characterized by a pruritic, recurrent, flexural, symmetric eczematous dermatosis. A personal or family history of allergic rhinitis, asthma or hay fever is often associated. Most patients have an increased ability to form IgE (reagin) to common environmental allergens.

ETIOLOGY AND PATHOGENESIS

Genetic

A genetic predisposition is very obvious in atopic dermatitis. The mode of inheritance is probably polygenic. A family history is present in about 70% of patients. If one parent has atopic diathesis, there is 60% chance of the child being an atopic. The figure increases to 80% if both parents are atopic. Monozygotic twins are concordant for the disease. Atopic diseases tend to run true to type within each family: in some families the affected members have eczema, while in others respiratory symptoms predominate. This is probably because the dermatitis and asthma are inherited through separate though closely related genetic pathways. HLA typing has, however, not supported the hypothesis of genetic inheritance.

Immunological Mechanisms

Raised IgE level (level of >200 µIU/mL in 80% patients) is the most consistent immunological finding in patients with atopic dermatitis. The levels of IgE may fluctuate with disease activity. The exact cause of the elevated level of IgE is not known. It could be due to a defect in the control of IgE production by T-lymphocytes. Atopics may also be over producing IgE to a variety of antigent challenges. Abnormalities of the lymphocytes have also been detected in the form of the following:
- Decereased delayed hypersensitivity
- Decreased number of circulating T-lymphocytes, especially suppressor T-cells associated with a decrease in T-cell activity

- Increased proportion of B-lymphocytes with surface-bound IgE.

Points of Focus

Pathogenesis of atopic dermatitis.
- A strong genetic predisposition is obvious
- Raised IgE levels are most consistent immunological finding
- Associated abnormalities of lymphocytes.

Clinical Features

Systemic steroids are often necessary when extensive involvement is present. Once the acute phase is brought under control with bland lotions, topical steroid lotions may be used.

Subacute

Topical steroid lotions or creams are highly effective. Potent steroids should be avoided over face and intertriginous areas for fear of causing atrophy or striae. Systemic steroids may occasionally by needed for extensive affections.

Chronic

Potent (fluocinolone or beclomethasone) or highly potent (clobetasol propionate or betamethasone dipropionate) topical steroids are usually effective. For resistant cases, efficary of steroids can be raised by combining them with a keratolytic agent (salicyclic acid) or the use of an occlusive plastic film (occlusive therapy) for a period of 4-8 hours following steroid application. Residual lesions can be injected with intralesional depot preparation of a steroid like triamcinolone acetonide 5 mg/mL. Intralesional injection may be repeated after 4-6 weeks, if needed.

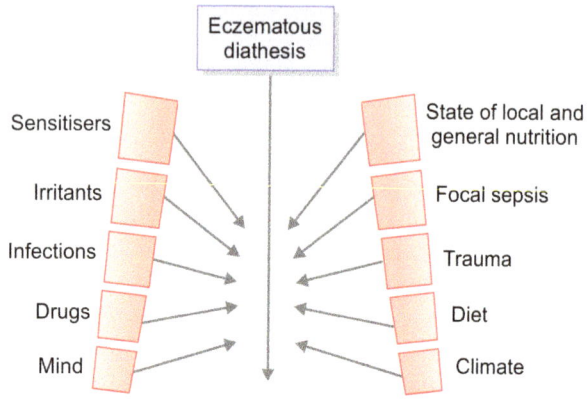

Fig. 10.7: Eczema and dermatitis

Clinical Implication

Topical use of potent or very potent corticosteroids with or without occlusive therapy or intralesional injection may lead to skin atrophy, striae, ulceration, hypopigmentation and telangiectasiae, especially on face and intertriginous (body folds) areas and in children. Frequent injections of intralesional steroids can lead to systemic absorption and consequent side effects of steroids especially in children.

Involvement of more than 20% body area is better treated with, drying and cooling, calamine lotion, etc. Soaps should be avoided while bathing.

Lichen simplex chronicus is a plaque of chronic lichenified dermatitis that results from persistent rubbing of an area, as an end result of any localized eczema or a habit tic. Prominence of skin markings, hyperpigmentation and thickening are features of lichenification. Potent topical steroids, if needed under plastic film occlusion, are effective. Resistant lesions respond to intralesional steroid injection.

Xerotic Eczema

Individuals with dry type of skin, especially elderly and children, tend to develop xerotic eczema during winter. Dry, hypopigmented, ill-defined patches with fine scales over extensors and face are typical. Oozing, crusting and fissuring, etc. occur later. Avoidance of soap and use of moisturizers improve most cases. Mild topical steroids may be used to bring it under control with rapidity.

- Nummular eczema
- Stasis eczema
- Bacterial eczema.

Superantigens and Eczema

This may induce or aggravate easily than intact skin. The presence of superantigens has two main implications for clinical practice.

COMMON PATTERNS OF ECZEMA

Common patterns of eczema are discussed below.

ATOPIC ECZEMA

The word atopy means 'strange or without place' and refers to a lack of niche for these problems in 'those early times'. Historically, the word 'atopy' was first used by for a group of hereditary disorders in people who had a tendency to develop an urticarial response to food and inhalant substances.

Azathioprine Dosed by Thiopurine-Methyltransferase Activity for Atopic Eczema

Azathioprine could be useful alternative for the treatment of severe atopic eczema in adults. In the absence of facilities for TPMT estimation, lower doses, found equally effective, could be used. However, regular monitoring of blood count and platelets estimation are essential.

CONTACT DERMATITIS

This dermatitis induced by contact with an external agent may be an irritant contact dermatitis (due to a direct irritant effect of the agent) or may be an allergic contact dermatitis (due to delayed, type IV hypersensitivity reaction).
- Contact irritant dermatitis
- Cumulative contact irritant dermatitis
- Contact allergic dermatitis
- Parthenium dermatitis.

SEBORRHEIC DERMATITIS

Seborrheic dermatitis is an endogenous eczema that is probably due to abnormal body response to the commensal yeast *Pityrosporum*. Young adult males are typically affected. Red papules topped by a yellowish greasy scale are characteristic. Lesions may coalesce to involve large areas or form thick scales. Face, scalp, central trunk and flexures are classically involved. Topically, mild steroids, antifungals and shampooing are useful. Systemic ketoconazole is occasionally needed to control the disease and steroids, only for erythrodermic disease.

ATOPIC DERMATITIS

Along with allergic rhinitis, bronchial asthma (endogenous) and hay fever, it constitutes atopy, a condition of altered reactivity to common and mild environmental stimuli.

Clinical Features

Infantile phase
Childhood phase

Adolescent and Adulthood Phase

Atopic dermatitis is a component of atopy, i.e. an abnormal reactivity to common environmental stimuli like contact with wool or synthetic fibers, dust, animal or plant products. These persons react with severe pruritus, acute weeping eczema of face in infancy and chronic lichenified eczema in adults. Extensor of limbs are involved during infancy and childhood. Therapy involves avoidance of irritants and precipitating factors and the use of moisturizers and mild topical steroids.

Dignostic Criteria for Atopic Dermatitis

Patient most have pruritus in the past 12 months, plus 3 or more of the following.
- History skin-crease dermatitis or cheek dermatitis (in infants)
- Personal history of asthma or hay fever (or first-degree relative if age < 4 years)
- History of generalized dray skin in past year.
- Visible skin-crease dermatitis (or dermatitis of the cheeks, forehead, or outer limbs if age < 4 years)
- Onset before age 2 years (not used in patients if age < 4 years).

Diagnosis

AD diagnosis is based on clinical criteria that require a history and physical findings confirming early onset of generalized dry skin with pruritus, predominantly on the face and flexural areas of the limbs. There are several validated instruments that are helpful for grading severity. In the defferential diagnosis, seborrheic dermatitis, psoriases, and allergic contact dermatitis can usually be excluded on clinical ground but occasionally require skin biopsy or patch testing. Other laboratory tests are rarely needed for diagnosis but may be helpful to detect bacterial, fungal, or viral comorbid conditions and to indentify contributory airborne and food sensitivities.

Treatment

First line of treatment of AD consists of daily non-prescription emollients for dry skin and low -potency topical corticosteroids (class 6 and 7) applied to facial and intertriginous active lesions. In adult and other children, lesions on other sites may be treated with limited courses of mid strength to superpotent (class 1-5) corticosteroids. Fissured and crusted areas frequently require topical or oral antibiotic therapy, based on culture and sensitivity results. Sedating antihistamines are indicated at bed time for patients whose sleep is disrupted by pruritus.

Second-line therapy includes topical calcineurin inhibitor, PUVA and other light treatment, and oral corticosteroids. The latter two modalities, as well as third line therapy for severe recalcitrant AD with such immunomodulators as cyclosporine, may be considered in collaboration with a dermatologist specializing in in inflammatory skin disorders.

INFANTILE ECZEMA (ECZEMA IN INFANTS)

- Atopic dermatitis
- Seborrheic dermatitis
- Xerotic eczema
- Napkin dermatitis
- Contact allergic dermatitis
- Secondary eczematization.

Eczema in infancy may be due to atopic dermatitis or seborrheic dermatitis or less frequently, xerotic eczema and napkin dermatis. Contact allergic dermatitis is rare in infancy but contact irritant dermatitis may be seen. Acute eczema of face and extremities with positive family history of atopy are seen with atopic dermatitis. Greasy scales over

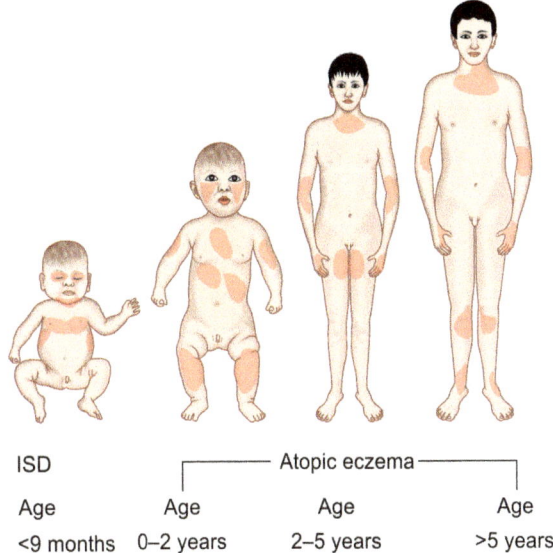

Fig. 10.8: Infantile eczema: Age-related pattern of involvement

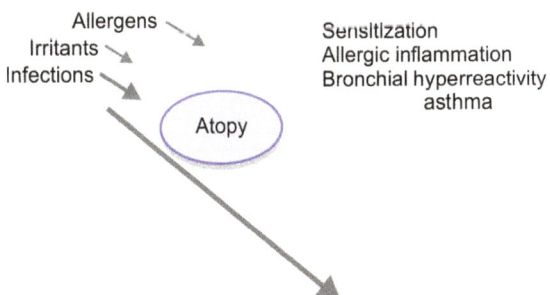

Fig. 10.9: Early diagnosis of the atopic eczema in child

erythema with accentuation in seborrheic distribution are features of seborrheic dermatitis. Xerotic eczema is a dry eczema of face and extensors that occurs in winter. Mild topical steroids should preferably be used. Stronger topical

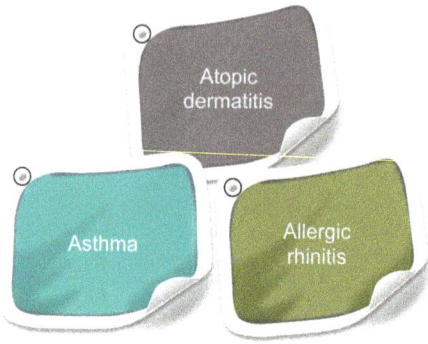

Fig. 10.10: Atopic triad

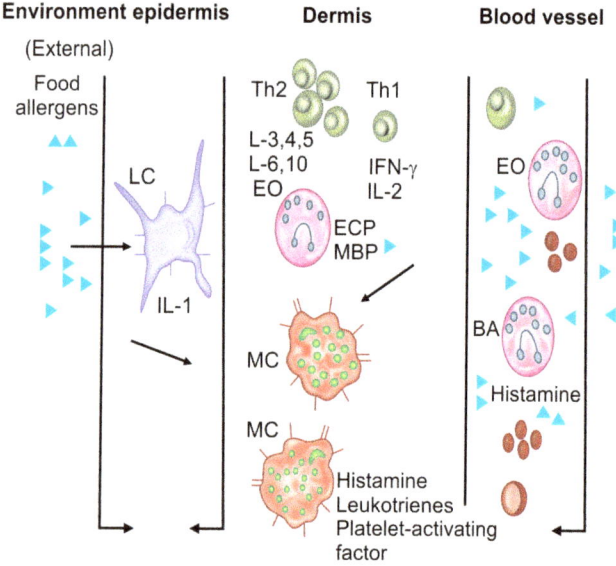

Fig. 10.11: Pathogenesis of atopic eczema in infants

steroids and systemic steroids may be used in short courses in unresponsive cases.

Incidence: Atopic eczema is seen in about 1–3% of all infants. It frequently begins before 6 months of age but is generally not seen in infants less than 3 months of age.

Presentation: Three distinct patterns of atopic eczema have been recognized depending on the age of the patient.

Atopic dermatitis in infancy (infanite eczema): In infancy, the lesions are intensely itchy papules and vesicles which soon become exudative. Secondary infection is common. Lesions begin on the face but can involve the rest of the body; usually there is sparing of the nappy (diaper) area. The disease runs a chronic course: about 40% of the cases clear by the age of 18 months. In the rest, the pattern changes into that of the childhood phase.

Childhood phase: The lesions are dry, leathery and extremely itchy being present mainly on the elbow and knee flexors. Sometimes a reversed (extensor) pattern may be seen.

Adult phase: The lesions of atopic dermatitis in adults are very itchy, lichenified plaques especially in the cubital and popliteal fossae and sometimes on the neck. A low grade involvement may be seen on the rest of the body. Often a discoid pattern of eczema is seen on the hands and feet.

Associated Features: Ichthyosis vulgaris.

Asthma, hay fever: These may see-saw with the dermatitis. Atopics also develop food allergies and urticaria more frequently.

Complications

Bacterial infections: These are frequent.

Viral infections: Atopics have a greater susceptibility to viral infections like herpes simplex and molluscum contagiosum

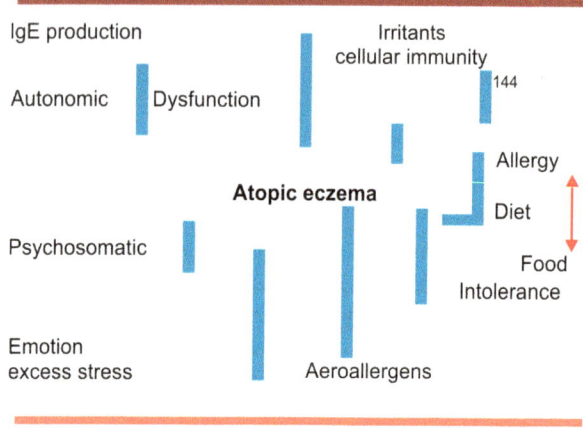

Fig. 10.12: Multifactorial genetic factors

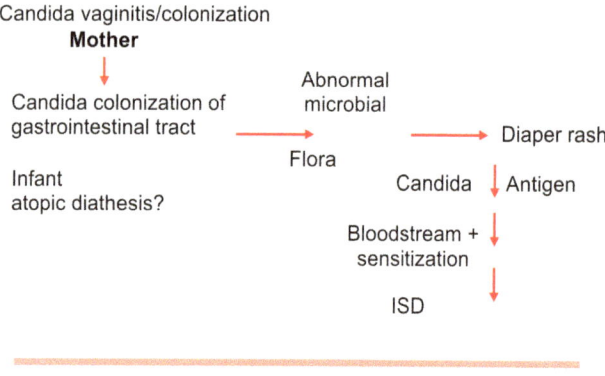

Infantile seborrheic dermatitis (ISD)

Fig. 10.13: Pathogenesis of infantile seborrheic dermatitis

due to impairment of cell-mediated immunity. In the presence of active eczema, herpes simplex infection may become generalized.

Disturbed sleep: Due to itching, these children may sleep poorly. Growth hormone levels generally rise during deep sleep and this may not happen in patients with atopic dermatitis due to disturbed sleep. Consequently, these children grow poorly.

The systemic absorption of topical steroids can cause several problems too !

Progress of the Disease

Points of focus: Clinical features of atopic dermatitis. Picture varies with the age of the patient.

Infinite: Begins at about 3 months, severely itchy exudative lesions on face and other parts, sparing diaper area. Clears in 40% by age of 18 months.

Childhood: Itchy, leathery flexural lesions.

Adult: Lichenified flexural lesions; sometimes a discoid pattern.

Associated features: Ichthyosis vulgaris, asthama, cataract.

Complications: Bacterial and viral infections.

Investigations

The value of prick testing in the diagnosis of atopic dermatitis is debatable. It may just about help in the diagnosis of a doubtful case, without assisting in the management.

Measurement of total serum IgE and IgE antibodies specific to certain antigens is useful in diagnosing the atopic state. It also helps in advising the patient on the role of dietary and environmental allergens in perpetuating their dermatitis.

Diagnosis

The diagnosis of typical cases is seldom dificult and is based on:

Family history of atopy/characteristic distribution and morphology of the lesions, depending on the age.

Itching is far more intense than what the dermatitis tends to suggest.

Differential Diagnosis

Depending on the age of the patient, atopic dermatitis would need to be differentiated from several disorders.

Infantile seborrheic dermatitis needs to be distinguished from infantile atopic eczema. Seborrheic dermatitis usually begins earlier, has a distribution on the scalp and proximal flexures (axillae and groins) and pruritus is absent. Atopic dermatitis, on the other hand, begins after the infant is

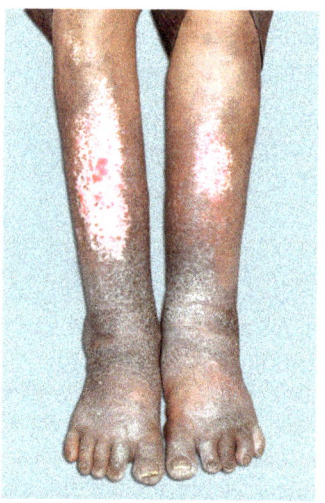

Fig. 10.14: Infective eczema—it shows scaling, edema, infection and due to itching inflammation. There is post-inflammatory depigmentation

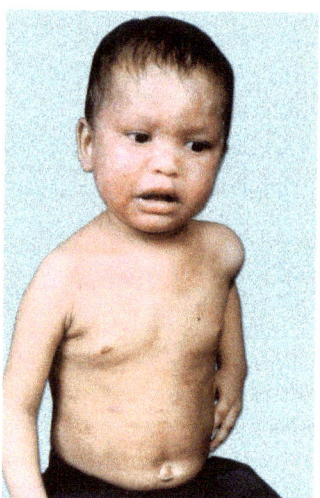

Fig. 10.15: Atopic dermatitis—face

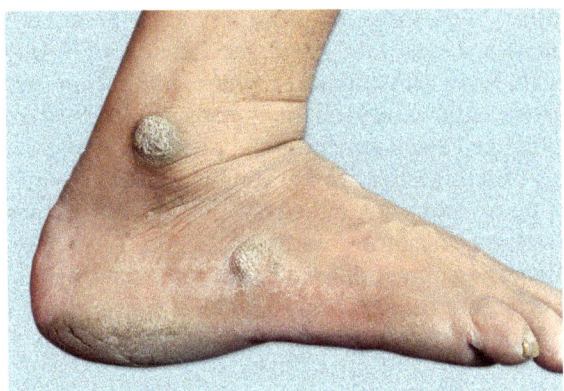

Fig. 10.16: Dry eczema on the foot—lateral and dorsal aspect: see the dry scale

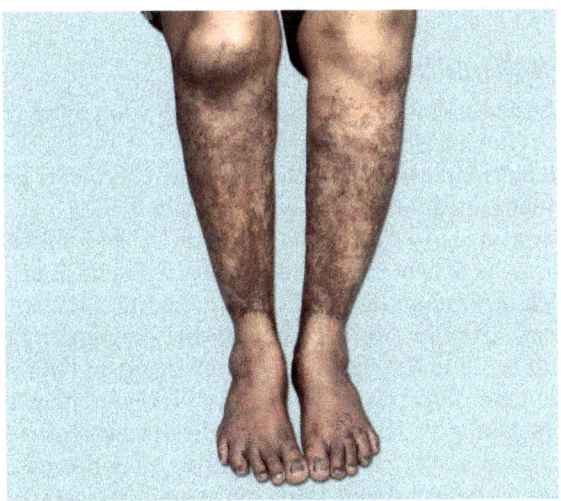

Fig. 10.17: Stasis eczema—see the hyperpigmentation because of poor venous return

3 months old and is an extremely itchy problem with papulovesicular lesions occurring predominantly on the face.

Scabies is a great mimicker, which in infants presents as exudative papulovesicular lesions on the face and extremities (eczematized scabies). These patients would also have a history of itchy lesions in other family members. Always look at the palms and soles of the child. Papulovesicular lesions here suggest a diagnosis of scabies.

Airborne contact dermatitis presents with lichenified plaques in the flexures and should be differentiated from adult variety of atopic dermatitis.

Treatment

General Measures

Explanation, reassurance and a bit of encouragement are necessary, both for the child and the parents.

What should be Avoided?

The basic thing is to avoid scratching. So, anything which triggers itching should be avoided.

Avoid irritants like woolen clothes, chemicals (occupational, recreational) as they may trigger itching.

Avoid excessive degreasing of the skin by using mild soaps.

The role of avoiding certain dietary items in controlling the itching in atopic dermatitis is controversial. Similarly, the evidence to support the hypothesis that pregnant mothers should avoid milk, eggs and other allergens to reduce the incidence of atopic disorders in the child is conflicting. There is some evidence to support the hypothesis that breastfeeding of children at risk of developing atopy, may decrease the chance of these children developing atopic dermatitis.

House dust mite avoidance: Many a time (not necessarily always) measures to reduce contact with house dust

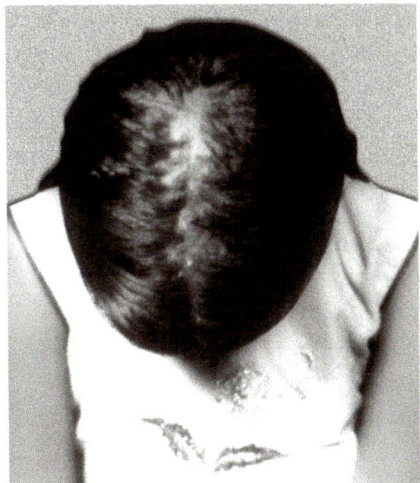

Fig. 10.18: Seborrheic dermatitis scalp

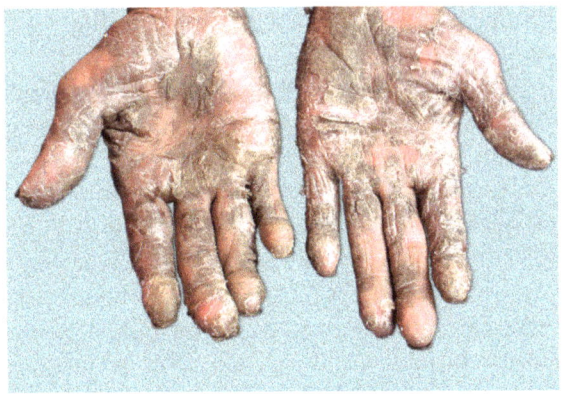

Fig. 10.19: Dry eczema—see the dryness scale on the both palms

mites (using barriers on mattresses, thorough and regular vacuuming of rooms, avoiding use of carpets, use of antimite sprays, etc.) may help patients with atopic diathesis.

Vaccinations: Routine vaccinations can be given during the quiescent phase of the disease. Children suspected to be allergic to eggs, should not be inoculated against measles, influenza and yellow fever.

Topical Therapy

The aims of the topical therapy are manifold:
- Protection of the skin from further scratching and from environmental factors
- Suppression of inflammatory changes and secondary infection, if present.

A variety of topical agents have been found useful.

Topical emollients: The role of emollients cannot be overemphasized. Emollients can be added to the bath or applied directly to the skin. Emollients are used to alleviate itching due to dry skin and in mild cases may suffice without any additional therapy.

Topical corticosteroids: These are used for localized exudative lesions, sometimes in combination with topical or systemic antibiotics. In extensive cases, it is best to dilute the corticosteroid with an emollient. In lichenified lesions, corticosteroids can be combined with keratolytic agents, with benefit.

Topical tacrolimus (non-steroidal topical immunomodulator): Tacrolimus treats the signs and symptoms of atopic dermatitis, reduces the incidence of flares, and offers the potential for long-term disease control.

Systemic therapy: Required in cases of atopic dermatitis, Systemic therapy includes antibiotics, corticosteroids and antihistamines.

Eczemas and Dermatitis

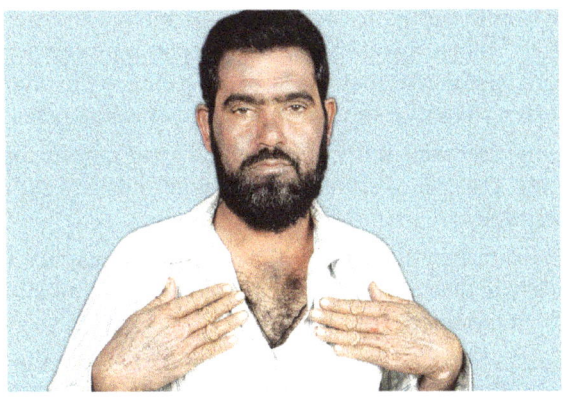

Fig. 10.20: Phytophotodermatitis showing the erythema and scales on the face and hands

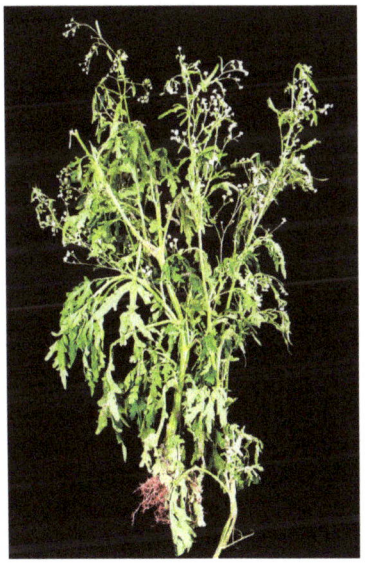

Fig. 10.21: Parthenium hysterophorus—also called "congress grass" is a wild composite which causes phytophotodermatitis

Systemic antibiotics are used in patients with extensive infected lesions. Even without frank sepsis, a proliferation of bacterial pathogens may exacerbate eczema so the rationale of empirically using systemic antibiotics in some cases.

Systemic steroids: With the availability of potent topical steroids, the use of systemic corticosteroids has reduced substantially.

Antihistamines: Especially the sedating ones, are used regularly to overcome the itching and are of value in those in whom the sleep is interrupted.

Newer therapies: In stubborn cases, UVB or PUVA is useful. A 3-month course of oral evening primrose oil may help. Cyclosporin (an immunosuppressive) may be used in stubborn cases.

Points of focus: Treatment of atopic dermatitis
- Multipronged approach
- Avoid triggers like woollens and excessive degreasing
- Topical and systemic therapy.

SEBORRHEIC DERMATITIS

Etiology

There is evidence to suggest that there is an overgrowth of Pityrosporum yeast in lesions of seborrheic dermatitis; this may play a part in the development of seborrheic eczema. The condition runs in some families, indicating a genetic predisposition.

Clinical Features

Epidermiology: If all cases of mild dandruff are also included, then the disease is fairly common (10-20% of general population). The incidence of seborrheic eczema in HIV-positive patients is much higher. It may be seen in infants (infantile seborrheic dermatitis) but is most common in adults.

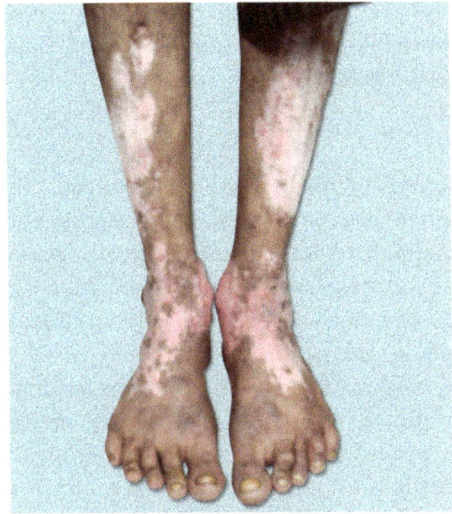

Fig. 10.22: Phytophotodermatitis due to *Psoralea corylifolia* plants

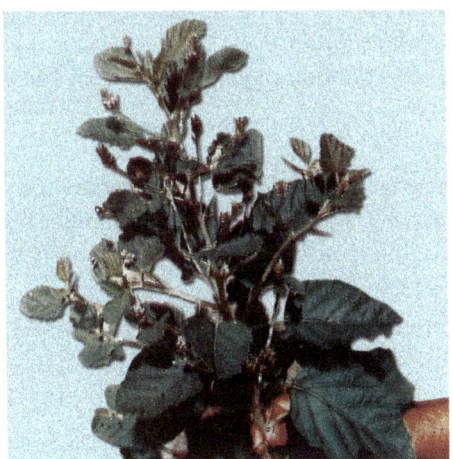

Fig. 10.23: *Psoralea corylifolia* plants commonly known as "bakuchi plants"

Morphology: The most characteristic lesion of seborrheic dermatitis is a follicular, dull or yellowish red papule which is covered with greasy scales.

Patterns

Several patterns of the disease are recognized.

An erythematous scaly or weeping eruption of the scalp (sharply marginated to the hairline), and eyebrows. There is a characteristics nasolabial scaling. Association with chronic blepharitis and otitis externa is frequent. Retroauricular involvement is also common.

Petaloid variant, so-called because the lesions are petal-shaped. In this nonexudative, scaly lesions are seen in the presternal and interscapular region. Sometimes, extensive erythematous follicular papules are seen on the trunk (seborrheic folliculitis).

Flexural seborrheic dermatitis which presents as sharply marginated erythema with greasy scales in axillae, groins and submammary region.

Severe seborrheic dermatitis occurs in patients with AIDS.

Distribution

The lesions originate in hairy skin and involve the scalp, face (nasolabial fold), presternal and interscapular regions and the flexures. This distribution of seborrheic dermatitis is very characterisitic.

Complications: Superadded bacterial infections (in the scalp) and candidal infections (in the flexures) are not infrequent.

Investigations

Usually no investigations are needed. However, always keep in mind the possibility of HIV infection in patients with seborrheic dermatitis.

Diagnosis

Diagnosis is based on:
- Typical distribution of the lesions
- Morphology (follicular papules with typical yellow, greasy scales).

Differential Diagnosis

The diagnosis is easy typical cases, but can be difficult in some cases. Seborrheic dermatitis needs to be differentiated from the following.

Psoriasis: The lesions in psoriasis are brightly erythematous and indurated and have silvery scales. Lesions of seborrheic dermatitis are yellowish, have greasy scales, are follicular and have a characteristic distribution.

Fungal infection: This needs to be differentiated from the flexural variant of seborrheic dermatitis.

Treatment

Patients should be informed that the therapy is not curative but would suppress the disease; recurrences are generally the rule once the treatment is stopped.

Treatment depends on:
- Site of disease
- Extent of disease.

Topical Treatment

This is the first line of therapy, especially when the lesions are localized.

Topical imidazoles: Based on the hypothesis that seborrheic dermatitis is caused by *Pityrosporum,* topical imidazoles are the first line of therapy. For the scalp, they may be used as a lotion or incorporated into a shampoo.

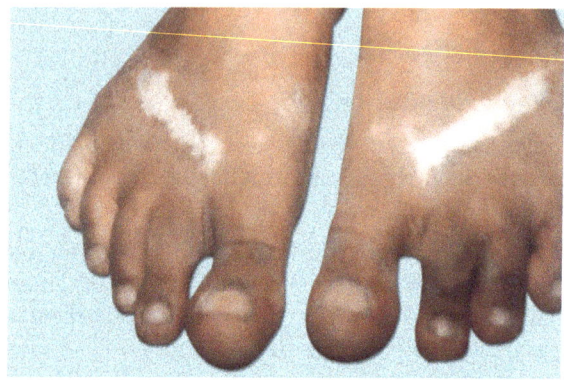

Fig. 10.24: Contact dermatitis—due to plastics rubber chapples causing dermatitis and depigmentation

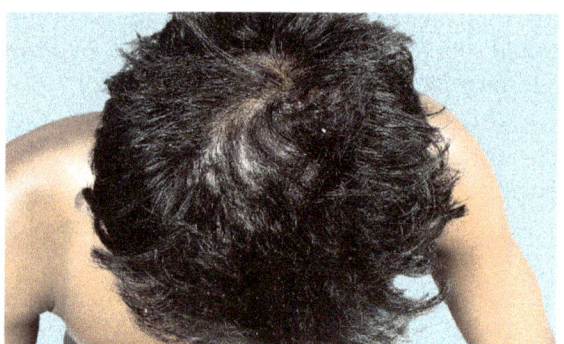

Fig. 10.25: Seborrheic dermatitis scalp

For the intertriginous areas, they are combined effectively with mild topical steroids.

Other topical therapies: A variety of other topical agents like 2% sulfur, 2% salicylic acid in aqueous cream and selenium sulfide incorporated into shampoos have been used. A topical lithium preparation has been successfully used in facial lesions.

Systemic Therapy

This takes the form of either antibiotics or antifungal agents (ketoconazole or itraconazole) and needs to be used for extensive lesions.

Points of Focus

- May be caused by a yeast, *Pityrosporum*
- Infrequently seen in infants, otherwise postpubertal
- *Clinical features:* Follicular papules with greasy scales
- *Characteristic distribution:* Scalp, nasolabial folds, retroauricular region, presternal and interscapular regions, squamous blepharitis, flexural lesions; can occur in isolation or in combination
- Responds to topical and systemic antifungal agents, sometimes along with topical antibiotics.

IRRITANT CONTACT DERMATITIS

Etiology

Most irritant dermatitis are occupational, be it an industrial contact or a household contact. Depending on the strength of the irritants, the dermatitis can either be an acute reaction (strong irritants) or a chronic reaction (weak irritants). Certain skin types (dry skins) and predisposed individuals (atopics) have a greater chance of developing irritant dermatitis.

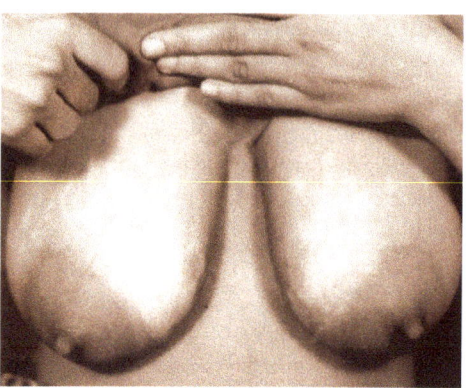

Fig. 10.26: Contact dermatitis due to braciers

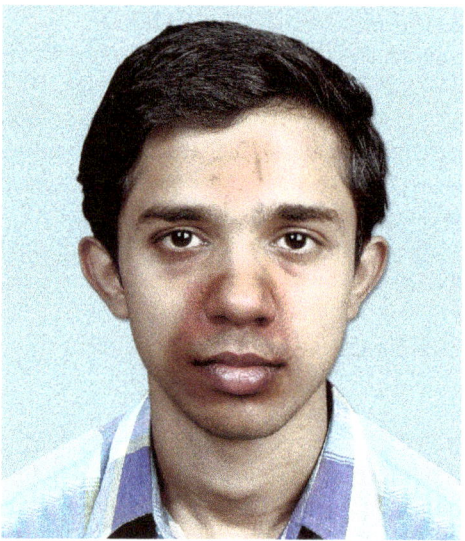

Fig. 10.27: Contact dermatitis due to topical cream massage

The common culprits causing irritant dermatitis.

Detergents	Alkalis
Solvents	Cutting oils
Abrasive dusts	

Clinical Features

Depending on the strength of the irritant, the patient presents with either acute exudative lesions or dry dermatitic plaques at the sites of contact (usually hands and forearms).

Diagnosis

It is important to differentiate irritant contact dermatitis from allergic contact dermatitis. Though this may be occasionally possible clinically, the confirmation comes by the patch test.

Treatment

Ideal to avoid exposure to the irritant. This may entail change of occupation, but this is not always possible. A reduced exposure by using protective gloves and clothing is then advocated. Barrier creams, however, are of little help.

In acute cases, moderately potent corticosteroids assist in quicker recovery.

In chronic cases, apart from topical steroids, emollients reverse the degreased state of the skin.

Points of focus: Irritant dermatitis

Occupational contact with irritants.

Acute (with strong irritants) or chronic (with weak irritants) dermatitis.

Treatment: Absolute or relative withdrawal of exposure to irritant and topical corticusteroids for acute stage.

ALLERGIC CONTACT DERMATITIS

Contact Sensitization in Very Young Children

Allergic contact dermatitis is an increasingly recognized clinical problem in children.

Two hundred children (62.3% 321 girls and 98 boys aged 3–36 month [mean age 27 ± 5.6 months]) developed at least one positive reaction. The most frequent reaction were to nickel sulfate (26.8%), followed by potassium dichromate (9%), cocamidopropyl betaine (7.2%), cobalt chloride (6.2%), neomycin sulfate (5%), and methylchloroisothiazolinone/methylisothiazolinone (4.4%). The prevalence of contact sensitization was similar in children with and without atopic dermatitis (61.3% and 63%, respectively).

Etiology

The list of potential allergens is very long.

Pathogenesis

Allergic contact dermatitis is a type IV delayed hypersensitivity reaction to antigens. The exogenous antigens are

Table 10.2: Agents causing contact dermatitis

	Agents	Sources
Plants	Parthenium	Air-borne exposure
Metals	Nickel chromates	Costume jewellery, clips Cement, leather goods, chromium plating
Cosmetics	Paraphenylenediamine	Hair dyes
	Fragrances	Cosmetics, perfumes, shampoos
	Formaldehyde	Preservative in cosmetics
	Parabens	Preservative in cosmetics
Medicines	Neomycin	Topical antibiotics
	Benzocaine	Local anesthetics
Rubber	Mercapto mix (aditives)	Shoe soles
	Thiuram mix (additives)	Rubber gloves

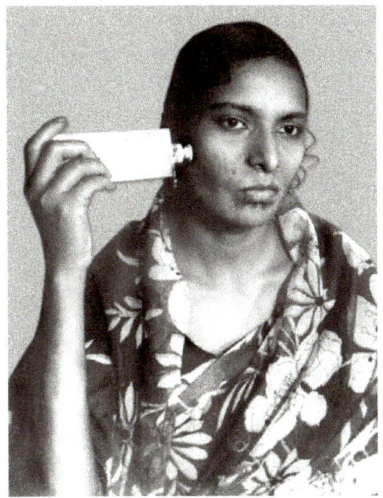

Fig. 10.28: Contact dermatitis due to hydroquinone cream

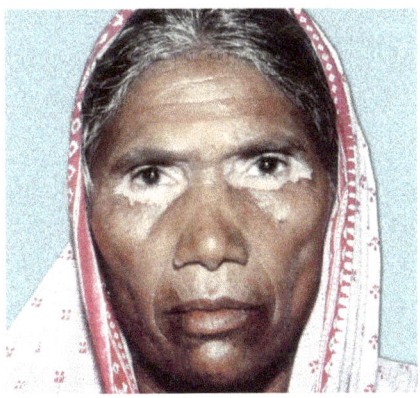

Fig. 10.29: Bindi dermatitis on forehead and the dermatitis due to spectacle frame resulting in to depigmentation and itching

processed by antigen-presenting cells (Langerhans cells). The processed antigen then interacts with sensitized lymphocytes. This lymphocyte population is stimulated to multiply and to secrete cytokines which cause tissue injury.

Clinical Features

Morphology

The patient can present with features of acute or chronic eczema.

Distribution

This depends on the allergen causing the eczema.

Table 10.3: Common patterns of distribution of lesions in allergic contact dermatitis

	Nickle Chromates	Feet (footwear)
Metals		Ear lobes, wrists, interscapular region
Plants	Pathenium	Airborne contact dermatitis:
Cosmetics	Hair dyes	Retroauricular area, neck, cubital and popliteal fossae Contact dermatitis: hands and forearms.
Medicines		Scalp face Neck, face,
Rubber	Perfumes	At sites of applications. Occupational: hands Contact sites : with gloves, shoe Soles, chappals, rubber bands

How to Investigate a Patient with Suspected Contact Allergy?

In depth questioning is the first step. This would indicate the nature of the domestic, occupational and recreational contact.

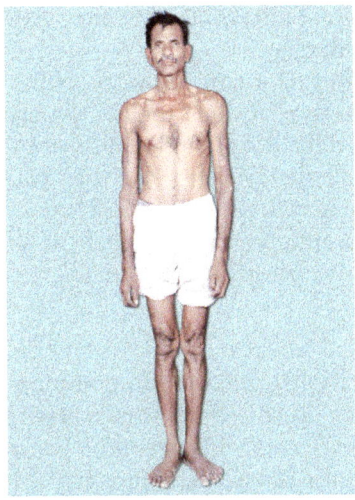

Fig. 10.30: Photodermatitis—hyperpigmention on the face, erythma on the face, chest and arms

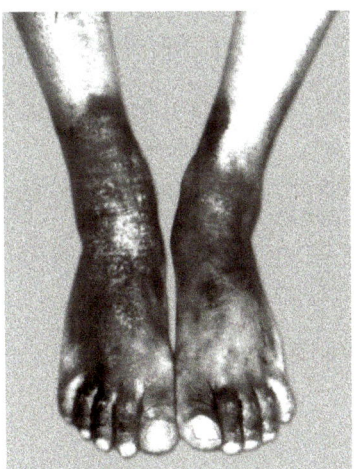

Fig. 10.31: Lichen simplex chronicus—thickening, and pigmentation of feet

Distribution of the skin lesions often gives a clue to the nature of the allergen.

Patch testing is a confirmatory. If the cause of the allergic dermatitis is obvious, then only suspected antigens (appropriately diluted in a bland vehicle) need to be tested. If, however, the allergen is not obvious, then it is prudent to test with the available battery of antigens. It is also recommended to test with the antigens which the patient is likely to use as substitutes to the sensitizing antigen.

Treatment

Avoid contact with the antigen completely. If irritant dermatitis, even decreased exposure to the irritant helps.

Topical corticosteroids are effective in most cases. Extensive airborne contact dermatitis may require treatment with a short course of oral corticosteroids.

Clinical manifestations: Could manifest as acute or chronic dermatitis, distribution characteristic.

History and distribution may indicate the allergen. Patch test.

Points of Focus: Allergic contact dermatitis

Common cause of dermatitis.

Common allergens: Plants, metals, cosmetics, medicines, rubber, confirmatory.

Removal of antigen essential to prevent recurrences. Treat the lesions symptomatically.

POMPHOLYX

Etiology

Unknown.

Summer aggravation well described and so the misnomer 'dyshidrosis' which wrongly implicates a dysfunction of sweat glands. The vesicles are not derived from the sweat glands.

There are a few patients of pompholyx who burst into a vesicular eruption on ingestion of even minute amounts of nickel.

Clinical Features

Recurrent episodes of deep seated, bland looking vesicles (sometimes blisters) on fingers ad palms and sometimes on soles. Though each episode of the disease is self-limiting, fresh crops of vericles keep developing, leaving the patient symptomatic for long periods. Lesions occasionally get secondarily infected.

Diagnosis

The lesions should be distinguished from vesicular lesions (called ide eruption) which occur associated with tinea pedis (fungal infection of the feet).

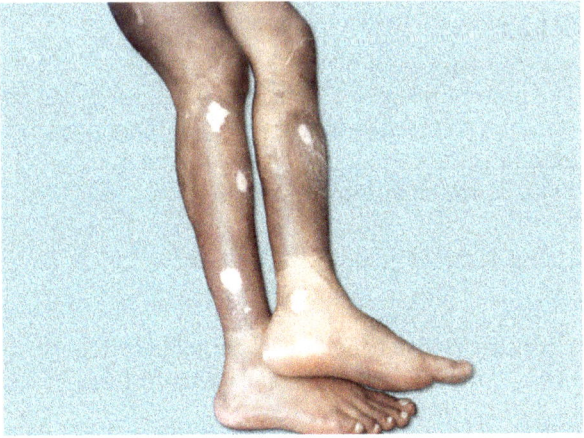

Fig. 10.32: Contact dermatitis—due to application of psoralen ointment on the vitiligo patches

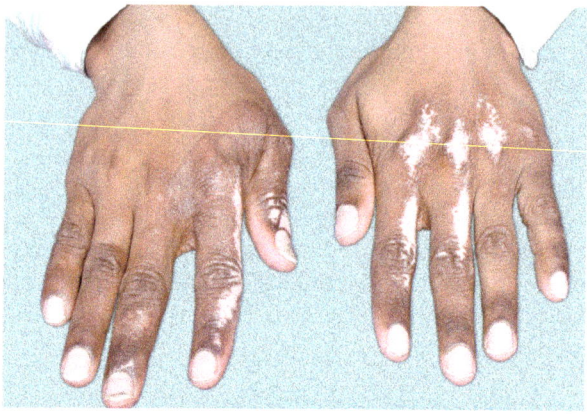

Fig. 10.33: Eczema on the hands

Treatment

Saline or other soaks are recommended followed by topical application of steroids. Appropriate antibiotics should be given for bacterial infection, if present.

Points of Focus: Pompholyx
   Unknown etiology.
   Recurrent episodes of deep-seated, bland vesicles on palms and soles.
   Soaks followed by topical steroid.

■ LICHEN SIMPLEX CHRONICUS

Etiology

This disorder is also called neurodermatitis. The change is induced in predisposed individuals by scratching.

Clinical Features

Single (occasionally more), thickened, hyperpigmented plaques with enhanced skin markings are seen (lichenification).

Many of these patients have an atopic diathesis. Sites frequently involved are nape of neck in women, legs in men and anogenital area in both.

Treatment

The basis of therapy is to break the itch-scratch cycle. This can be achieved by the use of topical corticosteroid and keratolytic agents under occlusion. Antihistamines may help. Lesion may reappear after treatment is stopped.

Topical Aspirin for Neurodermatitis

Topical aspirin might be a practical treatment for lichen

Points of focus: Lichen simplex chronicus.

Due to excessive scratching; may be associated with atopy.

Single (occasionally more) lichenified plaques on nape of neck, legs and anogenital region.

Topical corticosteroid combined with keratolytics used under occlusion.

NUMMULAR (DISCOID) ECZEMA

Definition

Discoid eczema is characterized by sharply demarcated, oval (disk-shaped), exudative plaques.

Etiology

Unknown in most cases, though discoid eczema is frequently seen in patients with atopy.

A reaction to bacterial antigens has also been suspected (positive yield of *Staphylococcus* on culture, better response of lesions to a combination of steriod and antibiotics than to either used alone).

Clinical Features

Usually seen on the extremities of middle-aged men as extremely itchy, multiple, coin-shaped vesicular or crusted plaques. The lesions run a chronic course.

Treatment

A combination of topical steroid and antibiotics gives the best results.

Points of focus: Nummular (discoid) eczema.

Unknown etiology; look for features of atopic dermatitis.

Multiple coin-shaped exudative plaques, on the limbs of middle-aged men.

Combine topical antibiotics with corticosteroids for a good response.

STASIS ECZEMA (GRAVITATION ECZEMA)

Etiology

This dermatitis is secondary to venous hypertension as a late sequel of previous deep vein thrombosis.

Clinical Features

A chronic patch of eczema with characteristic pigmentation.

Typically seen around the medial malleolus.

Look for venous varicosities, pigmentation and pedal edema.

Primary lesion may be complicated by contact sensitivity to topical agents.

Treatment

Eliminate edema by elevation of he foot-end of the bed and by pressure bandage.

Varicose veins need to be operated on, though stasis eczema is liable to persist, despite surgery.

Use mild topical steroids to relieve irritation but avoid potent corticosteroids. Bland applications like zinc cream help. Treat bacterial infection, if ulcer develops. Test for contact sensitivity, if there is aggravation after topical application.

Dobesil capsules and ointment is the drug of choice for varicose eczemas.

Table 10.4: Proposed criteria for the diagnosis of atopic dermatitis

Major criteria *Pruritus*	Minior criteria *Eyes*
Chronic or relapsing dermatitis	Contact, keratoconus intraorbital affected
Chronic or repeatedly occurring dermatitis/symptoms	Facial pallor Palmar hyperlinearity Xerosis
Personal or family history of atopic disease	Pityriasis alba White dermatographism
Typical distribution and morphology of atopic dermatitis rash:	Ichthyosis Keratosis pillaris
– Facial and extensor surface in children	Nonspecific dermatosis of hands and feets Nipple eczema
– Flexural lichenification and linearity in adults.	Positive type 1 hypersensitivity skin test
	Propensity of cutaneous infections Elevated serum IgE levels Food intolerance Impaired cell-mediated immunity Erythroderma Early age of onset

Points of focus: Stasis eczema

Secondary to venous hypertension.

Patch of eczema with pigmentation around the medial malleolus; pedal edema, varicosities associated.

Eliminate edema and varicosities. Rule out contact sensitivity; use mild topical corticosteroid.

ASTEATOTIC ECZEMA

Associated with old age; contributory factors included dry skin, low humidity as seen in the winter months; hypothyroidism; rarely associated with underlying malignancy.

The skin is generally dry; an itchy pattern of fine reticulated red, superficial fissures appears on the legs, an appearance quite akin to crazy paving.

Treatment of acute phase: Requires the use of mild topical corticosteroid in a greasy base.

Prevention

Regular use of any emollient and substituting an aqueous cream for soap usually prevents recurrences.

DIAPER DERMATITIS

Irritant dermatitis due to prolonged contact with feces and ammonia (produced by the action of urea-splitting microbes on urine). The problem has been aggravated by use of water-proof plastic diapers.

Moist, glazed erythema which affects the area of skin in contact with diapers. The depths of the skinfolds are spared.

Superadded infection with *Candida* is frequent.

Prevention

Essential to keep the area clean and dry. Best is to avoid use of the disposable napkins and if they have to be used, use the

Table 10.5: Atopic dermatitis: Algorithm for treatment
Initial assessment of diseases history, extent and severity
Include assessment of psychological distress, impact on family

	Emollients, education	
	Acute control of pruritus and inflammation	
Disease remission (No. signs or symptoms)	Topical corticosteroids or Topical calcineurin inhibitors 1,2 Tacrolimus bid Pimecrolimus bid or **Maintenance therapy** For disease persistence and/or frequent recurrences At earliest signs of local recurrence use topical calcineurin inhibitors to prevent disease progression Pimecroluims reduces the incidence of flares Long-term maintenance use of topical calcineurin inhibitors Intermittent use of topical corticosteroids Severe refractory disease Phototherapy Potent topical steroids Cyclosporine Methotrexate Oral Steroids Azathioprine Psychotherapeutics	Adjunctive therapy Avoidance of trigger factors Bacterial infections: Oral and/or topical antibiotics Viral infecations: antiviral therapy Psychological interventions Antihistamines

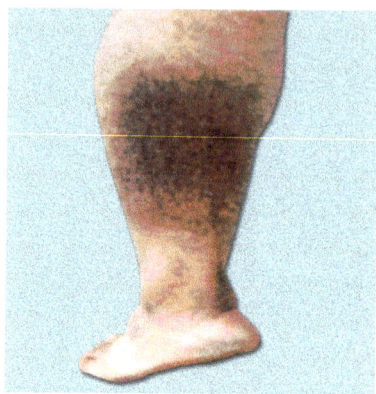

Fig. 10.34: Lichen simplex chronicus thickening and pigmentation of the leg

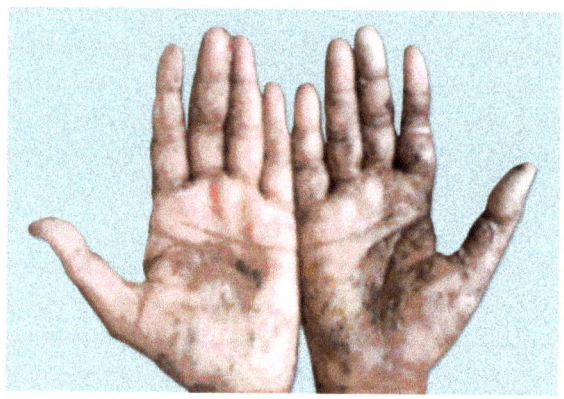

Fig. 10.35: Contact dermatitis of the palms

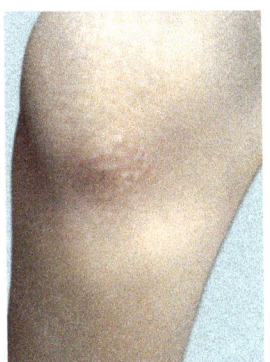

Fig. 10.36: Phrynoderma knees, spiny dry chronic knee

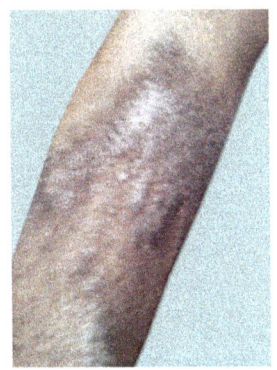

Fig. 10.37: Lichen planus—chronic thick lichenified lesions on the leg

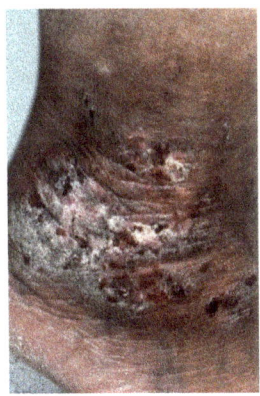

Fig. 10.38: Chronic lichenified eczema of leg

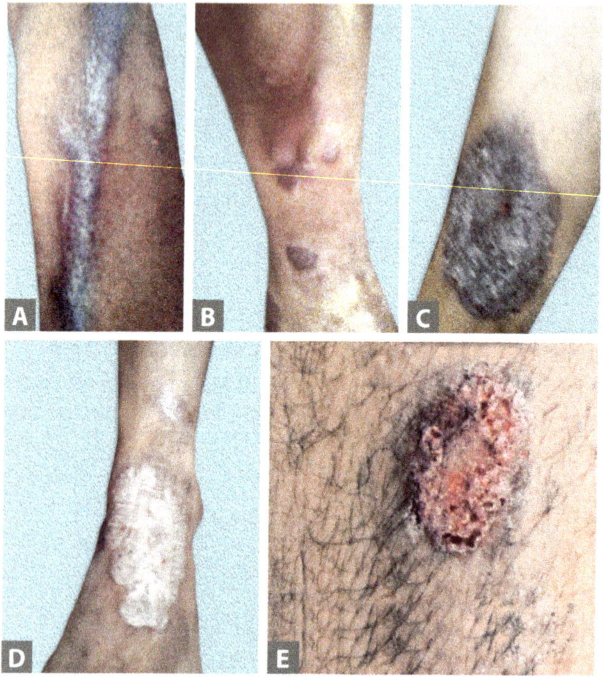

Figs 10.39A to E: Chronic eczema

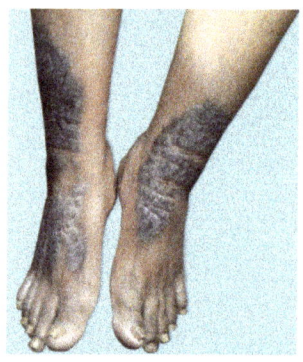

Fig. 10.40: Bilatral chronic eczema

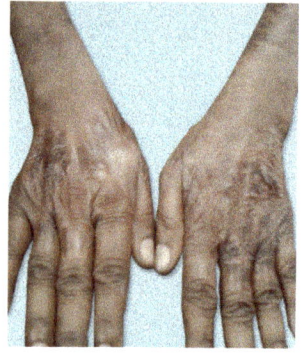

Fig. 10.41: Chemical eczema

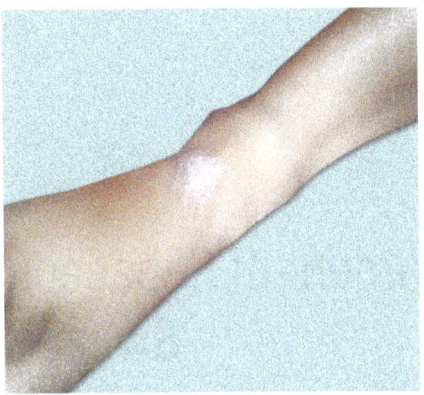

Fig. 10.42: Contact eczema due to wrist watch

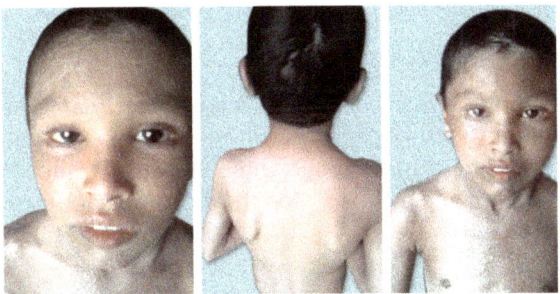

Fig. 10.43: Atopic dermatitis: face, back, etc.

superabsorbent ones. Use of towels and napkins is better, but these should be washed thoroughly and changed frequently.

Acute Phase

Mild corticosteroids (never stronger) with antifungal.

CHAPTER 11

Disorders of Sebaceous and Sweat Glands

ACNE VULGARIS

This condition is so common in adolescence that it may be considered physiological to have a few lesions is acne vulgaris at some time during adolescence and young adulthood. However, incidence of acne is low in some countries, e.g. Japan.

Etiology

Underlying factors include:
1. Androgens: Spurt in androgen production during puberty and adolescence is responsible for development of sebaceous glands.
2. Heredity: Excessive sebaceous gland activity is probably due to variation in end organ response to androgens and this may be genetically controlled.

3. Follicular keratinization: Abnormality of keratinization of the hair follicles plays an important role in the pathogenesis of acne. Mechanism of this abnormality is ill understood.
4. Propionibacterium acnes: This normal inhabitant of human skin is markedly increased in number, in subjects with acne.

Morphology

According to clinical severity, a simplified grading of acne is:

Grade I (non-inflammatory acne, comedonal acne): Skin colored papules (whiteheads, closed comedones), 1–2 mm in diameter, with a central whitish dot representing a follicular opening, are probably the earliest lesions of acne. Little larger, conical papules with a central dilated follicular pore that houses a black plug are called black heads or open comedones. A few erythematous papules may also be present at this stage.

Grade II (papulopustular acne): Multiple erythematous, conical, follicular papules, 2–4 mm in diameter, some of these topped by tiny pustules, are observed. Sometimes follicular pustules may predominate.

Grade III (papulonodular acne): A few larger (more than 5 mm) indurated erythematous papules and nodules are present. Larger and deeper pustules may also occur.

Grade IV (nodulocystic acne): Large skin colored and erythematous indurated nodules and their sequelae characterize this stage. Such painful nodules progress slowly to form painless cystic swellings that ultimately rupture and heal with scars.

Grade V (acne conglobata): Sometimes such scarring may be hypertrophic and be then associated with discharging sinuses with interconnecting sinus tracts. Large open comedones are common.

In severe grades of acne, lesions representing milder grades of acne are usually present.

Treatment

Table 11.1: Topical therapy of acne

Agent	%	Action	Side effect	Indication
Benzoyl peroxide	5%	Antibacterial	Irritation	Grade I–III
Retinoic acid	0.05%	Normalizes	Irritation, keratinization photosensitivity	Grade I–III
Erythromycin	3%	Antibacterial	Contact allergy	Grade II–III
Clindamycin	1%	Antibacterial	Contact allergy	Grade II–III
Calamine lotion or cream with added				
sulfur	2%	Peeling agents	Irritation	Grade I–III
salicylic acid	1%			
resorcinol	1%			
Antibacterials				
Retinoids				
Antiandrogens				

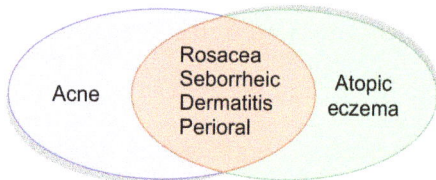

Fig. 11.1: Acne and other facial eruptions

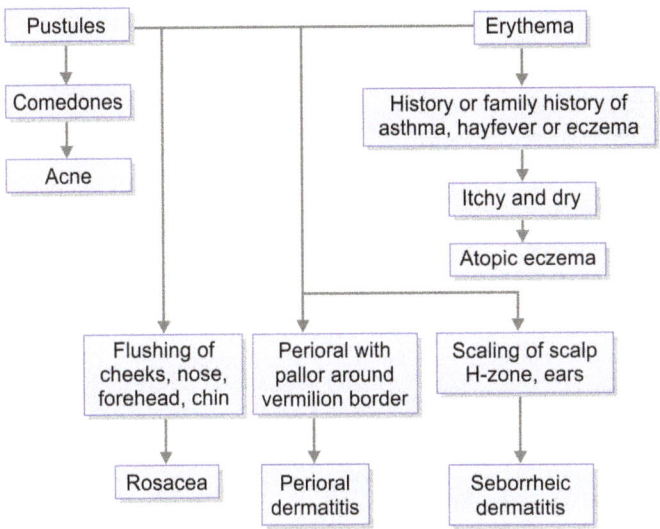

Fig. 11.2: Characteristics of facial lesions

Other Modalities of Therapy

These are used occasionally and include aspiration of acne cysts and their injection with triamcinolone acetonide suspension, application of dry ice (CO_2) or exposure to ultraviolet light to induce peeling. Scars that follow acne can be dealt with, once control of the disease is achieved. Dermabrasion, excision, collagen injection are some of the methods used to improve acne scars.

Acne vulgaris is a common disorder of adolescence and young adults. Heredity, androgens, follicular occlusion, excess sebum production and proliferation of *propionibacterium* acnes, all play their role in its pathogenesis. Skin colored follicular papules with central pulgs (comedones),

Table 11.2: Systemic therapy of acne

	Dose	Main side effects	Indication
Antibacterials			
Tetracycline	250 mg QDS	Gastritis, candidiasis diarrhea, drug eruptions	Grade II–V
Doxycycline	100 mg OD	Gastrtitis	
Erythromycin	250 mg QDS	Gastritis, hepatitis	
Minocycline	50 mg BD	Hyperpigmentation	
Co-trimoxazole	1 tab BD	Drug eruptions	
Anti-inflammatory antibacterial			
Dapsone	100–200 mg OD	Anemia, drug eruptions	Grade IV–V
Sebostatic (antiandrogens)			
Cyproterone	2 mg with cyclical estrogen	Breakthrough bleeding, vaginal candidiasis	Grade III–V in women
Sebostatic, keratostatic and anti-inflammatory (retinoids)			
Isotretinoin	20–40 mg OD	Teratogenicity, hyperlipidemia,	Grade IV–V in men
	For 4–8 weeks	Dry skin and mucosae, expensive	

erythematous papules, nodules, pustules and pseudocysts characterize the disease. Cheeks, forehead, chin, nose, neck, back and chest are the sites involved.

Topical antibacterials like benzoyl peroxide, erythromycin, clindamycin, and topical retinoic acid (0.05%) are effective in the control of mild to moderate acne. Oral antibacterials like tetracycline, doxycycline, co-trimoxazole or erythromycin,

Disorders of Sebaceous and Sweat Glands

given over many weeks, are added for unresponsive or severe grades of the disease. Oral contraceptive pills, antiandrogens are options in females whereas oral isotretinoin is reserved for males with severe acne.

Predictive Markers of Response to Isotretinoin in Female Acne

Acne vulgaris is a common and chronic disorder of the pilosebaceous unit. Female acne may be a subtype differing

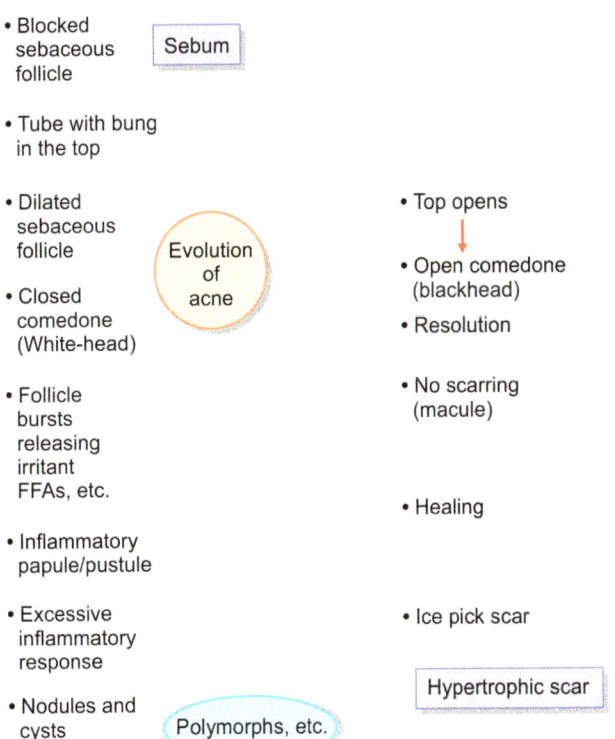

Fig. 11.3: Pathogenesis of acne

from teenager acne. Isotretinoin is the only therapy impacting on all the major acne-related etiological factors. All clinical studies demonstrating isotretinoin efficacy in acne patients have been performed either in teenagers or in a mixed population of teenagers and adults.

Isotretinoin at 0.5 mg/kg is effective and well tolerated in mild-to-moderate acne in females over 20 years old and results were similar to those of teenagers and men. We can propose positive predictive markers of response to isotretinoin in female acne, including a low body mass index, low glycemic-load diet, no tobacco, absence of early acne onset and of lesions on the neck.

Table 11.3: Global assessment of acne lesions by the dermatologist

0. No lesion	Residual pigmentation and erythema could be present
1. Almost no lesion	Rare scattered comedons and rare papules
2. Mild	Less than half of the face is affected
3. Moderate	More than half of the face is affected. A nodule can be present
4. Severe	The whole face is affected. Rare nodules
5. Very Severe	Very inflammatory acne affecting the whole face

Evaluation of Self-treatment of Mild-to-moderate Facial Acne with a Blue Light Treatment System

Many topical and oral medications are used in the treatment of acne vulgaris but their clinical utility is often suboptimal as a result of a slow onset of action, a lack of efficacy in some patients. Tolerability problems or the risk of other adverse effects such as the development of bacterial resistance to antibiotics. Blue light therapy can offer a valuabal additional treatment option. Therefore, a study has been performed to evaluate efficacy and tolerability of treating mild-to-moderate facial acne using a new, hand-held, light emitting diode blue light device in conjunction with a foam cleanser containing 5% glycolic acid and 2% salicylic acid plus a skin rebuilding serum containing 1.25% salicylic acid, 0.5% niacinamide, 0.08% liposomal-based azelaic acid and superoxide dismutase.

ACNE SCARRING

Classification of Acne Scars

A new simple classification system for acne scars that includes three scar types [icepick, rolling and boxcar] has been proposed keeping therapeutic options in mind others scars as sinus tracts, hypertrophic scars and keloidal scars are less common.

Treatment of Acne Scarring

A variety of approaches are available for revision of these scar types. Nonsurgical methods include subcutaneous or dermal fillers. Topical approaches include chemical peels and microdermabrasion or particulate resurfacing. Surgical modalities include primary elliptical excision punch elevation, punch autografting, dermal grafting planning, subcutaneous incision (subcosion) dermabrasion, and laser skin resurfacing.

Syndromes Associated with Acne

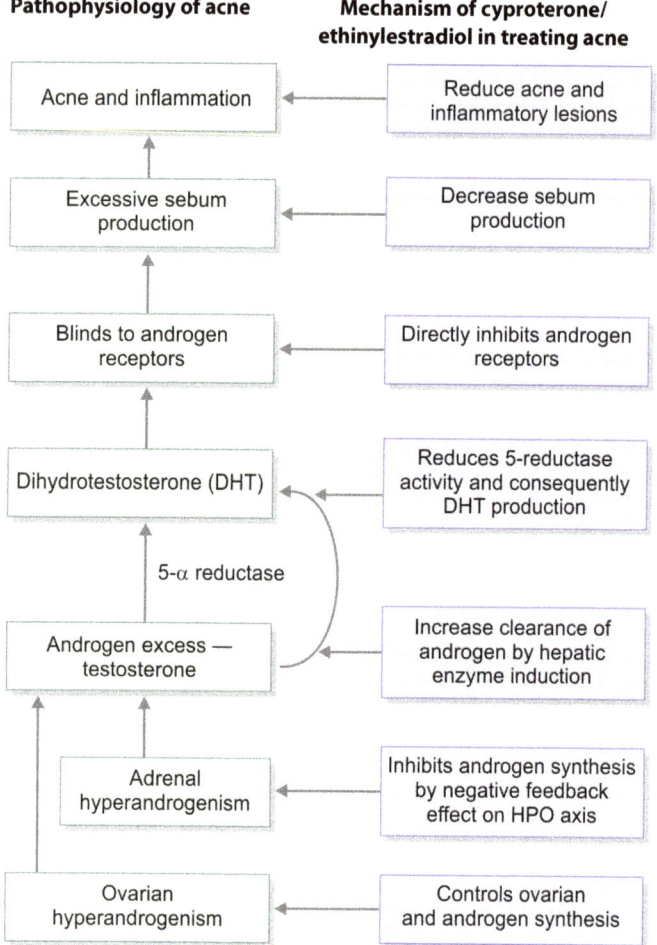

Cyproterone acetate/ethinylestradiol effectively controls hyperandrogenism

Acne is a multifactorials disease and may also be associated with various syndromes such as:
- Nonclassical adrenal hyperplasia
- Hyperandrogenism (HA), insulin resistance (IR), and acanthosis nigricans(AN) i.e HAIR-AN syndrome
- Polycystic ovary syndrome(PCOS)
- Seborrhea, acne,hirsutism and androgenetic alopecia (SAHA) syndrome
- SAPHO syndrome (synovitis, acne, pustulosis, hyperostosis and osteitis)
- PAPA syndrome (pyogenic arthritis,pyoderma gangrenosum, and acne).

Tips for Acne Prevention

- **Keep it clean:** Wash your face gently with warm water and mild face wash or acne wash.
- **Be gentle:** Instead of scrubbing , use gentle, circling motion for cleaning your face.
- **Don't rub:** Avoid rubbing your skin with towel ,and always completely rinse your skin after you wash it, and gently pat it dry.
- **Moisturize the skin:** Use moisturizing lotion , if your face feels dry after washing. Select "noncomedogenic" skin care products.
- Shower as soon as you can after any activity that causes heavy sweating, especially sports.
- **Tie your hair:** Try keeping your hair off your face . washing your hair every day may help.
- **Never pick your acne or blackheads:** Try not to scrub or pick at your pimples. This can make them worse and can causes scars.
- **Detoxify yourself:** Drink at least 64 ounces of water every day.

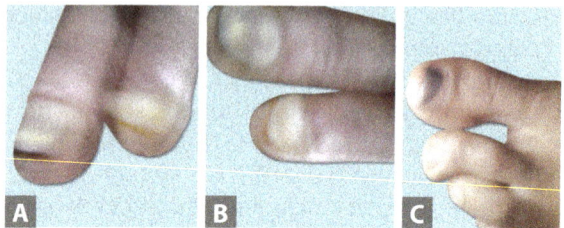

Figs 11.4A to C: Psoriasis of the nails

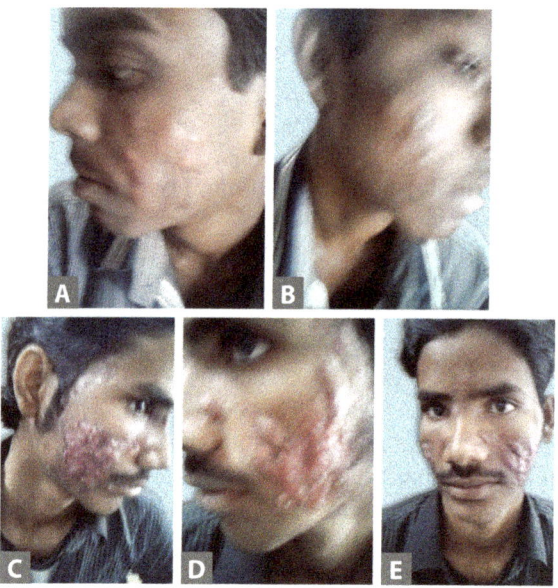

Figs 11.5A to E: Acne vulgaris – lesions showing papulo-pustulo and cysts of acne

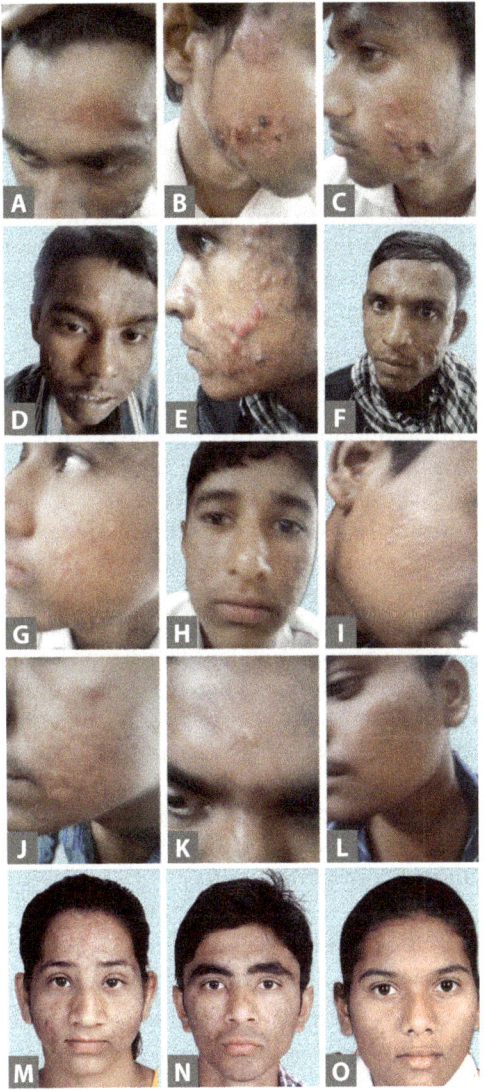

Figs 11.6A to O: Acne vulgaris

ROSACEA (ACNE ROSACEA)

A predominantly facial eruption of middle aged women, rosacea is quite unrelated to acne vulgaris. Facial flushing is a forerunner of rosacea in many instances. Etiology of rosacea is not fully known. However, in addition to the role played by the mite '*Demodex folliculorum*, factors that induce facial flushing also play a part in the pathogenesis of rosacea. *Demodex folliculorum*, a normal inhabitant of the follicular canal in humans, is increased in number in patients with rosacea. An associated change in the bacterial flora is also noted.

Rosacea is unrelated to acne. Typically, it affects middle aged ladies. A facial eruption of bright red papules with a flare of erythema and topped by tiny pustules characterizes the disease. Avoidance of sunlight, hot spicy foods, caffeinated and alcoholic beverages is helpful. Topical benzoyl peroxide or metronidazole can control milder disease whereas systemic antibacterial like tetracycline for many weeks is needed for severe cases. Topical 1% hydrocortisone may be used but stronger steroids are contraindicated due to the fear of rebound phenomenon and skin atrophy. For flushing and burning—propranolol 40 mg, twice daily or nadalol 40 mg daily, clonidine 50 µg twice daily, and rilmenidine 1 mg daily. Telangiectasia—vascular laser and intense pulsed light source.

Rhinophyma—surgical treatment, electrocoagulation, crysurgery, carbon dioxide or neodymium-doped yttrium aluminum garnet (Nd:YAG) lasers.

PERIORAL DERMATITIS

It effects the perioral region. Perioral dermatitis is also seen of applications of lipistics, hydroquinone creams common use for removing the hyperpigmentation.

Common Disorders of the Sweat Apparatus

Functional	— Hyperhidrosis, anhidrosis, bromhidrosis, chromhidrosis, dyshidrosis.
Infections	— Periporitis, abscesses, hidradenitis suppurativa.
Inflammatory and sweat	— Miliaria, fox-fordyce's disease, dyshidrosis exfoliativa.
Tumors	— Cystic—hydrocystoma. Nevoid syringoma—rare. Malignant tumors.

CHAPTER 12

Papulosquamous Diseases

PSORIASIS

A skin and joint disease with multifactorial etiology, psoriasis affects 1-2% of the general population. Pustular and erythrodermic psoriasis may pose a threat to life whereas wide spread skin and joint affection is disabling. However, these complications are uncommon.

Etiology

Exact cause is unknown. Familial incidence suggests genetic predisposition. Mechanical, chemical or radiation trauma can initiate or worsen psoriasis (Koebner phenomenon). Drugs like chloroquine, lithium, beta blockers, and NSAIDs can worsen or induce psoriasis. Withdrawal of systemic corticosteroids in a patient of psoriasis can precipitate an attack of erythrodermic or generalized pustular psoriasis. Summer improves psoriasis and winter worsens it.

Pathology

Hyperplasia and neutrophilic infiltration of the epidermis as well as papillary vascular dilatation and congestion are seen in classic plaque type psoriasis. Accelerated epidermal turnover and deficient keratinocyte maturation result in visible exfoliation of the skin (scaling). Vascular changes lead to erythema whereas dense neutrophilic infiltrate may lead to sterile (non-infective) intraepidermal pustules in pustular psoriasis.

Current Understanding

Psoriasis is now considered as the most prevalent T cell mediated inflammatory skin disease. Generalized immunosuppressants were found to improve psoriasis. This led to further research on T cells, the major component of

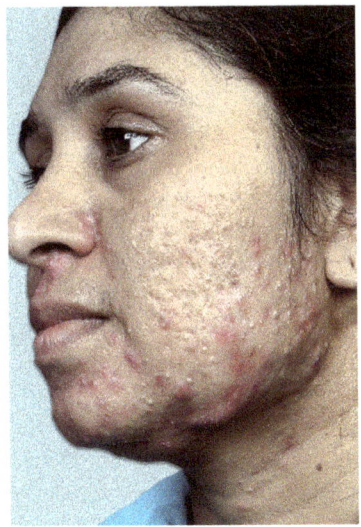

Fig. 12.1: Acne vulgaris—face showing comedones, papules, pustules, and nodules and scars

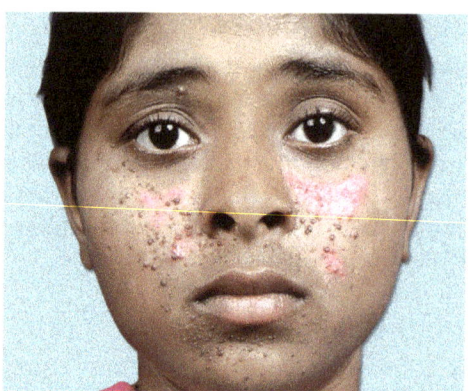

Fig. 12.2: Acne vulgaris—face showing comedones, papules, and pustules

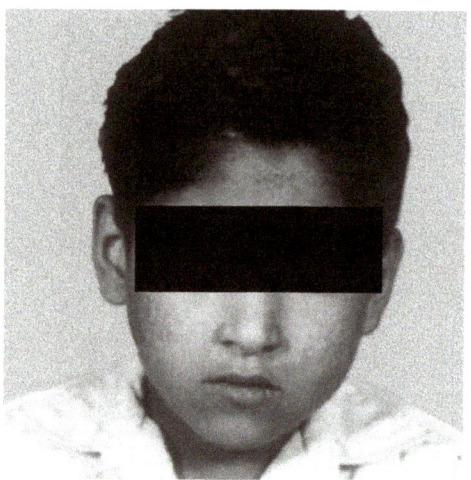

Fig. 12.3: Juvenile acne showing small papular lesions on cheeks and forehead

Table 12.1: Practice management guideline

Acne	Mild		Moderate			Severe
	Comedonal	Papular/pustular	Papular/pustular	Nodular	Nodular 2	Nodular/conglobate
1st choice	Topical retinoid	Topical retinoid + Topical antimicrobial	Oral antibiotic + Topical retinoid +/– BPO	Oral antibiotic + Topical retinoid + BPO		Oral isotretinoin
Alternatives	Alternative topical retinoid or azelaic acid or salicylic acid	Alternative topical antimicrobial agent + Alternative topical retinoid or azelaic acid	Alternative oral antibiotic + Alternative topical retinoid +/– BPO	Oral isotretinoid or Alternative oral antibiotic + Alternative topical retinoid +/– BPO (azelaic acid)		High dose Oral antibiotic + Topical retinoid +BPO
Alternatives for females	See 1st choice	See 1st choice	Oral antibiotic + Topical retinoid/ azelaic acid +/– Topical antimicrobial	Oral antiandrogen + Topical retinoid +/– Oral antibiotic +/– Topical antimicrobial		High dose Oral antiangrogen + Topical retinoid +/– Alternative topical antimicrobial
Maintenance therapy	Topical retinoids	Topical retinoids	+/– BPO			

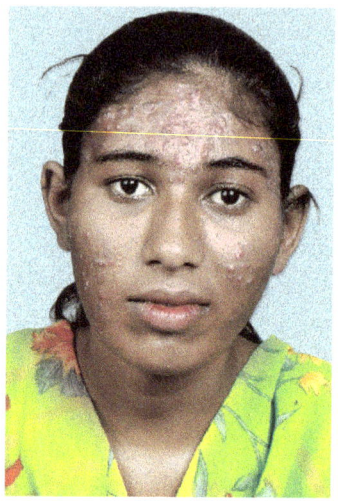

Fig. 12.4: Acne vulgaris—nodulocystic lesions and papules, nodules, and cheeks and forehead

the inflammatory infiltrate in psoriasis. Activated T cells enter the skin and release cytokines and chemokines which initiate and perpetuate the inflammatory cascade. Epidermal hyperplasia is a reaction of the immune system, mediated by $CD8^+$ and $Cd4^+$ T lymphocytes. Better understanding of molecular control in psoriasis has helped to design biological agents to treat psoriasis.

Morphology

Initial lesion of psoriasis is a barely elevated, erythematous papule topped by a whitish scale. Sometimes scales may not be evident unless the surface is stroked or scratched.

Distribution

Classic plaque type of psoriasis (psoriasis vulgaris) affects elbows, knees, extensors of extremities, scalp and sacral region in a symmetric pattern. Palms and soles are involved commonly.

Variations in Morphology and Distribution

Sebopsoriasis

Lesions occur in the distribution pattern of seborrheic dermatitis and tend to have yellowish rather than silvery scales.

Erythrodermic Psoriasis

Affection of most or all of the body seen as widespread or whole body erythema and scaling.

Pustular Psoriasis

Crops of pustules based on erythema. Distributional subtypes include : Localized palmoplantar pustular psoriasis.

Generalized Pustular Psoriasis

This is the life-threatening variant, the patient being febrile and toxic as waves of pustules based on tender erythema appear all over the body. Hypocalcemia may occur.

Guttate Psoriasis

This variant is common in children and has the best prognosis. Guttate (drop-like) papules topped with white scale appear all over the body, especially the trunk.

Psoriatic Arthritis

About 5% of psoriatics have arthritis. Although classic psoriatic arthritis affects distal interphalangeal joints, this variety is uncommon. More commonly, psoriatic arthritis involves few large joints or may mimic rheumatoid arthritis.

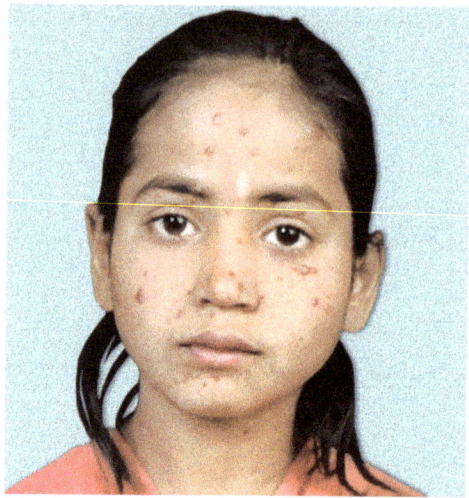

Fig. 12.5: Acne vulgaris—papules and pustules on cheeks and forehead. Scattered lesions and few warts all over the face of a adolescent girl

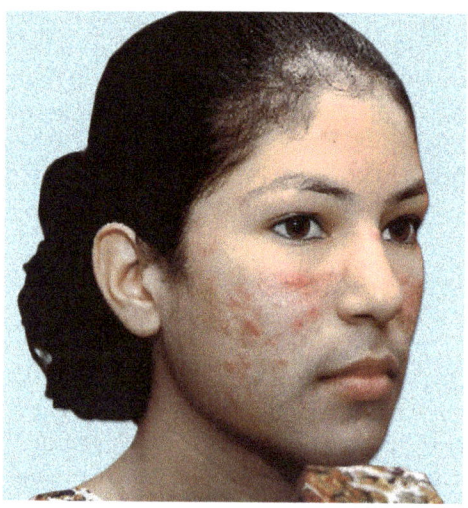

Fig. 12.6: Acne vulgaris—papules and pustules on cheeks

Papulosquamous Diseases

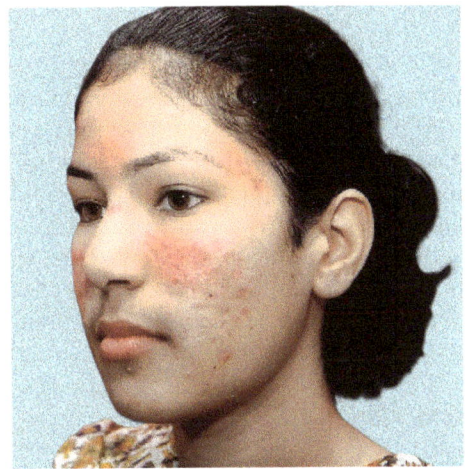

Fig. 12.7: Acne vulgaris—face showing comedones, papules and pustules

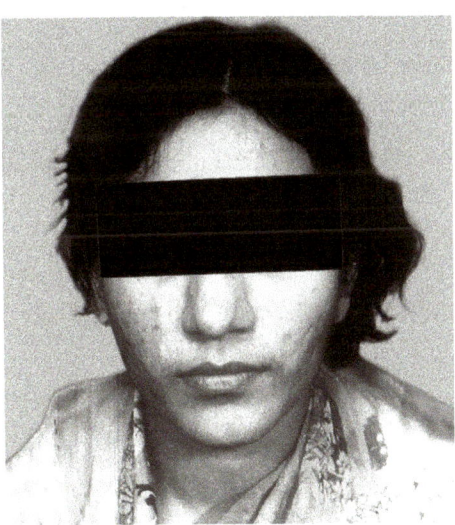

Fig. 12.8: Acne vulgaris—showing mild papules and pustules

Complications

Complications of psoriasis are eminently those of erythroderma. Psoriasis is a papulosquamous disorder that represents an inflammation pattern of the skin to external (trauma) or internal (drugs) stimuli in a predisposed (genetic) individual. Erythematous papules and plaques covered with thick silvery white scales which are the classical lesions. Koebner's phenomenon and Auspitz sign are present. Extensors of limbs and trunk, and scalp are preferentially affected. Nails and joints may be affected. Important variants of psoriasis include guttate (in children, widespread but self-limiting), annular, erythrodermic, sebopsoriasis, pustular psoriasis and arthropathic psoriasis.

Retinoids

Retinoids are analogs of vitamin A. The two retinoids commonly used in psoriasis are etretinate and acitretin. They act in a multipronged way in psoriasis, resulting in thinning down of the thick hyperkeratotic plaques.

The latest compound of retinoids is *Acitretin*. The 1st specific and proven therapy for psoriasis. The tablets are available by various pharmaceutical companies as Acrotac, Acitrin, Soriac.

Indications for Retinoids

Retinoids are very effective in pustular psoriasis and have also been used in psoriatic erythroderma. These drugs are used in the doses 20–50 mg daily.

Retinoids can be combined with PUVA because they act synergistically (this regime has been named Re1-PUVA). This reduces the cumulative toxicities of both the drugs, but one should continue to observe standard precautions.

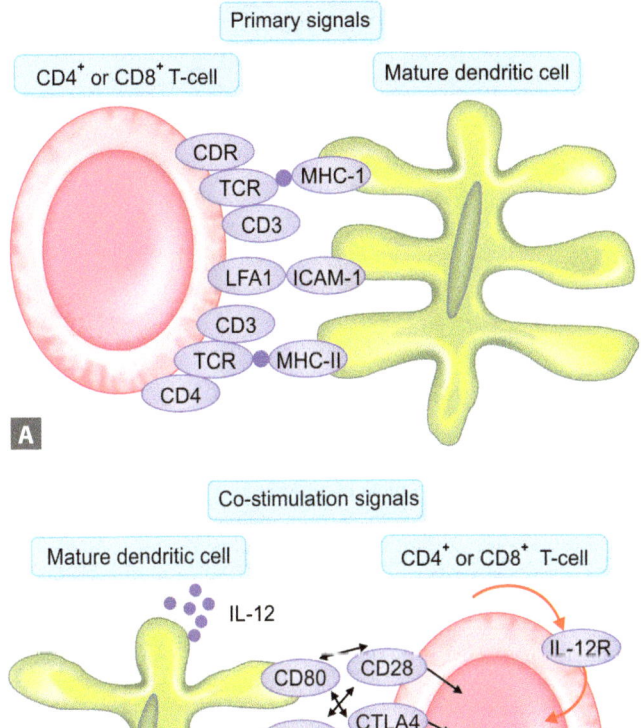

Figs 12.9A and B: Current understanding

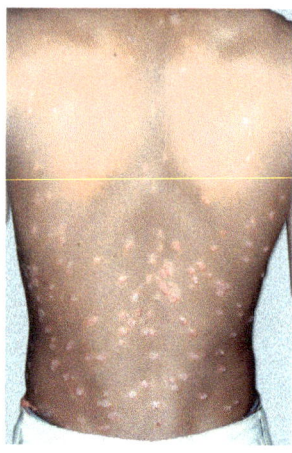

Fig. 12.10: Psoriasis vulgaris—plaque lesions over the extensor surface of limbs and trunk

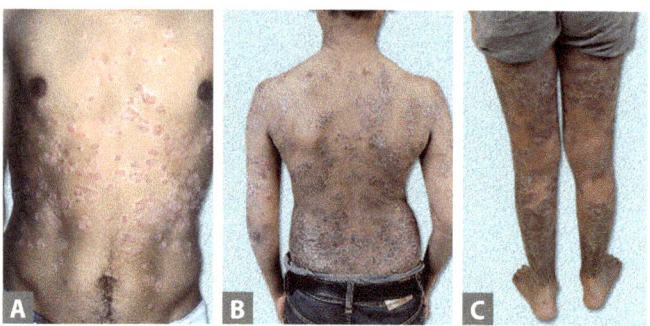

Fig. 12.11A to C: Psoriasis vulgaris—showing classical silvery scaly lesions [(A) front view (B and C) back view]

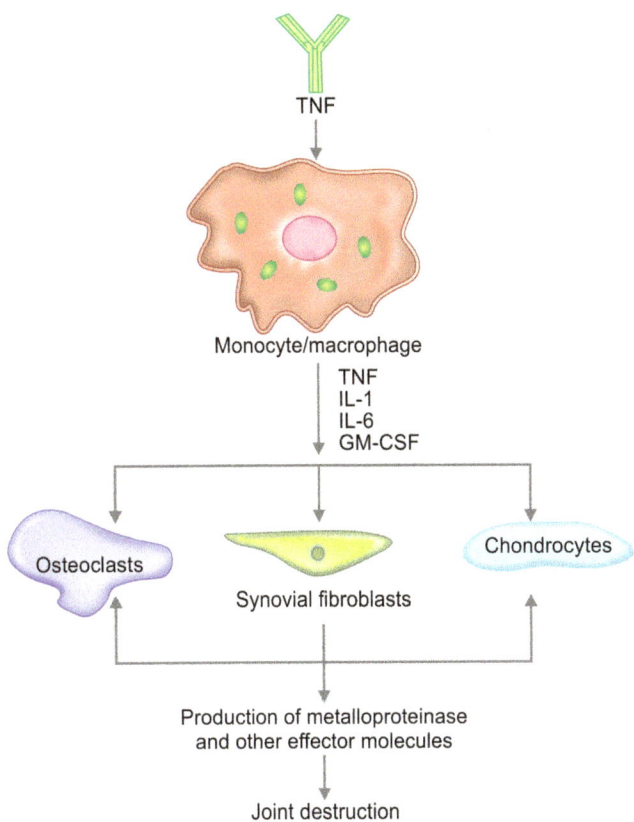

Fig. 12.12: Tumor necrosis factor (TNF)-mediated cascade that leads to inflammtory responses and subsequent joint destruction

Side Effects and How to Monitor Patients on Retinoids

The most important side effect of retinoids is teratogenicity. So retinoids are best avoided in women of childbearing age. If at all they have to be prescribed in them, concomitant

Table 12.2: Treatment options in psoriasis

Type of psoriasis	Treatment of choice	Alternative treatments
Localized stable plaque	Short-contact dithranol Tar	Topical steroids
Extensive stable plaque (>30% surface area)	UVB PUVA	Methotrexate Cyclosporin A
Widespread small plaque	UVB, PUVA	Tar
Guttate	Antibiotics and emollients while erupting; PUVA	Weak tar preparations Mild local steroids
Facial	Mild topical steroids	
Flexural	Mild to moderately potent topical steroids + antifungal	
Pustular psoriasis of hands and feet	Topical moderately potent or potent steroids	Methotrexate (small doses)
Acute erythrodermic, unstable or generalized pustular	Methotrexate + Topical band application	Acitretin (if available) Cyclosporin A

contraception is mandatory for a reasonable period after treatment is withdrawn (because of the long half-life of the drug).

Retinoids may cause elevation of triglycerides and sometimes of cholesterol; so monitoring serum lipids is essential. Abnormalities of liver function have also been observed and should be monitored.

Cyclosporin

Mode of action: Cyclosporin inhibits cell mediated immune reactons due to inhibition of lymphocyte, mitosis and inhibition of release of lymphokines. It also has a direct antiproliferative effect on the keratinocyte.

Indications: Use should be restricted to patients with severe psoriasis because the drug is toxic. The initial daily dose used is 3 mg/kg (up to 5 mg/kg) and with improvement the dose can be reduced.

Caution: Cyclosporin should be used with great caution.

Hypertension (mild-moderate) is a frequent side effect (seen in 50% of patients). It responds to calcium-channel blockers or angiotensin converting enzyme inhibitors. Diuretics (because they worsen renal function) and beta blockers (they worsen psoriasis) are best avoided.

Nephrotoxicity is another serious side effect. Initially weekly and later monthly monitoring of serum creatinine is recommended. Dose titration of cyclosporin is advocated if serum creatinine levels rise to 30% above the baseline levels. Drug may need to be withdrawn if high levels of serum creatinine persist despite dose reduction.

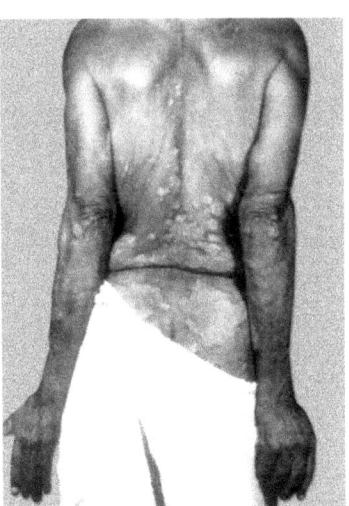

Fig. 12.13: Psoriasis: The lesions varying in shape and size coalesce to form large gyrate or geographical lesions on buttocks on back

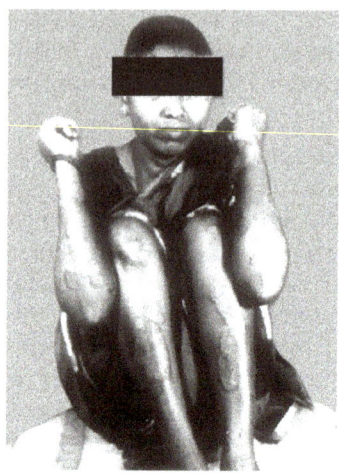

Fig. 12.14: Psoriasis lessions appearing as well demarcated, erythematous patches covered with silvery scales

Table 12.3: Genetic, immunologic and environmental factors in the pathogenesis of psoriatic arthritis

Genetic factors	Immunologic factors	Environmental factors
50 times greater risk in first-degree relatives	Higher serum IgA and IgG levels	Bacterial infection
Associated with HLA loci B27, B17, Cw6, DR4, and DR7	Antinuclear, keratin, and heat-shock protein antibodies	HIV infection
Other loci include MICA PSORS2 and TNF	Activated clonal and oligoclonal CD8$^+$ and CD$^+$ T-cell	Drugs
	Higher circulating levels of TNF	Stress

HLA, Human leukocyte antigen; Ig, immunoglobulin; MICA, MHC class I-related chain gene A; PSORS2, psoriasis locus at chromosome 17q24q25; TNF, tumor necrosis factor

Papulosquamous Diseases

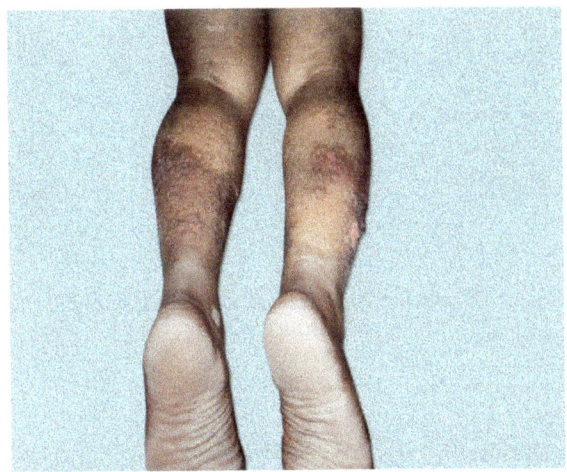

Fig. 12.15: Psoriasis—associated with vitiligo lesions (back view)

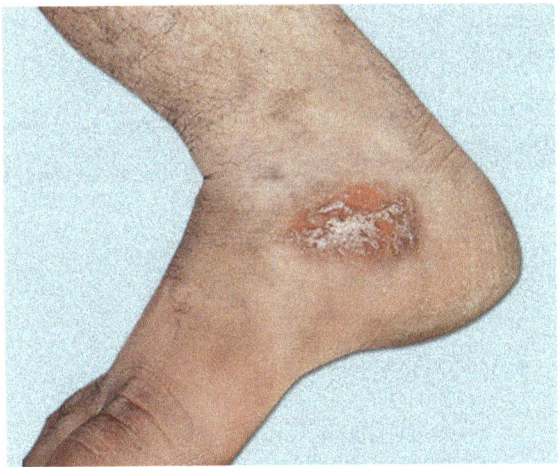

Fig. 12.16: Psoriasis—circular, scaly, solitary lesion on foot

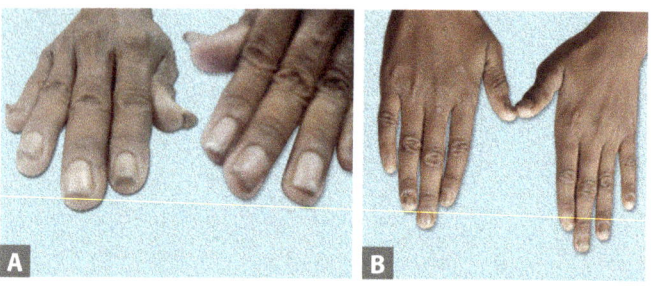

Figs 12.17A and B: Psoriasis of nail both hands nail piting and nail destruction seen

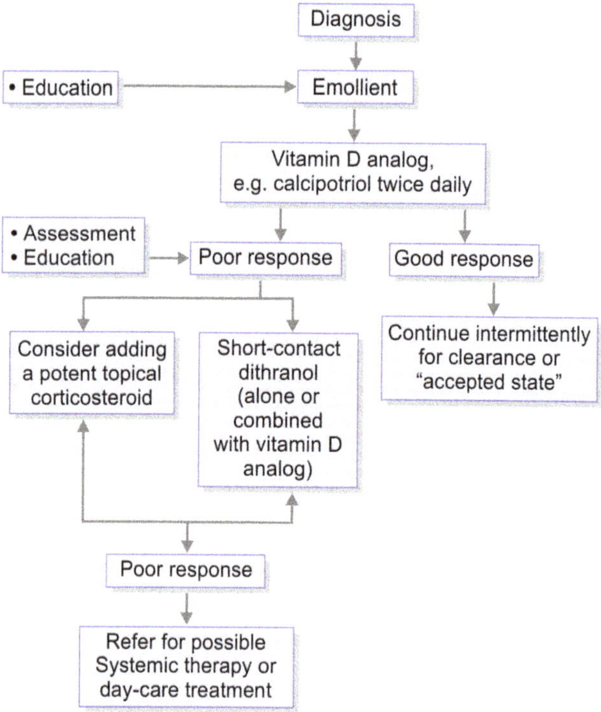

Fig. 12.18: Management algorithm for plaque psoriasis

Papulosquamous Diseases

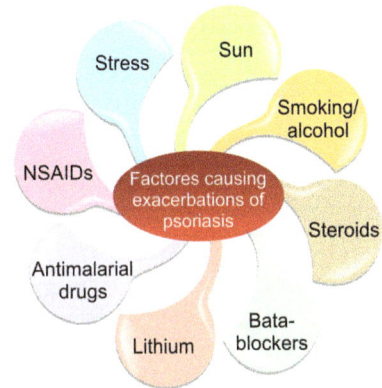

Fig. 12.19: Factors causing exacerbations of psoriasis

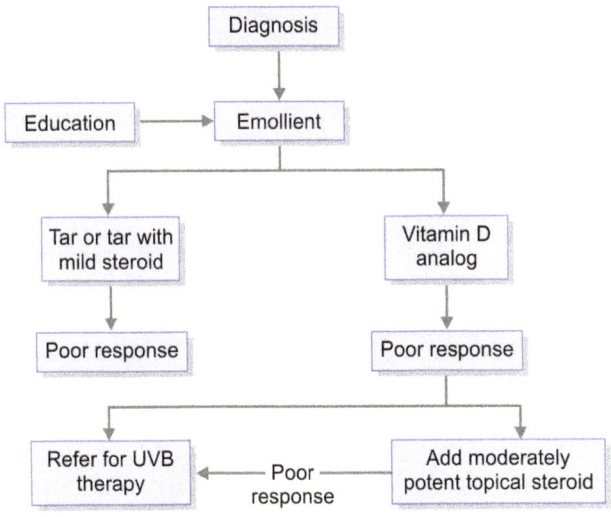

- Penicillin V may be required in the early stages
- Recurrent attacks may be reduced by tonsillectomy

Fig. 12.20: Management algorithm for guttate psoriasis

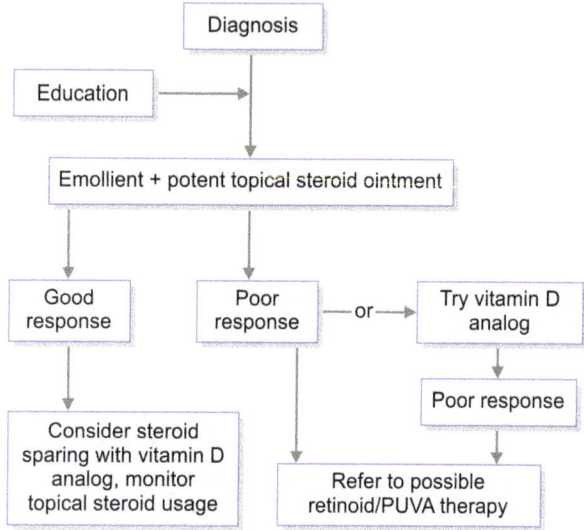

Fig. 12.21: Management algorithm for palmoplantar psoriasis

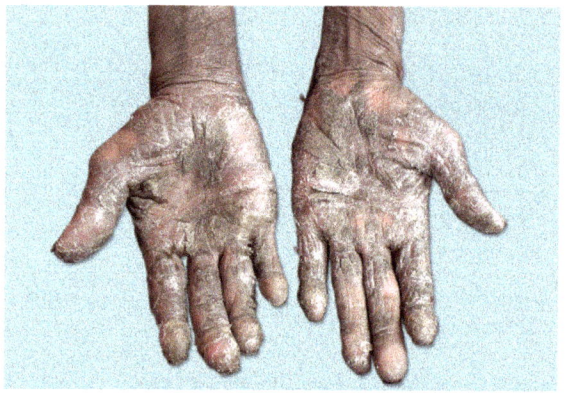

Fig. 12.22: Psoriasis of the palms: Both hands showing excessive scaling

Treatment of Severe Scalp Psoriasis from the Medical Board of the National Psoriasis Foundation

Treatment Algorithm

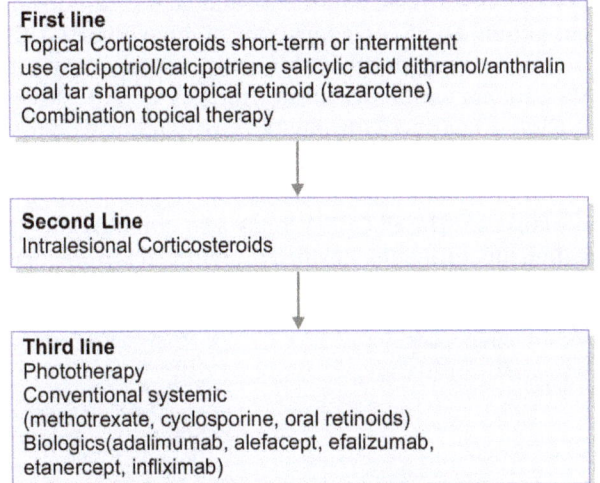

First line
Topical Corticosteroids short-term or intermittent use calcipotriol/calcipotriene salicylic acid dithranol/anthralin coal tar shampoo topical retinoid (tazarotene)
Combination topical therapy

Second Line
Intralesional Corticosteroids

Third line
Phototherapy
Conventional systemic (methotrexate, cyclosporine, oral retinoids)
Biologics(adalimumab, alefacept, efalizumab, etanercept, infliximab)

Etiopathogenesis

Psoriasis is a complex disorder with a polygenic and multifactorial etiology. It is likely that psoriasis may not be a single disorder but group of disorder with a common phenotype. this contention is supported by observed variations in the age of onset, severity, type and distribution of lesions as well as variation in affection of nails and joints. There is enough evidence that that in a genetically predisposed individual, phenotype is brought about by the interplay of various environmental factors like injury, friction, mental stress, infections [streptococcal, HIV] and drugs [blockers, lithium, systemic steroids, chloroquin].

Remissions and exacerbation may, however, occur without any obvious reason.

Psoriasis is not a single-gene disorder. At least nine chromosomal loci [named PSORS 1 to PSORS 9] have been identified to be associated with psoriasis. The strongest association is with PSORS 1 locus situated on chromosomal 6p containing about ten genes. One of them, the HLA-CW6 is strongly associated with early onset psoriasis in one study, 85.3% patients with early onset psoriasis were positive for HLA-CW6 in contrast with only 14.7% patients with late onset psoriasis. Caucasians who carry HLA-CW6 gene have a lower age of onset, guttate type of lesions and more extensive and severe disease. The PSORS 1 locus also contains the gene encoding for corneodesmosin, a protein that is upregulated in psoriatic epidermis.

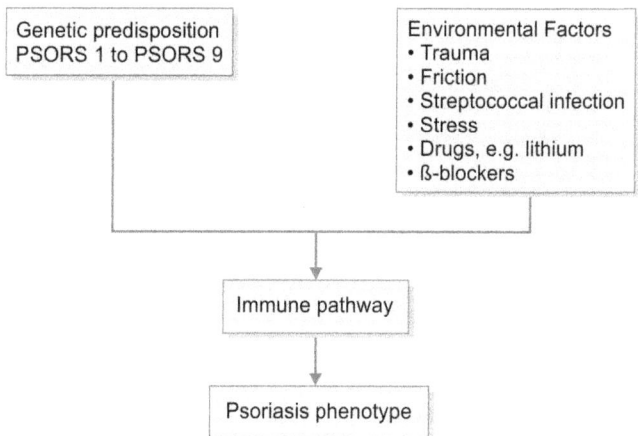

The currently accepted model of pathogenesis of psoriasis involves the interaction of 3 immunocytes viz. the antigen presenting cells [APCs], $CD4^+$ T-cells and $CD8^+$ T-cells. The APCs involved are the langerhans cells in the epidermis and the dermal dendritic cells in the dermis. The interactions may be summarized as below:

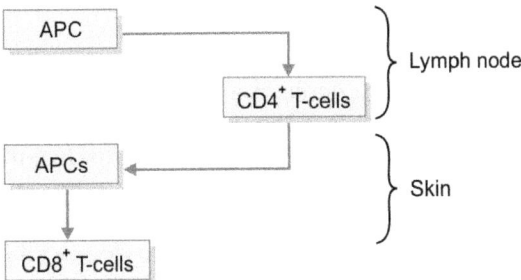

This is the simplistic version of the pathophysiology. Several more cells [e.g. plasmacytoid dendritic cells, natural killer NK cells, etc.] and soluble cytokines are involved in the pathogenesis.

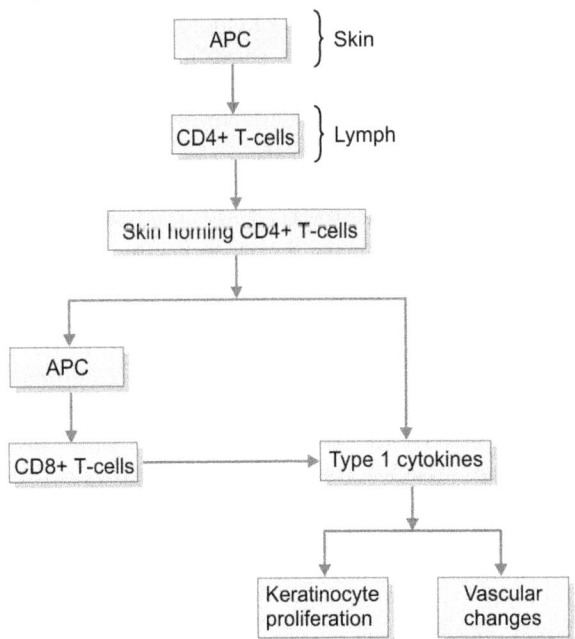

HIV and Psoriasis

The increased occurrence and exacerbation of psoriasis of HIV infection which depletes a patient of CD4 cells CD4 cells appears to be a paradox. But this apparent paradox is explained by the role of memory CD8+ T-cells. In advanced HIV infection the memory CD8+ T-cells subpopulation comprises over 85-90% of total CD8+ T-cells count because the naive CD8+ T-cells are infected and destroyed by the imbalance in favor of memory CD8+ T cells is responsible for psoriasis occurring in HIV infected patients.

Phototherapy for the Treatment of Plaque Psoriasis

In conclusion, the high levels of clinical efficacy and local tolerance demonstrated in this study indicate that calcitriol in combination with UVB has considerable potential for the management of patients with chronic plaque psoriasis, particularly on a long-term basis.

Decreased quality of life, type 2 diabetes mellitus, Crohn's disease, depression, psoriatic arthritis, and cardiovascular associated with psoriasis. Apparently, the risk of non-melanoma cancer has also been associated with phototherapy and immunosuppressive therapy. Specifically the risk of cardiovascular diseases is very significant in patients with psoriasis. Diseases such as coronary calcification, dyslipidemia, increased highly sensitive C-reactive protein (CRP), and hyperhomocysteinemia are highly prevalent in psoriatic patients. The role of proinflammatory cytokines and endothelial activation are hypothesized behind this association. Further, the inflammatory mechanisms in psoriasis also lead to deficiency of omega-3 fatty acid, folate, and vitamin B12 deficiencies, which is also significant in cardiovascular diseases.

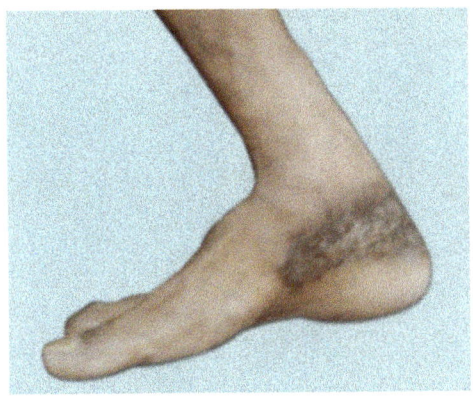

Fig. 12.23: Psoriasis of foot

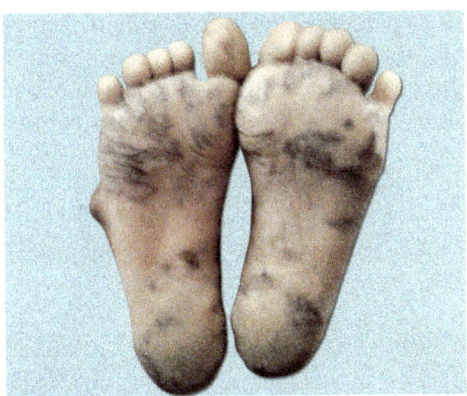

Fig. 12.24: Psoriasis of feet showing dryness roughness scaleness and thickness on both the feet

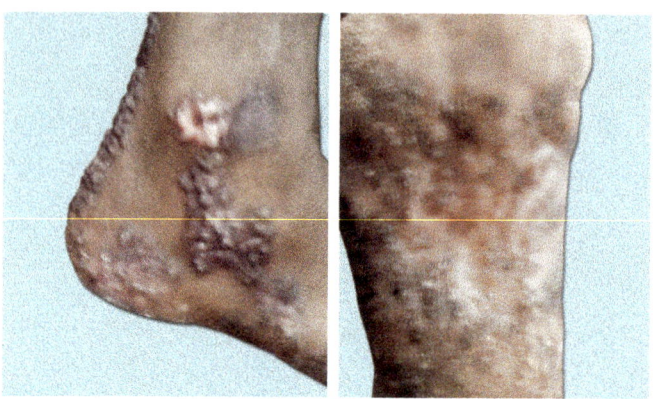

Fig. 12.25: Psoriasis of foot

A clinical condition known as psoriatic arthritis occurs in as many as 25 percent of individuals afflicted with psoriasis. Incidentally, the arthritic symptoms precede the skin lesion in approximately 10 percent of this population. A seronegative inflammatory arthritis, psoriatic arthritis is presented as

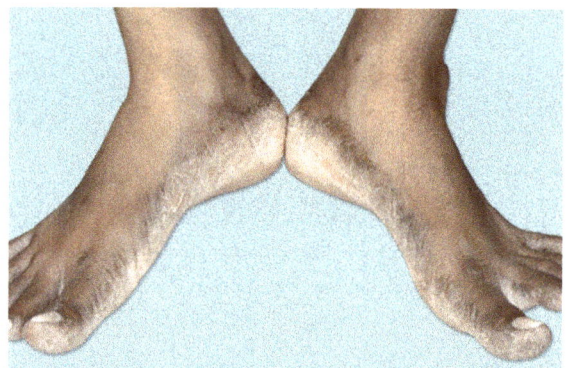

Fig. 12.26: Psoriasis of the feet showing dryness roughness scaleness and thickness on both the feet

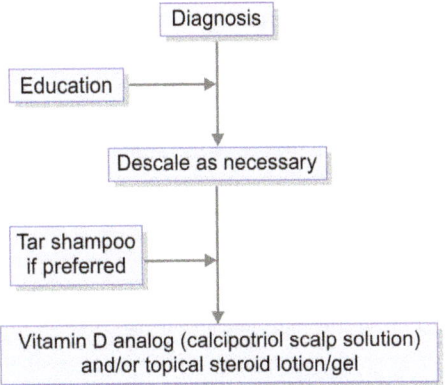

Fig. 12.27: Management algorithm for scalp psoriasis

oligoarthritis distal interphalangeal joint involvement, dactylitis (inflammation of the digits), and calcaneal inflammation. Whether, the arthritis and skin disease remains debatable however; genetic evidence, immunological studies, and treatment response variability is suggestive of the fact that they may be two different conditions, possibly with similar underlying inflammation and immune irregularity.

SYMPATHETIC RECEPTION

Initially, it may be helpful to agree on simple reception protocol for urgent initial presentations of skin disease, paying particular attention to the patients psychological distress, which may appear disproportionate to the perceived severity of the disease, for example, a sympathetic advice regarding emollient therapy is safe and often very beneficial, and may allow future education and treatment to be arranged with less stress for both patient and doctor.

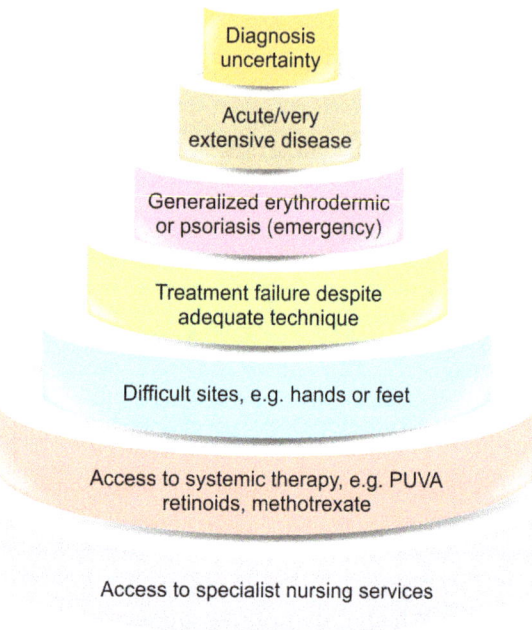

Fig. 12.28: Referral criteria for psoriasis patient

Table 12.4: Diagnostic signs and symptoms of arthritis

Signs to examine for	Symptoms to ask about
Tender or swollen joints	Morning stiffness
Asymmetric inflammatory arthrits	Persistent joint pain or other arthritic symptoms
Dactylitis or "sausage digits"	Fluctuation of joint pain with psoriasis exacerbations
Enthesitis	Family history

Treatment of Psoriasis

Psoriasis is widely believed to be incurable. However, it can be brought under control and, usually heals with prolonged remissions. Correction of overweight, avoidance of trauma or irritating agents including strong soaps and detergents and reducing intake of alcoholic beverages helps in halting progression. Sunlight and sea bathing improve psoriasis except in the photosensitive patients.

Psoriasis is said to be unstable based on the presence of Koebner phenomenon, bright erythema, pustules or occurrence of many new lesions.

Clinical Implication

Topical tar, anthralin, potent steroids and PUVA therapy are relatively contraindicated for unstable psoriasis for fear of worsening it or precipitating pustular psoriasis.

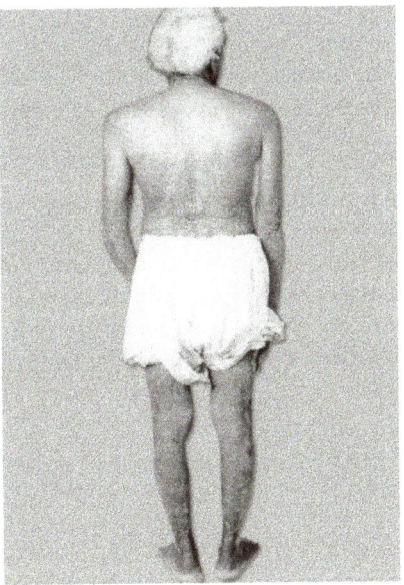

Fig. 12.29: Psoriasis vulgaris—plaque over the extensor surface of limbs and trunk (back view)

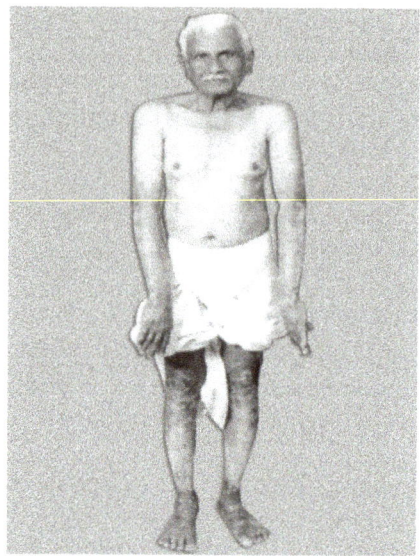

Fig. 12.30: Psoriasis vulgaris—plaque over the extensor surface of limbs and trunk (front view)

Unstable psoriasis may be brought under control with liberal applications of topical bland emollients (white soft paraffin) and supportive therapy. Oral methotrexate, retinoids, cyclosporin and even systemic steroids can control unstable psoriasis. However, systemic steroids are usually avoided for the fear of precipitating pustular psoriasis upon withdrawal.

Topical Therapy

Emollients

White soft paraffin soothes the skin, traps moisture, restores barrier function to some extent and helps in removal of thick scales by softening them.

Table 12.5: Differential diagnosis among psoriatic arthritis, rheumatoid arthritis, osteoarthritis, and ankylosing spondylitis

Signs and symptoms	Psoriatic arthritis	RA	OA	AS
Peripheral disease	Asymmetric	Symmetric	Varies	—
DIP involvement	+	—	+, Heberden nodes	—
Sacroiliitis	Asymmetric	—	—	Symmetric
Stiffness	Peripheral joints, some spine, morning	Morning	With activity	Significant spine
Gender bias	1:1 male to female	3:1 female to male	Hand and toe OA more frequent in females	3:1 male to female
Enthesitis	+	—	—	+
RF	—	+	—	—
HLA association*	B27, Cw6	DR4	—	B27
Radiographic changes	Erosions, paramarginal absence of osteopenia	Erosions, osteopenia pencil-in-cup, asymmetric syndesmophytes	Osteophytes, erosions spinal	Squaring of vertebral bodies, symmetric syndesmophytes osteopenia

Steroids

Potent topical steroids like fluocinolone acetonide, betamethasone dipropionate or clobetasol propionate from the first line of therapy for localized plaques of psoriasis.

Coal Tar

Stable but resistant plaques are best managed with 5-10% coal tar with or without UV-B exposure (sunlight).

Dithranol

Alternatively, 0.1-1% dithranol, applied carefully over the plaques and lift only for 30-60 minutes, can be used with good results.

Clinical Implication

Dithranol is highly irritant if applied over normal skin or on lesions of unstable psoriasis and hence it should be used under close medical supervision.

Keratolytics and Humectants

Salicylic acid 3-10% and urea 10-20% help in resolution of stable plaques by their keratolytic and humectant properties.

Calcipotriol, Calcitriol, Tacalcitol, Maxacalcitol

This vitamin D analog is effective in inducing remissions of localized plauqes.

Systemic Therapy

Widespread psoriasis needs systemic agents in addition to topical therapy.

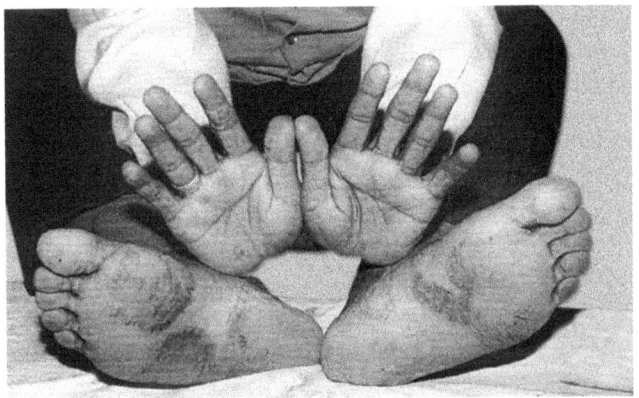

Fig. 12.31: Psoriasis of the palms on the soles the thick plaque lesions

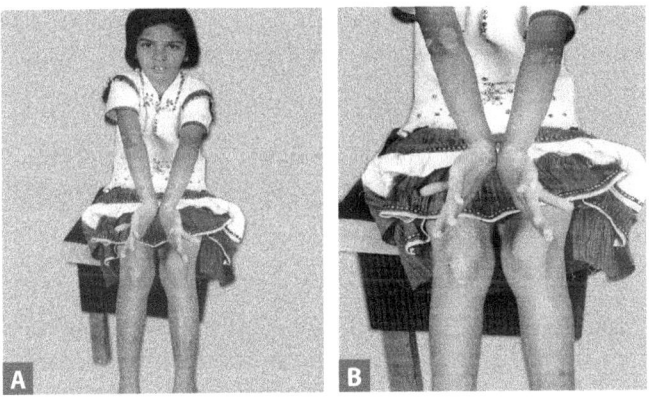

Fig. 12.32: Psoriasis vulgaris (in children)—plaque lesions all over the extensor surface of limbs and trunk

Methotrexate

Three doses of 2.5–5 mg oral methotrexate at 12 hourly intervals administered every week are extremely effective.

Hepatic and renal disease are relative contraindications. Close monitoring of blood counts and hepatic function are essential.

PUVA Therapy

Oral 8 methoxy psoralen 30 mg on alternate days followed up with UVA (320–400) exposure constitutes PUVA therapy.

Steroids

Systemic steroids should only be used in life-threatening situations in erythrodermic and pustular psoriasis to bring them under control with rapidity.

Retinoids

Etretinate 50 mg per day orally, is another option for the treatment of recalcitrant widespread psoriasis. It is absolutely contraindicated in pregnancy and must be avoided in women of childbearing age.

Cyclosporin

This immune modulator is useful in controlling erythrodermic and resistant psoriasis.

Newer Evolution in Psoriasis Management

Tazarotene is a novel molecule. It is a selective retinoid receptor and belongs to the third generation retinoids. It has the following structure formula, which is ethyl 6 nicotinate.

Mechanism of Action

- Tazarotene is converted in the skin to its active metabolite tazarotenic acid
- Tazarotenic acid has a high affinity for RAR beta and RAR-gamma receptors

- By binding with RAR receptors, tazarotenic acid regulates (AP-1 dependent) gene expression
- RAR and PXR down regulate API and INF γ.

Tazarotene is rapidly converted by the esterases present in the skin to the active metabolite tazarotene acid and sulfoxide, which is inactive metabolite. Tazarotene acid has high affinity for the retinoic acid receptors namely, the beta and the gamma receptors. Tazarotenic acid regulates the activator protein dependent gene expression, which is responsible for psoriasis, and it also down regulates the interferon alpha, which is responsible for the expression of the ICAM and HLA-DR.

Tazarotene Action in Psoriasis

Tazarotene normalizes all the threee basic pathogenic mechanisms involved in psoriasis, that is

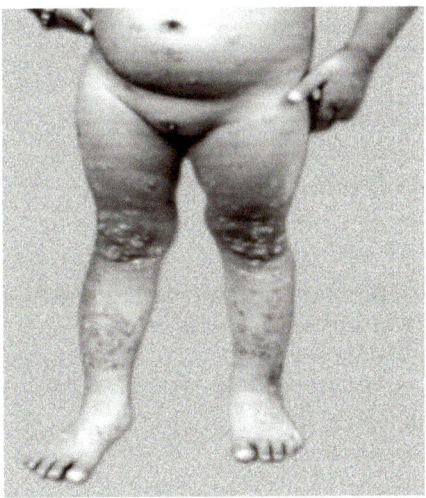

Fig. 12.33: Psoriasis vulgaris (in children)—plaque lesions all over the extensor surface of limbs and trunk (front view)

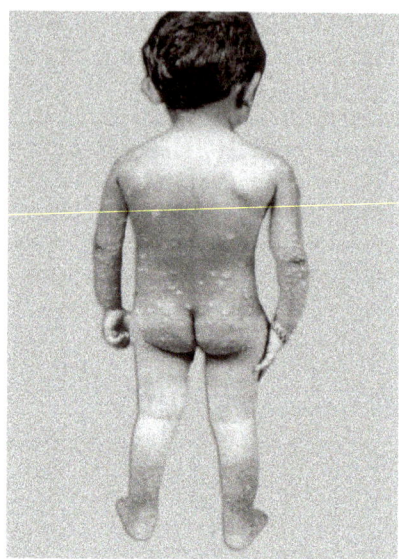

Fig. 12.34: Psoriasis vulgaris (in children)—plaque lesions all over the extensor surface of limbs and trunk (back view)

- Abnormal differentiation
- Hytperproliferation
- Dermal inflammation.

Benefits of Tazarotene

Tazarotene is receptor specific retinoid, inhibits all the three pathological factors in psoriasis.

It has a limited percutaneous penetration and is rapidly metabolized into tazarotenic acid and other metabolites, which are quickly eliminated from the body, hence there are no systemic side effects.

- Since less than 6% of the applied tazarotene enter into the bloodstream, one need not be afraid of adverse effects associated with systemic retinoid

- It has longer remission, better compliance
- It is compatible with many other therapies of psoriasis
- Since it is applied once daily and the therapeutic efficacy that is sustained even after 12 weeks of treatment, it gives the patient a cost-effective treatment option
- There is increased confidence in treatment
- This is a non-steroidal drug especially in an era in which there is steroid phobia.

Unstable psoriasis is managed with topical emollients and supportive therapy. If erythroderma or pustular lesions supervene, systemic methotrexate, steroids, etretinate and cyclosporin are the available options. Stable plaque type psoriasis responds to topical potent steroids or coal tar or anthralin or, if extensive, to systemic PUVA therapy. Emollients, weight reduction and, avoidance of trauma, detergents and alcohol are helpful in control of psoriasis.

Hair Regrowth following TNF-α Blockade in Coexisting Psoriasis Vulgaris and Alopecia Areata

Tumor necrosis factor (TNF-α) can modulate hair cycles, as well as mediate immunological diseases. TNF-α blockade is thought to effective for psoriasis vulgarisis(PS) but not for alopecia areata (AA).

Long-term Oral Azithromycin in Chronic Plaque Psoriasis

Most azithromycin treated patients showed a significant improvement in their PASI score from 12 weeks onwards.

A measurement of the stigma among vitiligo and psoriasis patients in India.

Both psoriasis and vitiligo patients suffered moderate to severe restriction while participating in their domestic and social life. Psoriasis patients faced significantly more restrictions in a number of day to day life situations. The Indian population of this study was predominantly dark-skinned and hypopigmentation as seen in vitiligo is much more noticeable than psoriatic red patches. However, the result showed that the component of hypo or hyperpigmentation of skin was not the only factor leading to participation restrictions.

Psoriatic Arthritis is a Strong Predictor of Sleep Interference in Patients with Psoriasis

This study presents evident that history of arthritis, pruritus and pain of psoriasis lesions, and emotional factors are predictive of sleep interference in patients with psoriasis. Physicians treating patients with sporiatic disease need to incorporate this life altering comorbidity into their assessment of disease and selection of treatment.

Increasing Use of More Potent Treatment for Psoriasis

Guidelines of Care for the Management of Psoriasis and Psoriatic Arthritis

Table 12.6: Use of topical agents : The fingertip unit and how to assess quantity of topical agents needed to cover a given body surface area.

Area to be treated	No. of Fingertip units	Approximate body surface area (%)
Scalp	3	6
Face and neck	2.5	5
One hand (front and back) including finger	1	2
One entire arm including entire hand	4	8

Contd...

Contd...

Area to be treated	No. of Fingertip units	Approximate body surface area (%)
Elbows (large plaque)	1	2
Both soles	1.5	3
One foot (dorsum and sole), including toes	1.5	3
One entire leg including entire foot	8	16
Buttocks	4	8
Knees (large plaque)	1	2
Trunk (anterior)	8	16
Trunk (posterior)	8	16
Genitalia	0.5	1

Table 12.7: Strength of recommendations for the treatment of psoriasis using topical the therapies

Agent
Class I corticosteroids
Class II corticosteroids
Class III/IV corticosteroids
Class III/VI/VII corticosteroids
D analogues vitamin
Tazarotene
Tacrolimus and pimecrolimus
Anthralin
Coal tar
Combination corticosteroids and salicylic acid
Combination corticosteroids and D analogues vitamin
Combination corticosteroids and tazarotene
Combination corticosteroids and salicylic acid

Intertriginous Pustular Psoriasis

Psoriasis presents in childhood in up to a third of cases. Plaque and guttate types of psoriasis are most often the initial manifestation, although the so-called " napkin" psoriasis is a common feature of infantile disease. Pustular psoriasis is particularly rare in childhood.

Drugs that Aggravate Acne

Certain medications can aggravate acne. The following mnemonic for drugs that may aggravate acne is helpful:
- **P** (phenytoin), (isoniazid),
- **M** (moisturizers),
- **P** (phenobarbital), **L** (lithium),
- **E** (ethionamide), and
- **S** (steroids).

Adapalene is more photostable than retinoic acid. When combined with benzoyl.

Topical Dapsone

Dapsone is a potent antibiotic with anti-inflammatory activity. It is highly lipophilic and has only been available as an oral tablet.

Azithromycin

Antibiotic-resistant propionibacterium acnes—a growing problem.

Pityriasis Rosea

Though presumed to be a viral infection, the causative organism has not been demonstrated. Its seasonal occurrence in young adults and children, presence of a primary lesion, occasional prodromal symptoms, spontaneous resolution within 6 weeks and rarity of second attacks are all pointers to a viral etiology.

Variations in morphology or distribution of pityriasis rosea include
1. Papular—no or scanty scales.
2. Psoriasiform—thick scales resembling psoriasis.
3. Vesicular—vesicles are also present.
4. Localized—only one region (e.g. axilla) is involved.
5. Inverse—extremities and face involved, trunk spared.

Therapy

Being a self-limiting viral infection (presumably) therapy is supportive. Avoidance of irritating agents and soaps, use of soothing creams and, if pruritus is present, topical steroids are helpful. The eruption resolves without any therapy within 4–6 weeks.

Pityriasis rosea is a viral exanthem with minimal prodromal symptoms. If affects the young and is seasonal. Initial lesion (mother plaque) is an annular erythematous plaque with fine collarette scales. Within a few days, it is followed by numerous smaller but similar lesions, round or oval, arranged along the ribs. Lesions are non-pruritic and occur over the trunk or proximal extremities. Self-healing within 4–6 weeks is a rule.

Lichen Planus

A common inflammatory disorder of the skin, lichen planus is an autoimmune disease.

Patient Profile

Young adults are common victims. However, no age is exempt. Both sexes are affected equally.

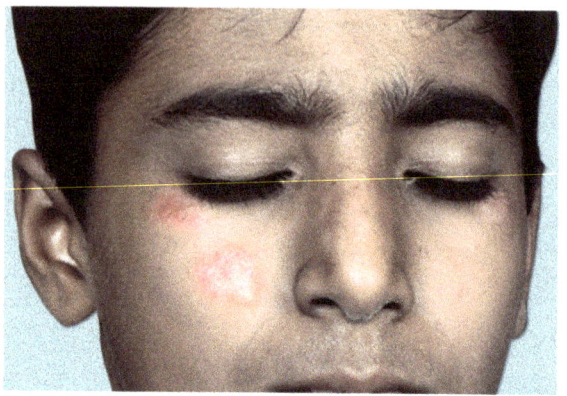

Fig. 12.35: Inverse pityriasis rosea—lesions over the face

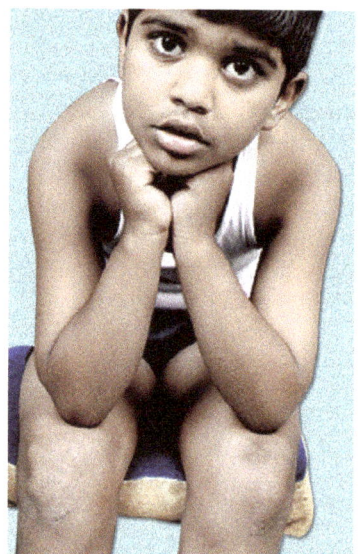

Fig. 12.36: Lichen nitidus—knees and elbow fine spiny and shiny lesions

Variations in the morphology of lichen planus include:
1. Annular—ring like
2. Vesicular and bullous
3. Linear—due to Koebner phenomenon
4. Hypertrophic—large thick plaque on shin, ankle or foot.
5. Atrophic—macular (flat) lesions
6. Follicular—conical papules with central keratin plug. A common consequence is scarring alopecia of scalp (Graham-Little syndrome).

Distribution

Flexor aspects of wrists and forearms, shins, ankles, dorsa of feet, anterior thighs and flanks are sites of predilection. Oral, especially buccal mucosa, lips and genitalia are also commonly affected.

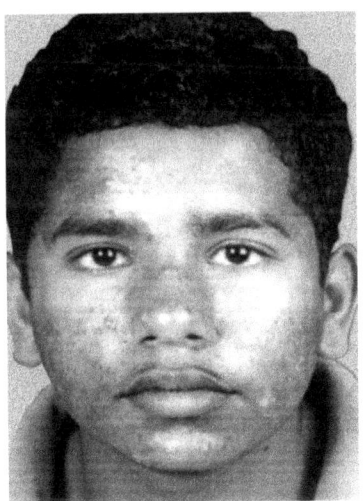

Fig. 12.37: Acne vulgaris—nodulocystic lesions in addition to other acne lesions over the cheek, forehead and nose

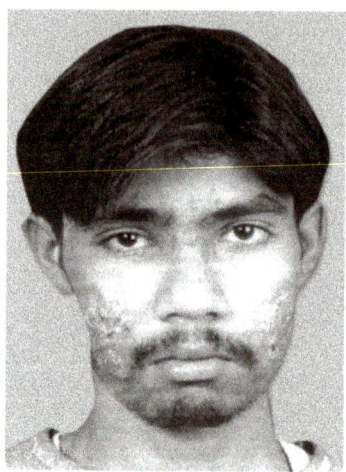

Fig. 12.38: Nodulocystis acne on both the cheeks also forehead and scars on the cheeks

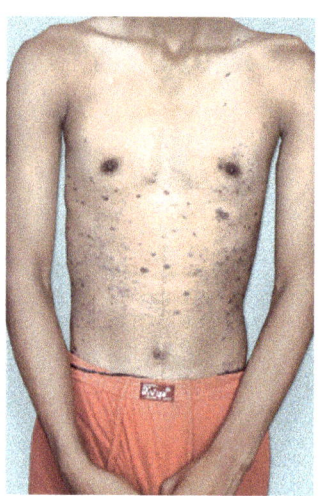

Fig. 12.39: Lichen planus—flat topped violaceous papular lesions on the chest and arms (front view)

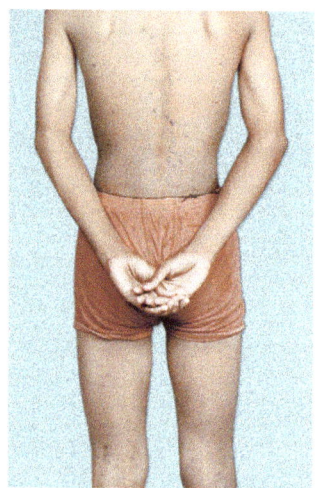

Fig. 12.40: Lichen planus—flat topped violaceous papular lesions on the chest and arms on the back

Variations based on distribution include:
1. Acute widespread—involving most of the area mentioned.
2. Chronic localized—common around ankles and wrists.
3. Segmental—involves one nerve segment.
4. Oral—papules arranged in an annular or lacelike pattern.
5. Nail—thin striated nails with pterygium (extension of proximal nail fold on to the nail plate) formation.

Therapy

Oral antihistaminics like pheniramine maleate or cetirizine are needed to relieve pruritus. Other than this, topical therapy sufices for localized lesions. Potent corticosteroids like fluocinolone acetonide, betamethasone valerate are effective for ordinary lesions. Hypertrophic lesions need stronger steroids like clobetasol propionate or intralesional injections of triamcinolone acetonide.

Lichen planus is an autoimmune disease that affects the young-and middle-aged adults. An eruption of pruritic, erythematous, polygonal, flat topped papules with a violaceous hue and scanty scale characterizes the disease. A typical case has Wickham's striae (crisscross whites lines) and Koebner phenomenon (induction of lesions by trauma). Flexors of wrists and forearms, thighs, shins, ankles, oral and genital mucosae are affected frequently. Variants include hypertrophic, annular and linear lesions. Biopsy is diagnostic. Topical and intralesional steroids are effective for localized lesions. Widespread disease frequently required systemic steroid therapy.

Increased Serum Apelin-12 and Lipid Profile in Patients with and without Psoriasis

Our finding indicate that apelin-12 concentration were significantly higher in subject with psoriasis, supporting the hypothesis that overproduction of apelin-12 might play a role in the etiopathology of psoriasis.

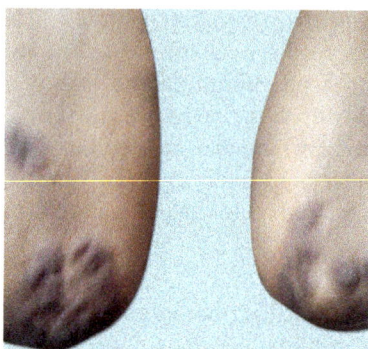

Fig. 12.41: Psoriasis of the arms elbows

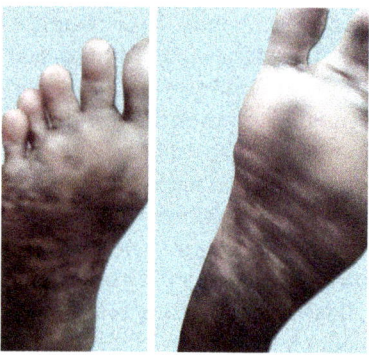

Fig. 12.42: Psoriasis of the sole of the feet

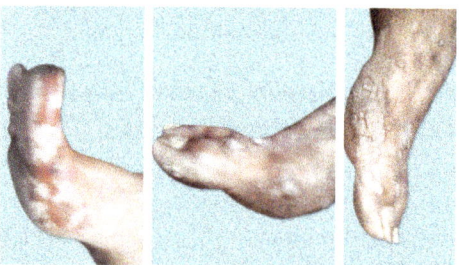

Fig. 12.43: Psoriasis of feet and sole

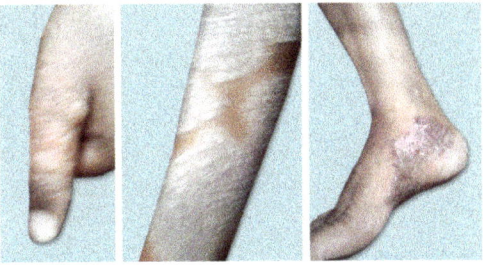

Fig. 12.44: Psoriasis—typical silvery scale lesions

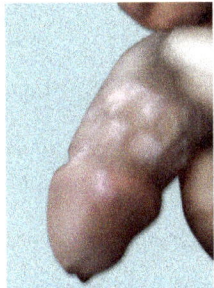

Fig. 12.45: Lichen planus on the penis

Planus

Sulfasalazine is effective and alternative therapy of generalized lichen planus.

CHAPTER 13

Disorders of Pigmentation

Color of the skin largely depends on the number and distribution of the four biochromes present in the skin.

Flowchart 13.1: Color of skin

- Skin color
  - Epidermis
    - Melanin (brown)
    - Carotenoids (yellow)
  - Dermis
    - Oxyhemoglobin (bright red)
    - Reduced hemoglobine (bluish red)

ALBINISM

Oculocutaneous albinism is an autosomal recessively transmitted defect in melanin synthesis. Skin and hair are white and irides, red. Nystagmus, refractive errors and photophobia are usual. Over the years, the skin develops solar keratoses and elastosis due to sun damage. Management comprises photoprotection of skin and eyes, correction of refractive errors and genetic counseling.

VITILIGO

This pigmentary disorder of unknown cause is characterized by depigmented or hypopigmented patches that result from reduced or absent mylanocytes. Leukoderma, a term used

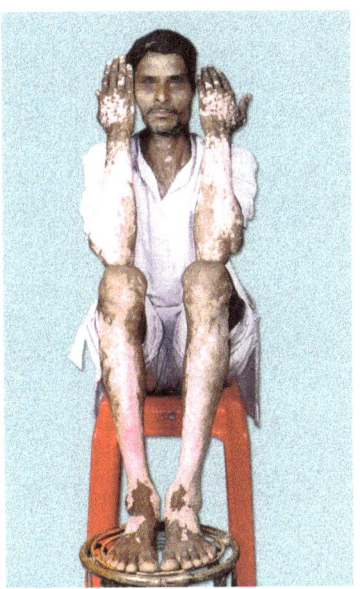

Fig. 13.1: A typical case of vitiligo: Bilateral symmetrical vitiligo vulgaris

Flowchart 13.2: Etiology of vitiligo (Punshi, SK 2005)

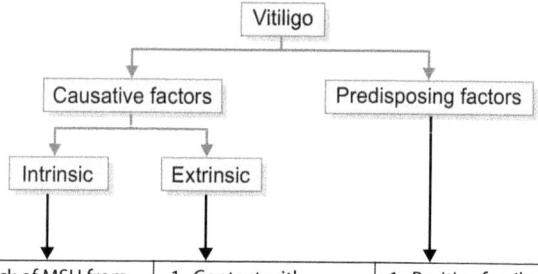

Intrinsic	Extrinsic	Predisposing factors
1. Lack of MSH from pituitary 2. Increase in melatonin like substance at nerve endings 3. Autoimmune response directed against the enzyme process forming melanin 4. Humoral factors 5. Allergy and atopy 6. Oxidants (free radicals) 7. Vitiligo is a form of apoptosis	1. Contact with rubber and nylon articles, photographic developers, hydroquinones guanofuracin (kitamura) 2. Pressure due to tight wearing of sarees, dhoties and elastic undergarments 3. Indiscriminate use of broad sprectrum antibiotics, streptomycin, oxytetracycline, ciprofloxin, etc. 4. Photographic developing solutions 5. Blood groups B and AB 6. Hypochlorhydria and achlorhydria	1. Positive family history 2. Septic foci 3. Gastrointestinal and hepatic disturbances 4. Physical and emotional trauma 5. Diet deficient in cupraminerals, zinc and proteins

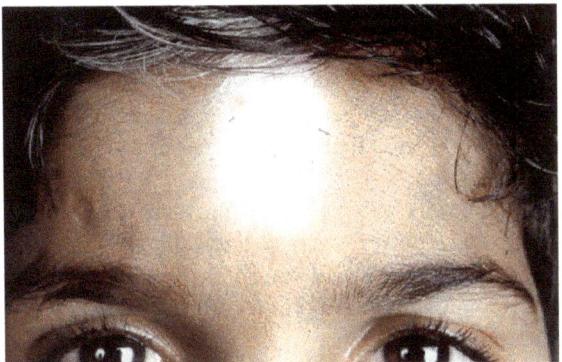

Fig. 13.2: Piebaldism—typical white forelock

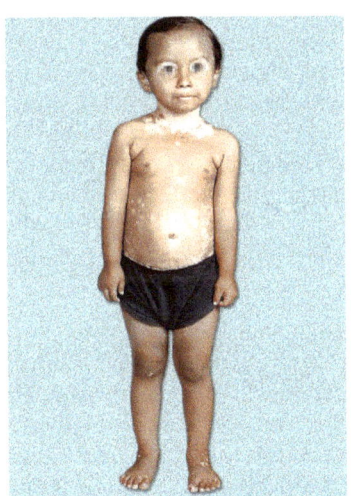

Fig. 13.3: Vitiligo in children

for vitiligo in nonmedical literature, is different from vitiligo. The term leukoderma is applied to depigmented patches of known causes, e.g. following burns, contact with chemicals like phenols or catechols or following an inflammatory skin disease. As opposed to vitiligo, it does not progress after the cause is removed.

Piebaldism is an uncommon, autosomal dominate, congenital, stable leukoderma characterized by a white forelock and vitiligo like amelanotic macules, usually containing a few normally pigmented or hyperpigmented macules.

Clinical Profile

About 1-2% of the general population has vitiligo. Vitiligo begins commonly in the 2nd to 4th decades. It is uncommon in children and the elderly. Both sexes are affected equally. Family history of vitiligo is present in only about 25% of cases. Most patients with vitiligo are otherwise normal and do not need any investigations. However, there is an increased incidence of diabetes mellitus, thyroid dysfunction, Addison's disease, alopecia areata, and lichen planus in patients with vitiligo.

Morphology

Depigmented (milky white) or hypopigmented (light colored) macules and patches that are sharply demarcated from the surrounding normal skin typify the disease. The affected skin is otherwise normal except for a little erythema of patches on sun exposed regions due to heightened sensitivity. Hair within a patch may turn white (leukotrichia). Margins of the patches may occasionally be hyperpigmented or hypopigmented. Hyperpigmentation may also be seen around follicles within a patch and this is a sign of recovery.

Disorders of Pigmentation

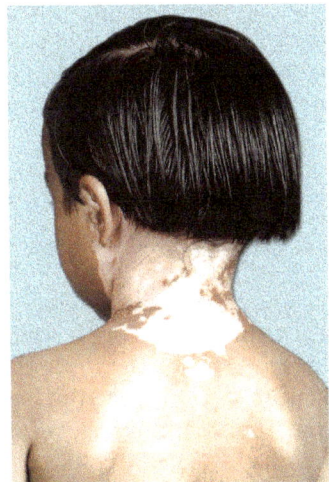

Fig. 13.4: Vitiligo in a child on backside

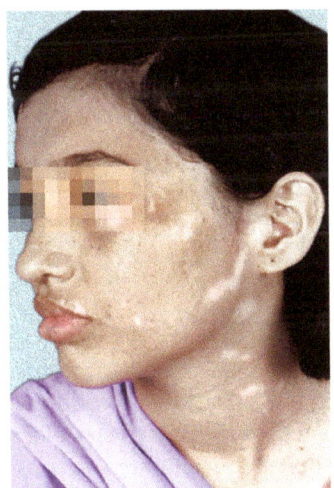

Fig. 13.5: Vitiligo on the face

"Punshi's sign"—In menstruating girls and ladies there is change of color in the vitiligo lesions every month during the menstrual period. From white to pink and vice versa after the period is over that shows, it is a hormonal independent disease.

Distribution

According to the extent of involvement, vitiligo can be classified into:
1. Localized: A few patches over one body region.
2. Dermatomal: Patches limited to the region of one or two nerve segments.
3. Vulgaris: Widespread and symmetrical patches involving extremities and trunk. Common sites of affection include shins, forearms, palms, soles, elbows, knees, lips, eyelids, upper trunk, genitals, axillae and groins.
4. Acro-orificial: Involves acral (fingers, toes, palms, soles) and periorificial (lips, perioral, periocular, glans penis) areas, carries poor prognosis.
5. Universal: Total or near total affection of the while body.

Flowchart 13.3: Color of skin

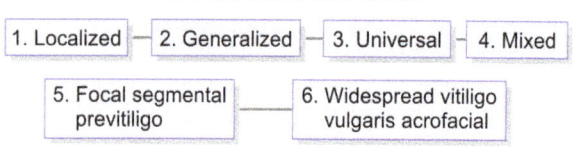

Differential Diagnosis

Leprosy patches rarely become depigmented (milky white) and have impaired sensations. Hypopigmented (but not depigmented) patches of pityriasis versicolor are covered with powdery scales that get accentuated on stroking the affected skin. Leukoderma due to contactants can be suspected based on its characteristic sites, e.g. dorsa of feet due to chappals, central forehead due to bindi.

Treatment of Vitiligo

Small and solitary patches of short duration may respond to apotent topical steroid like fluocinolone acetonide. Topical PUVA therapy is also useful for such patches.
1. General measures
2. Medical
3. Surgical
4. Alternative/camouflage
5. Psychological counseling
6. Social counseling
7. Lasers in vitiligo
8. Local basic fibroblast growth factors in vitiligo
    a. Natural—placental extract
    b. Synthetic—melanin.
9. Tacrolimus, tacravate

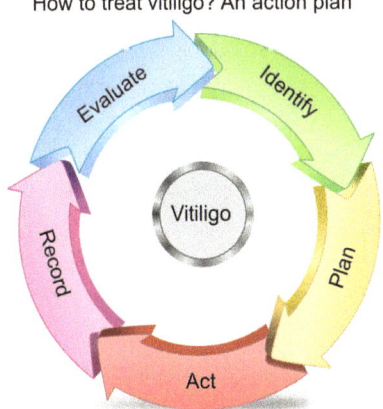

Fig. 13.6: Treatment of vitiligo

Drugs introduced by author in the treatment of vitiligo:
1. Placental extract in vitiligo acts as a biogenous stimulator. It stimulates the melanocyte to form the melanin acting on the theory of self exhaustion or self destruction of melanocytes.
2. B 665 (Clofazimine) in vitiligo.
3. Geriforte and Liv 52 herbal preparations act as adjunct to psoralen in vitiligo.
4. Pigmento in vitiligo
5. Topical application of annacarcin oil (extract of semicarpus anacardium) in vitiligo.
6. It is proposed that more than one type of vitiligo exists and certainly the nondermatomal type with its allergic disturbances improves with (a) corticosteroids (b) antihistamines (c) immunotherapy with levamisol, histamine-gammaglobulin complex in addition to usual melanising agents.

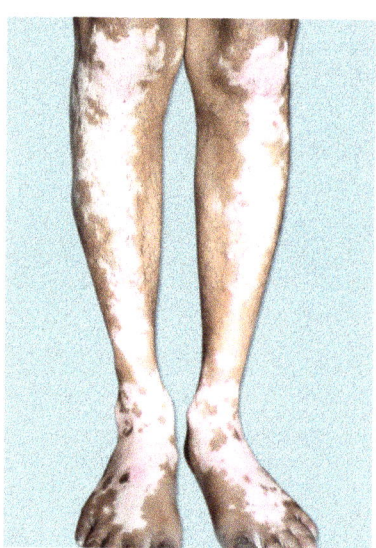

Fig. 13.7: Vitiligo vulgaris lesions on the legs and the feet almost symmetrical lesions

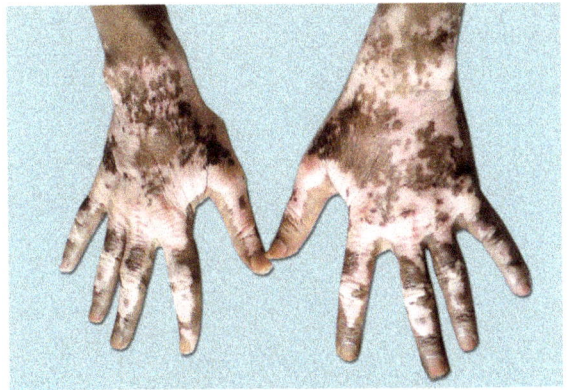

Fig. 13.8: Vitiligo on the hands

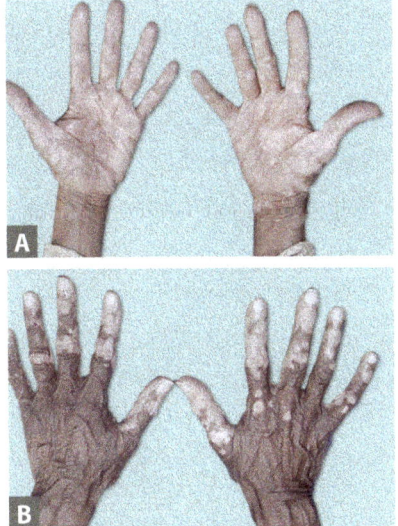

Fig. 13.9A and B: Vitiligo of palms and fingers

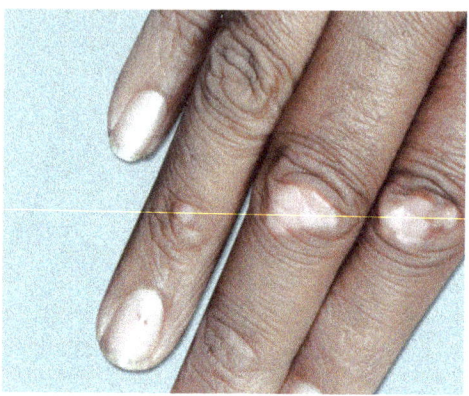

Fig. 13.10: Vitiligo on the fingures (knuckles)

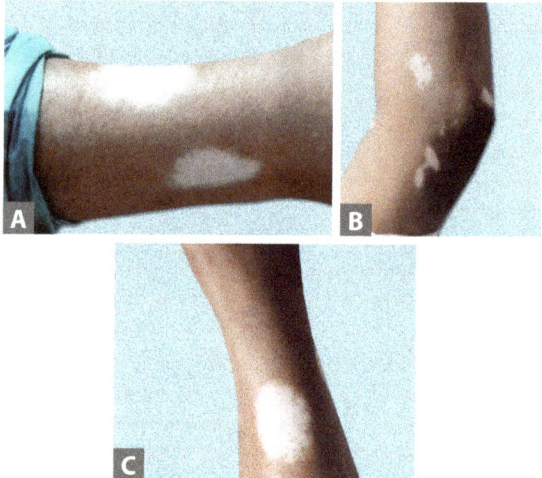

Fig. 13.11A to C: Vitiligo of arms

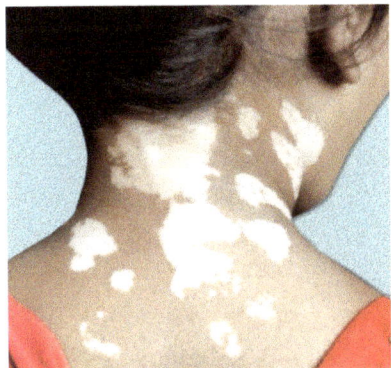

Fig. 13.12: Vitiligo on the back

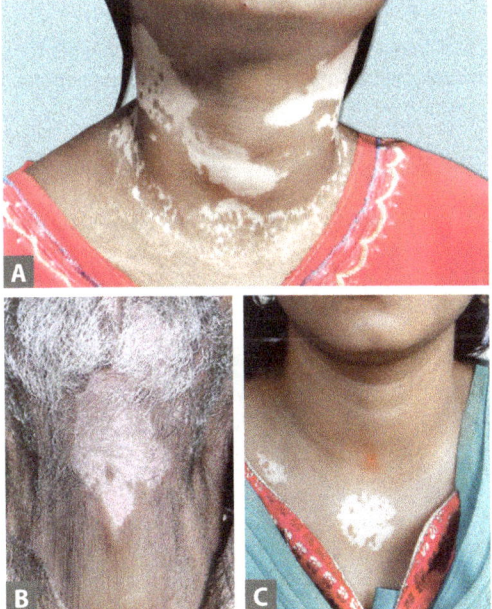

Fig. 13.13A to C: Vitiligo on the neck

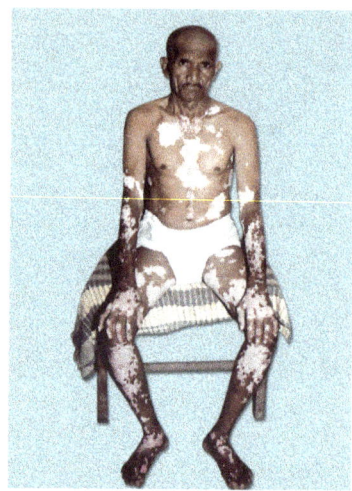

Fig. 13.14: Generalized vitiligo—multiple depigmented and hypopigmented macules over the chest and abdomen

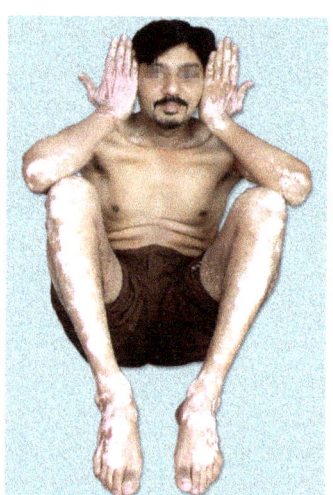

Fig. 13.15: Generalized vitiligo

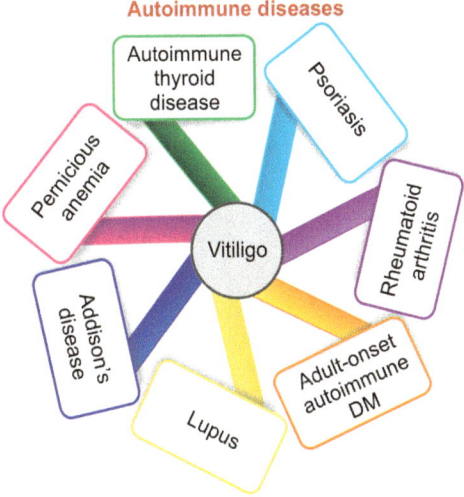

Fig. 13.16: Autoimmune diseases epidemiologically and genetically associated with vitiligo

7. Herbomineral therapy of vitiligo.
8. Antioxidants in vitiligo.

Recent Advances in Genetic Studies in Vitiligo
- Gene on chromosome 17
- Linkage signals especially chromosome 7, 8, 9 and 17
- CTLA4
- PTPN22
- FOXD3
- (Fain PR et al. Am J Hum Genet. 2003;72:1560-4) (Spritz RA et al. Am J Hum Genet. 2004;74:188-91).

Systemic steroids may help in arresting the progress of rapidly spreading disease. However, caution must be exercised to avoid their adverse effects. Once the disease stops spreading, multiple patches, with >20% body area

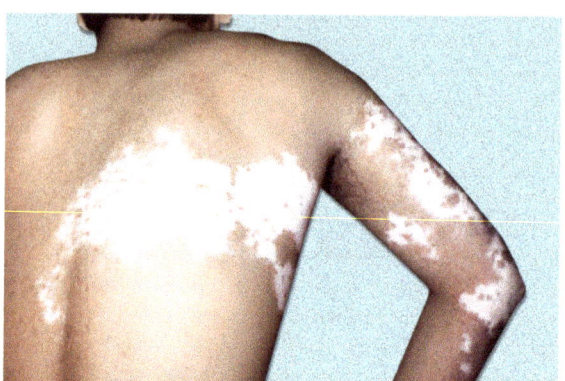

Fig. 13.17: Segmental vitiligo

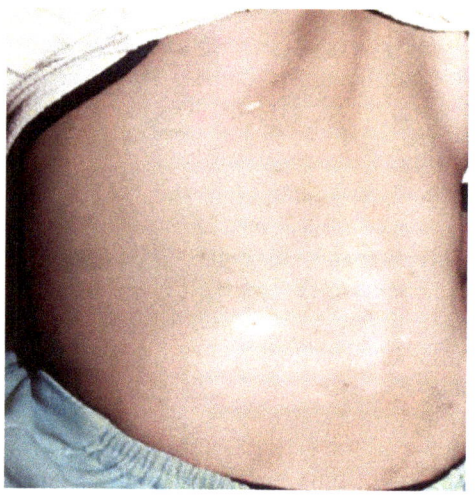

Fig. 13.18: Halo nevus

Disorders of Pigmentation

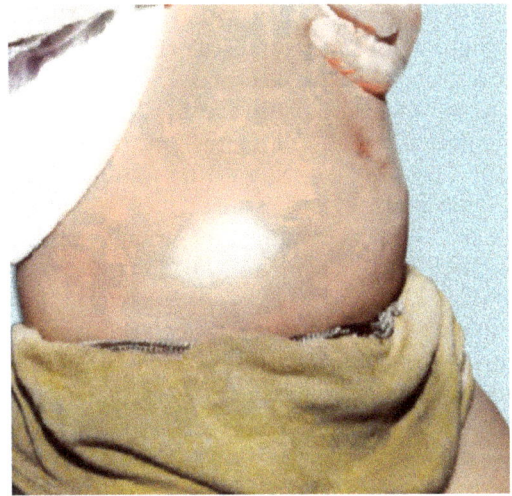

Fig. 13.19: Nevus achromicus

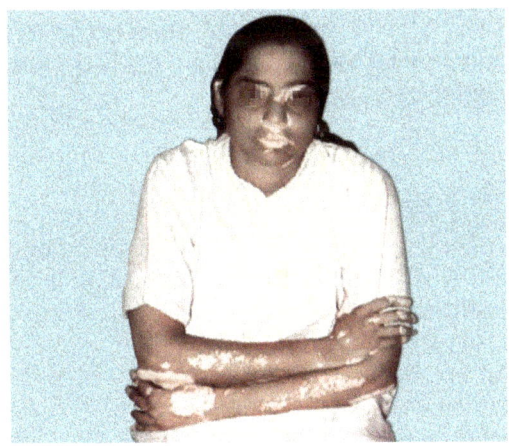

Fig. 13.20: Vitiligo on lips and tips

involvement, are best managed with systemic PUVA therapy. Topical applications and intramuscular injections of placental extract are also claimed to be useful.

Once the disease is static and only small areas of depigmentation remain, dermatosurgical techniques like minipunch grafting, shave grafting and suction blister grafting or tattoing can be used to treat these residual patches. Melanocyte culture and autografts probably offer a ray of hope to cases with widespread vitiligo that are resistant to other therapies.

Vitiligo is an autoimmune disease that kills melanocytes. Common age of onset is between 15 years and 35 years. Lesions are well defined, milky white (depigmented) macules or patches. Vitiligo may be localized, regional (or segmental), generalized, universal (affecting all the skin surface) or acromucosal. Because of the social stigma it carries, treatment of this benign condition is important. Unstable (rapidly spreading) vitiligo is controlled with systemic steroids. Once static, localized patches can be treated with topical steroids or topical PUVA and then residual areas surgically grafted whereas generalized lesions need systemic PUVA therapy for repigmentation.

PUVA THERAPY

PUVA Therapy for Vitiligo

PUVA (Psoralen + Ultraviolet A) therapy comprises of topical or systemic administration of psoralen followed up with ultraviolet A (320 – 400 nm) light. Psoralens are a group of plant derived chemicals (furocoumarins) that sensitize the skin to ultraviolet rays thereby stimulating melanocyte function and their regeneration. PUVA therapy is contraindicated in pregnant women and young children as well as in individuals with hepatic or renal damage.

Sunlight can also be used instead of an artificial source of UVA (PUVASOL therapy). However, due to variables like time of day, clouds and inadvertent exposure, it is difficult to monitor the exact exposure dose with sunlight. This increases the chances of phototoxicity (sunburn). In spite of this, sunlight remains the cheapest and easily available source of UVA.

Topical PUVA therapy comprises careful application of 0.01 - 0.1% solution of trimethylpsoralen over the affected skin, protecting the surrounding skin with a sunscreen. Ultraviolet exposure is given after 20-30 minutes of application. Avoidance of further exposure is necessary to avoid sunburn. Therapy is repeated every alternate or third day with gradual increase of exposure. A few small patches of vitiligo respond well to topical PUVA therapy over 2-4 months.

Systemic PUVA therapy consists of oral ingestion of trimethylpsoralen or methoxalen 20-30 mg to be followed, after 2 hours, by ultraviolet exposure. It is important to avoid further sun exposure as also to protect eyes with sunglasses (ultraviolet protective glasses). Therapy is repeated on alternate days with a graded increase in UV exposure. Widespread stable vitiligo takes 6 - 12 months to respond to this treatment.

Side Effects of PUVA Therapy

Topical Therapy

1. Photoprotection: It prevents sunburn and Koebner phenomenon, prevents tanning of uninvolved skin and therefore lessens contrast between normal and depigmented skin.
2. Topical potent corticosteroids.
3. Intralesional corticosteroids: (Triamcinolone acetinide) especially for leukotrichia on scalp.

4. Human placental extract.
5. Topical immunomodulators: Such as tacrolimus (0.1%, 0.03%), pimecrolimus or tacrolimus (0.1%) combined with narrow band UVB, three times a week.
6. Calcipotriol: Can be used as monotherapy or combined therapy (sunlight, PUVA, or narrow band UVB, clobetasol).

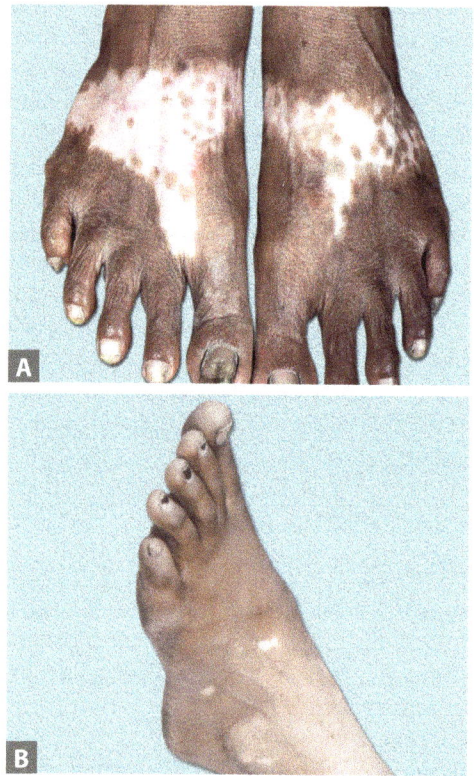

Fig. 13.21A and B: Chemical leukoderma due to plastic and rubber chappals

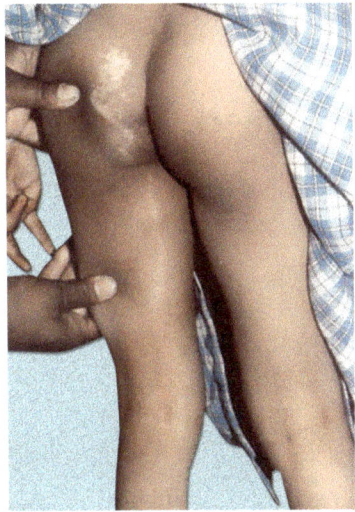

Fig. 13.22: Linear vitiligo extending from thigh to whole legs

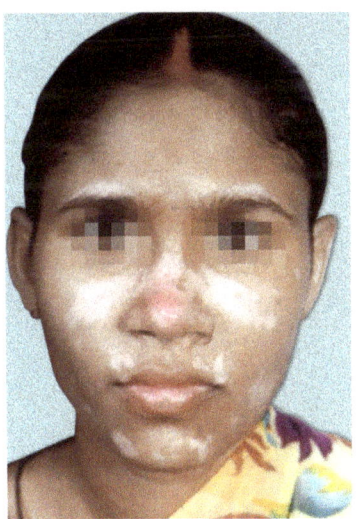

Fig. 13.23: Vitiligo on the face butterfly appearance

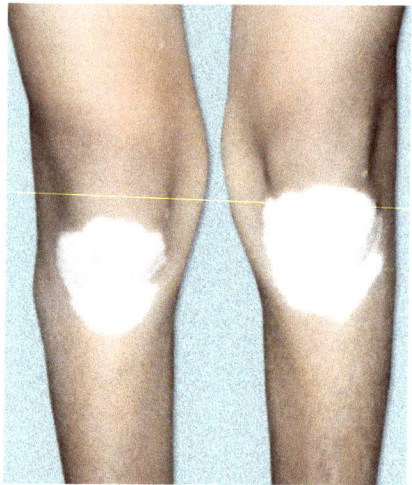

Fig. 13.24: Mirror image on the vitiligo on both the knees

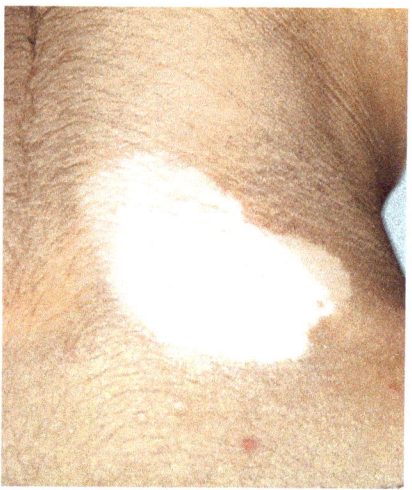

Fig. 13.25: Bichrome vitiligo: Two shade of colors localized patch

Disorders of Pigmentation

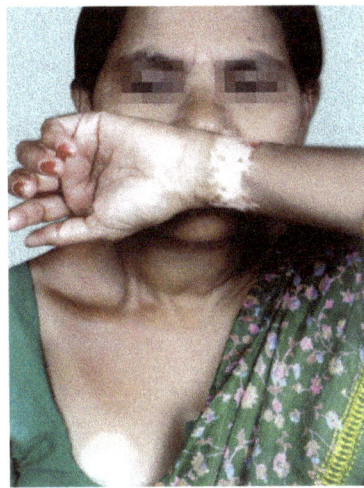

Fig. 13.26: Postchemical leukoderma due to wrist watch strap and on the breast due to pressure on the money purse

7. Topical pseudocatalase + calcium + UVB.
8. Vitix: Formulation containing superoxide dismutase and catalase. It removes hydrogen peroxide from skin, thereby helps in repigmentation.
9. Phenytoin local application: It inhibits release of norepinephrine and activity of monoamine oxidase, inhibits the production of superoxide anion and suppresses cytotoxic T - lymphocyte activity and induce type 2 like cytokine profile.
10. Dead sea climatotherapy in combination with pseudocatalase: Here patients take bath in dead sea for 15 minutes twice daily followed by a shower to wash off salt followed by applications of pseudocatalase cream prior to sun exposure.
11. Topical prostaglandin analogs (PGE2).
12. Cosmetic camouflage where nothing works or when on treatment.

Systemic Therapy

1. Low dose oral corticosteroids—prednisolone 0.3 mg/kg body weight daily.
2. Oral dexamethasone or betamethasone pulse therapy—0.5 mg/every 5 kg body weight for two consecutive days in a week.
3. High dose methylprednisolone pulse therapy 8 mg/kg/day IV over 30 minutes for three consecutive days every 4–8 weeks.
4. Multivitamine therapy (folic acid/vitamin B_{12}/vitamin C).
5. Antioxidants (B-carotene, α-tocopherol, methionine, ubiquinone, vitamin C).
6. Immunomodulates—levamisole 150 mg on two consecutive days every week; cyclophosphamide 50 mg twice daily; cyclosporine 6 mg/kg/day; azathioprine.
7. Quinoline compounds—chloroquine 250 mg/day and hydroxychloroquine 400 mg/day. They can be combined with psoralen therapy.
8. Stem cell therapy.

Oral psoralens may cause nausea and vomiting. Over exposure (phototoxicity) to UVA leads to erythema, edema, vesication, pain and tenderness of the involved skin. Hyperpigmentation of the surrounding normal skin is the most common side effect. In white skinned people, after many months or years of use, skin damage due to UV radiation may lead to solar elastosis, solar keratoses and squamous cell carcinoma. Long-term use is also fraught with the danger of developing cataracts, unless eyes are protected during therapy.

PUVA Therapy in Other Disorders

Systemic PUVA therapy constitutes an important therapeutic option in psoriasis. It is indicated in patients with chronic, stable, plaque type psoriasis involving >25% body surface area that is unresponsive to topical therapy. Oral psoralen tablets are followed up with UVA exposure as in vitiligo, on alternate days.

Topical as well as systemic PUVA therapy has been used successful in unresponsive alopecia areata, especially when whole scalp or whole body is affected. Other disorders in which PUVA therapy is occasionally used are pityriasis rosea, atopic dermatitis, mycosis fungoides and parapsoriasis.

PUVA stands for psoralen with ultraviolet A (320-400 nm) irradiation. Sunlight can be substituted as a source of UVA light (PUVASOL therapy). For localized lesions of vitiligo, psoralens may be administered locally and then followed up with local UVA irradiation (Local PUVA). Systemic PUVA therapy consists of oral psoralens (20-30 mg/dose), followed 2 hours later with UVA irradiation. PUVA therapy is quite effective in inducing pigmentation in vitiligo and causing resolution of psoriasis plaques in cases unresponsive to topical agents. Alopecia areata, parapsoriasis, mycosis fungoides and pityriasis rosea also respond to PUVA therapy. Side effects of PUVA include photoxicity, hyperpigmentation, solar elastosis, cataracts and, in white skinned individuals, squamous cell carcinoma.

Differential diagnosis of a hypopigmented patch includes leprosy, vitiligo, pityriasis alba, pityriasis versicolor and postinflammatory hypopigmentation. Leprosy patches can be distinguished by their atrophy and reduced or absent sensations and sweating as well as enlarged nerves. Biopsy is confirmatory. Vitiligo patches are frequently

Table 13.1: Differential diagnosis of a hypopigmented patch

- Leprosy
- Vitiligo
- Nevus depigmentation
- Pityriasis versicolor
- Postinflammatory hypopigmentation
- Pityriasis alba

depigmented (as against leprosy) but the skin is otherwise normal. Pityriasis versicolor presents as scaly hypopigmented macules and patches on the trunk of young adults. Scaling becomes prominent on scratching the lesions and fungi can be demonstrated under the microscope. Postinflammatory hypopigmentation follows an inflammatory process and lacks scaling. Pityriasis alba affects the face of children as ill defined hypopigmented macules and patches with fine scaling.

A Measurement of the Stigma among Vitiligo and Psoriasis Patients of India

Both psoriasis and vitiligo patients suffered moderate to severe restriction while participating in their domestic and social life. Psoriasis patients faced significantly more restrictions in

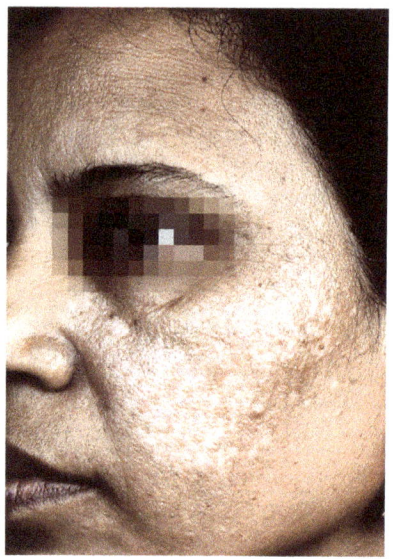

Fig. 13.27: Depigmentation due to application of hydroquinone compound

Disorders of Pigmentation

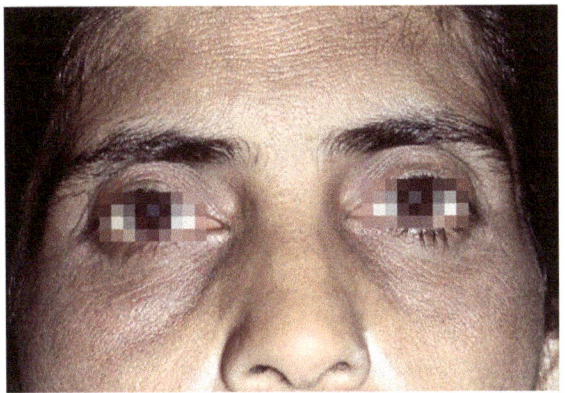

Fig. 13.28: Periorbital melanosis

a number of day-to-day life situations. The Indian population of this study was predominantly dark-skinnned and hypopigmentation as seen in vitiligo is much more noticeable than psoriatic red patches. However, that result show that the component of hypo or hyperpigmentation of the skin was not the only factor leading to participation restrictions.

Table 13.2: Classification of melasma

Type	Features
Epidermal	Light brown, with enhancement of pigmentation under Wood's light. Histologically, it is characterized by a melanin increase in the basel, suprabasel, stratum corneum layers.
Dermal	Ashen or bluish-gray. There is no enhancement of pigmentation under Wood's light. Histologically, there is a preponderance of melanophages in the superficial and deep dermis
Mixed	Dark-brown. Enhancement of pigmentation is present under Wood's light in the some areas and not in the others
Indeterminate	Not apparent under wood's light.

Table 13.3: Mechanism of action of different treatment options

Mechanism of action	Therapy
Tyrosinase inhibitor	Hydroquinone, tretinoin azelaic acid, kojic acid
Nonselective suppression of melanogenesis	Corticosteroids
Inhibition of reactive oxygen species	Azelaic acid
Removal of melanin	Chemical peels
Thermal damage	Laser treatments

Hyperpigmentation

Differential diagnosis of hyperpigmentation

Hyperpigmentation may be due to increased melanin in the epidermis or in the dermis. Epidermal melanin appears brown or brownish black whereas dermal melanin appears blue or bluish black.

Localised:

Epidermal: Melasma—face, during or after pregnancy
Cafe au lait spots – any part of the body.
Freckles—face, in very fair skinned persons.
Junctional melanocytic nevi—palms, soles, genitalia, in children and young adults.
Postinflammatory hyperpigmentation following eczema, dermatophytosis.

Dermal: Mongolian spots—sacrum, back, infants and young children.
Postinflammatory hyperpigmentation following lichen planus, fixed drug eruption.

Combined: Congenital melanocytic nevi—any part, present at birth.
Melanoma—hands and feet, variegated color, slow growing, adults—young or old, nodule may ulcerate.

Disorders of Pigmentation

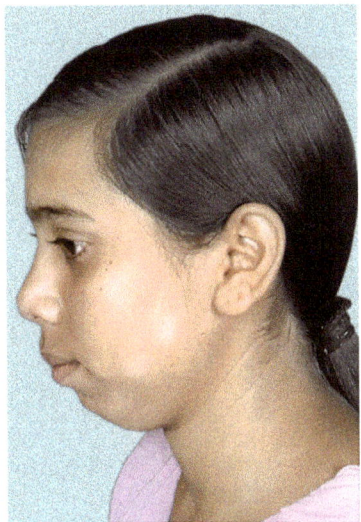

Fig. 13.29: Pityriasis alba

Widespread (involving more than one region):

Epidermal: Cafe au lait spots of neurofibromatosis—presence of more than 5 café au lait spots suggests the diagnosis of neurofibromatosis. Postinflammatory hyperpigmentation following a widespread dermatosis, e.g. psoriasis.

Dermal: Postinflammatory hyperpigmentation following widespread lichen planus, fixed drug druption.

Combined: Giant congenital melanocytic nevus—involves large part of body, present at birth.

Multiple poorly defined hypopigmented, slightly scalp patches can occur on the face of children.

In Caucasians, they may only be visible in the summer when the normal skin tans. In dark-skinned individuals, it is relatively common. It is considered to be a form of post-inflammatory hypopigmentation following mild eczema.

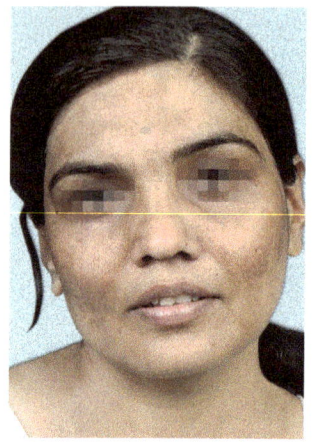 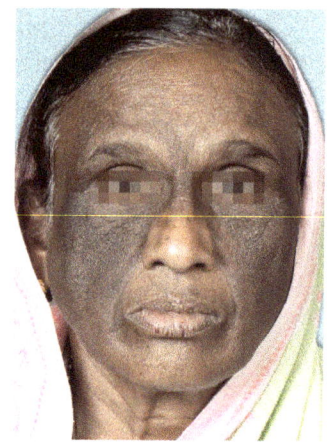

Fig. 13.30: Melasma—hyperpigmentation light brown macules over the cheeks

Fig. 13.31: Hyperpigmentation on the face

Hyperpigmentation of skin may be generalized or localized. It may also be classified as epidermal, dermal or combined. Common causes of hyperpigmentation include melanocytic nevi, cafe au lait spots, mongolian spots, freckles, melasma, postinflammatory hyperpigmentation and the diffuse pigmentation involving sunexposed regions due to suntan or in Addison's disease.

Melasma (Pregnancy Mark)

This is the most common cause of hyperpigmentation of face in women.

Patient Profile

Although most patients are women, men are occasionally affected. Hormonal changes are thought to underlie this disorder which frequently appears in the latter half of pregnancy or postpartum. Oral contraceptives have also been implicated in its causation in some cases.

Morphology

Grouped, well defined, 2-5 mm, light to dark brown macules tend to coalesce in the center resulting in bigger brown patches. Macules remain more or less discrete at the periphery which becomes irregular in outline.

Symmetrical affection of malar regions and nose is typical. Sides of face, forehead and chin are involved in severer cases.

Therapy

Avoidance of sunlight and application of a sunscreen (e.g. amino benzoic acid – PABA) is helpful. Topical application of 2 – 5 % hydroquinone cream over many months leads to lightening of the dark patches. However, complete clearing is exceptional. Chemical peels, claimed to be useful, should be used with caution since they may, by themselves induce hyperpigmentation in some cases.

TREATMENT

Different treatment options are currently available for melasma. Specific treatments include:
1. Pharmacological treatment
2. Chemical peeling
3. Physical treatment.

Various mechanisms of hypopigmenting agents are as follows:
- Destroying or decharacterizing melanocytes.
- Interfering the biosynthesis of melanin and precusor
- Inactivating the biosynthesis of enzyme tyrosinase
- Interfering with the transfer of melanin granule to malpigian cell
- Changing dark color melanin to light color melanin.

These approaches should take in account of the following aspects:
 (i) Synergistic effects of combined therapies
 (ii) Stability of whitening formulation
 (iii) Toxicity and skin penetration; and
 (iv) Definition of markers and targets for evaluating depigmenting properties *in vitro* and *in vivo*.

Pigmentation demarcation lines over the face
A. On the lateral aspect of the upper arm extending over the pectoral areas.

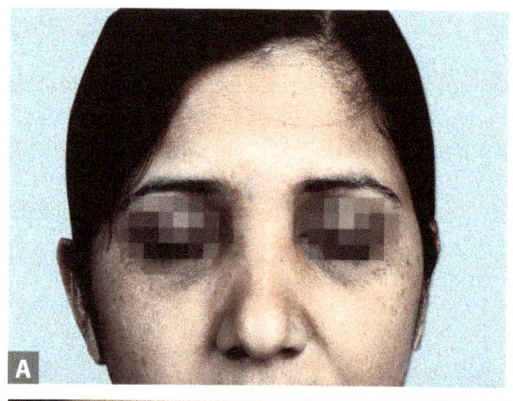

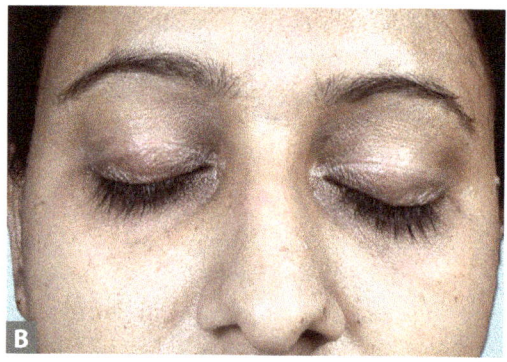

Figs 13.32A and B: Periorbital melanosis

Table 13.4: Summary of hyperpigmentation conditions

Hyperpigmentation disorder	Causative factors	Clinical features	Cellular characteristics	Modular markers modified
Solar lentigines (SL)	Induced by UR - R	Circumscribed, brown to black macules Range from <1 mm to serve l cm Occur in epidermis Found on UV exposed areas of the body, such as the face, dorsum of the hand, extensor forearm, upper back.	Increased melanin production Slight increase in number of melanocyte	Increased TYR-positive cells per length of the dermal/epidermal interface compared with unaffected skin. Keratinocytes potential to produce ET-1 is significantly higher compared with unaffected skin. TNF-alpha is up-regulated in SL lesional epidermis.
Melasma	Exacerbated by sun exposure pregnancy, oral contraceptives, certain antiepileptics, etc.	Symmetric facial hyperpigmentation May invole epidermis dermis or both	Increased melanin production. Normal numbers of melanocytes. Melanocytes are larger, more dendritic.	High level of progesterone, estrogen, and MSH. Increased transcription of genes encoding DCT, TYR.
Solar lentigines (SL)	Develops after resolution of acne, contact dermatitis	Discrete hyperpigmented macules with hazy margins May involve epidermis, dermis or both	Increased melanin production. Normal number of melanocytes.	PGE_2 and PGF_2 alpha synthesis is upregulated. They act as paracrine factors which stimulate melanocyte dendricity. Leukotrienes and thromboxanes may be responsible for the inflammatory hyperpigmentation.

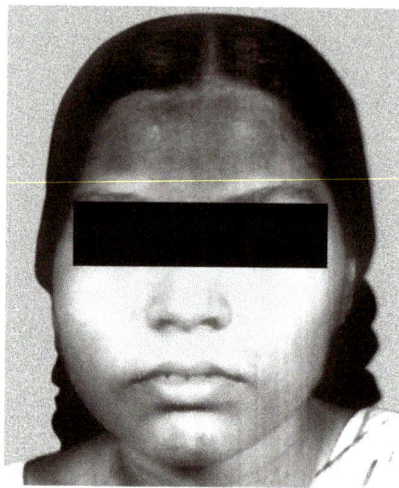

Fig. 13.33: Hyperpigmentation due to constant application of balm on forehead on the complaint of headache

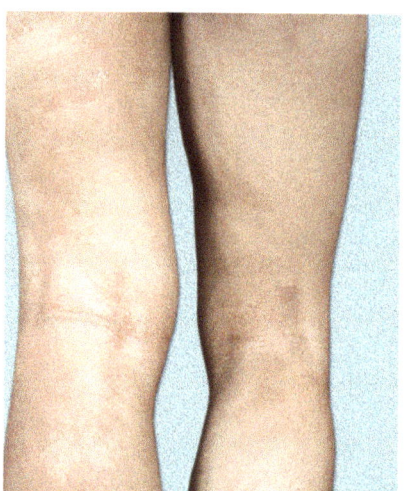

Fig. 13.34: Hyperpigmentation on the back of the legs

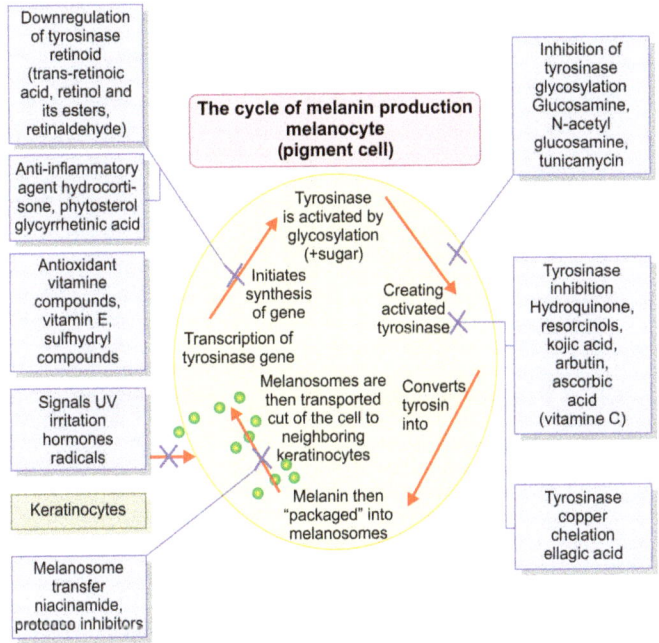

Fig. 13.35: Genomics and proteomics of pigmentation

- B. On the posteromedial portion of the lower limb.
- C. Mediosternal line, a vertical hypopigmented line in the pre and parasternal area,
- D. On the posteromedical area of the spin, and
- E. Bilateral hypopigmented streaks, bands or lanceolate areas over the chest in the zone between the mild-third of the clavicle and the periareolar skin.
- F. 'V' shaped hyperpigmented lines between the malar prominence and the temple.
- G. 'W' shaped hyperpigmented lines between the malar prominence and the temple.
- H. Linear bands of hyperpigmentation from the angle of the mouth to the lateral aspects of the chin.

Table 13.5: Classification of melasma

Type	Normal light	Wood's light	Histology
Epidermal	Light brown	Enhancement of color contrast	Melanin deposition basal and suprabasal layers of epidermis
Dermal	Ashen/bluish gray	No enhancement of color contrast	Melanin-laden macrophages in a pervesicular location fund in superficial and middermis
Mixed	Deep brown	Enhancement of color contrast in some areas, while not in others	Melanin deposition is found in the epidermis and dermis
Wood's light not apparent (in patients with dark skin-skin types V and VI)	Ashen gray or unrecognized	Not evident under Wood's light	Melanin deposition is found in the dermis

Table 13.6: Mechanism of action of various pigmentation control targets and effective agents

Pigmentation control targets and effective agents	
Pigmentation control target	*Effective agent*
Tyrosinase inhibition	Hydroquinone resorcinols, kojic acid, arbutin, ascorbic acid (vitamin C), deoxyarbutin
Tyrosinase copper chelation	Ellagic acid
Inhibition of tyrosinase glycosylation	Glucosamine, N-acetyl glucosmaine, tunicamycin
Melanosome transfer	Niacinamide, protease inhibitors
Downregulation of tyrosinase	Retinoid (trans-retinoic acid, retinol and its esters, retinaldehyde)
Antioxidant	Vitamin C compounds, vitamin E, Sulfhydryl compounds
Antiinflammatory agent	Hydrocortisone, phytosterol, glycyrrhetinic acid.
Increase epidermal turnover	Retinoids, salicyclic acid

Melasma commonly begins in young ladies during pregnancy. Multiple, brown, coalescing macules over cheeks and nose in symetric fashion are characteristic. Avoidance of sunlight, use of a sunscreen and 2–5% hydroquinone, vitamine C, vitamin E helps in improving the pigmentation.

Topical Agents
- Hydroquinone (HQ)
- Isotretinoin (ISOTRET)
- Adapalene (AD)
- Topical corticosteroids (TS)
- Azelaic acid (AA)
- Arbutin
- Melatonin

Flowchart 13.4: Management of melasma

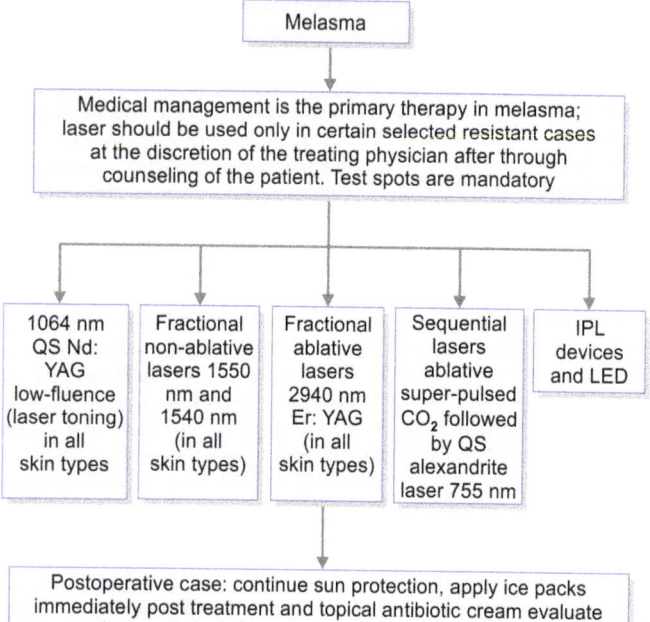

- Kojic acid (KA)
- Licorice extract (Glabridin)
- Glycolic acid (GA)
- Aloesin
- Niacinamide
- Paper mulberry

Classification of Melasma

- Retinol
- Soy extracts
- Vitamin C

- Flavonoid extracts
- Emblica
- Unsaturated fatty acids—oleic acid and linoleic acid extract from Chilean snail—SP helix
- Aspersa Muller
- Tyrostat
- N-acetyl-4-S- cysteaminylphenol
- Liquitrim
- Dioic acid
- Pidobenzone (4%)

Oral Therapy

Pycnogenol: French maritime pine bark extract (Pinus Pinaster) Grape seed extracts proantocyanidins vitamin C.

Chemical Peels

- GA 20–70%
- Trichloroacetic acid TCA-10-25%
- Jessener's peel
- (SA+LA+ resorcinol+ethanol)
- Salicylic acid (SA) 20–30%
- Retinoic acid peel (RA) 1–5%
- KA 2–5%
- Pyruvic acid (50%)
- Combinations
- GA (50%)+KA (10%)
- SA (20%)+mandelic acid (MA)(20%)
- Retinol peel 5%
- SA (20%)+GA (30%)

Laser Treatments

- Pigment specific lasers—Q switched lasers
- Resurfacing laser—CO_2 and Er:YAG

- Fractional laser—nonablative lasers
- (Er: Glass 1550 nm) and ablative lasers(CO_2 and Er:YAG)
- Intense pulse light—IPL
- Combination technique—ablative laser followed by Q switched laser.

Reliability Assessment and Validation of the Melasma Area and Severity Index (MASI) and a New Modified MASI Scoring Method

Melasma area and severity index, the most commonly used outcome measure for melasma, has not been validated. Hence, researchers sought to determine the reliability and validity of the MASI.

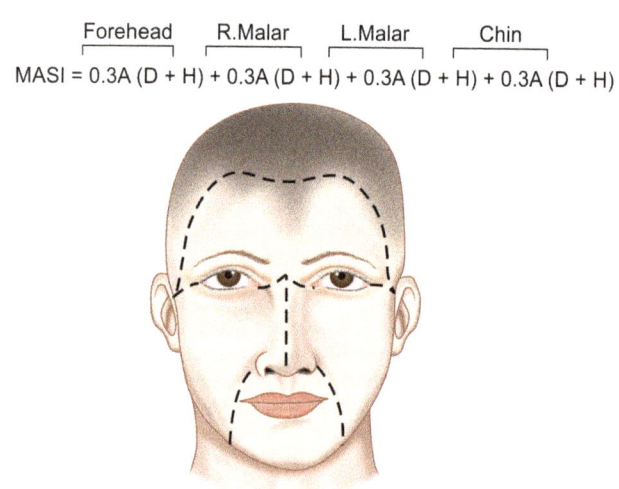

Fig. 13.36: Melasma area and severity index (MASI). A, area; D, darkness, H, homogeneity; L, left, R, right

- 694-nm FRx-QSRL for melasma
- Novel 1927-nm fractional thulium fiber laser for melasma
- All –trans retinoic acid and hydroquinone for epidermal melanosis.

Efficacy and Safety of Tacrolimus Cream 0.1% in the Treatment of Vitiligo

Phototherapy and application of topical corticosteroids are most commonly prescribed. Topical tacrolimus ointment is an effective and well-tolerated alternative therapy for vitiligo especially involving the head and neck. The combination with other therapeutic modalities could result in better response in repigmentation.

The effective role of topical tacrolimus in treatment of vitiligo may relate to its suppression of autoantibody recognition of cell surface melanocyte antigens and inhibition of subsequent cytotoxic T-lymphocyte reactions.

It is immunomodulatory properties and lack of cutaneous side effects seen with topical corticosteroids, tacrolimus is potential therapeutic alternative for vitiligo of the head and neck even in patient with an improved benefit risk ratio.

Impact of vitiligo on the health-related quality of life of 104 adult patients, using dermatology life quality index and stress score: First Egyptian report.

This is the first study to access the health related QOL in adult Egyptian vitiligo patient using both DLQI and SS. It revealed a significant deterioration of their health-related QOL, with younger, female, educated patient with darker skin Prototypes, visible lesions and positive family history being at higher risk. Even in country with limited resources like ours, it is important to recognized and address the psychological issues, as it would ultimately lead to improve health-related QOL and thereby treatment outcomes, due to well-known role played by psychological stress in initiation and progression of vitiligo.

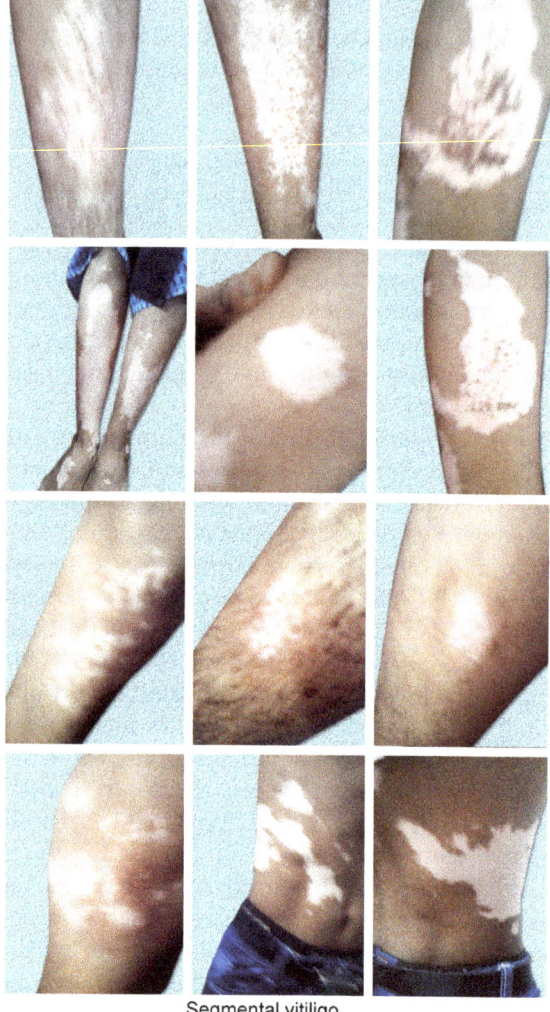

Segmental vitiligo

Fig. 13.37: Vitiligo lesions on the legs (after treatment); vitiligo lesions on the legs showing repigmentation

Disorders of Pigmentation

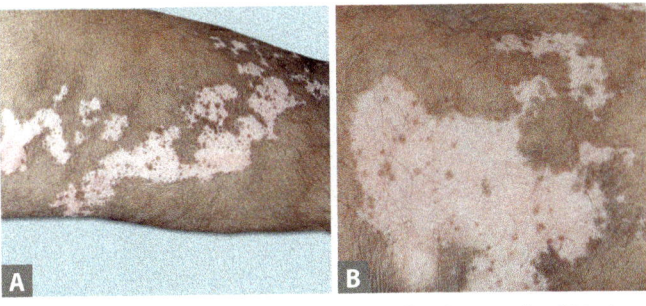

Fig. 13.38A and B: Vitiligo repigmenting showing specks of black pigmentation

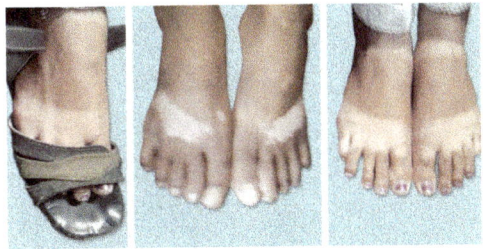

Fig. 13.39: Leukoderma due to chappals

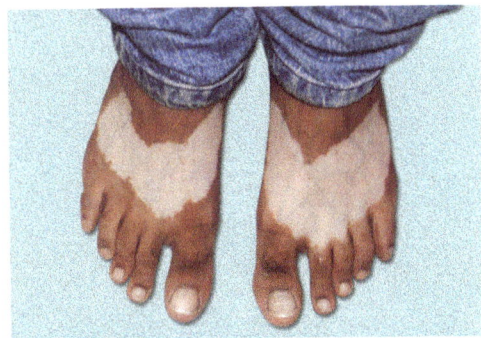

Fig. 13.40: Leukoderma due to plastic chappals

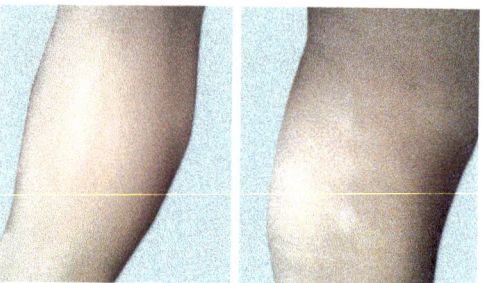

Fig. 13.41: Koeber's phenomon white scratch mark after itching

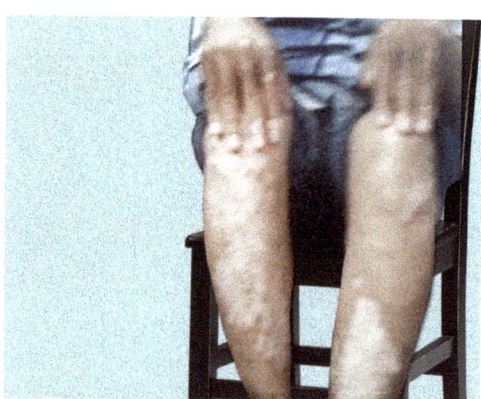

Fig. 13.42: Vitiligo of the legs and hands

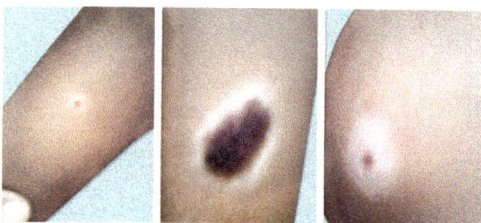

Fig. 13.43: Halo nevus

Disorders of Pigmentation

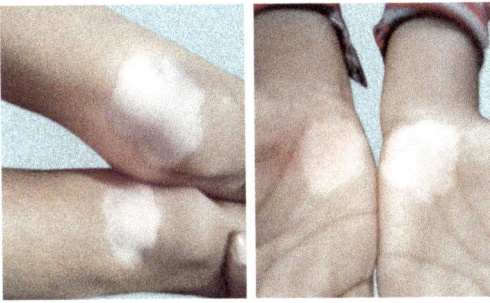

Fig. 13.44: Bilateral mirror image vitiligo

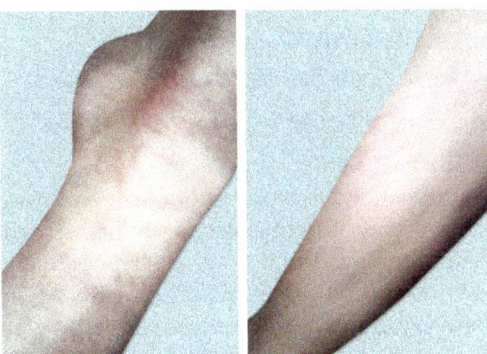

Fig. 13.45: Depigmentation due to hydroquine cream

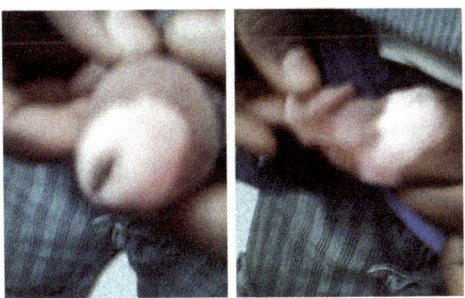

Fig. 13.46: Leukoderma due to rubber condom

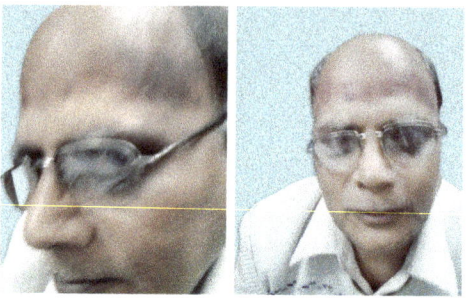

Fig. 13.47: Hyperpigmentation due to vicks-veporub and balm

Low-dose 1064-nm Q-switched Nd: YAG Laser for the Treatment of Melasma

308 nm Excimer Lamp vs laser for Vitiligo

Inflammatory vitiligo

Inflammatory vitiligo is a poorly understood but clinically recognizable syndrome that mimics hypigmented MF. In inflammatory vitiligo, the lesions are hypopigmented and annular, with an etythematous raised rim. When lesion inflametory vitiligo coalesce, they can achieve the size (>5 cm) of an early lesion of MF. These two entities also show several histopathologic similarities, including a dense lyphocytic infiltrate, and a predominance of CD8 T cells. In addition, a loss of melanoctyes can be seen in both vitiligo and hypopigmented MF. If the classic MF areas are involved it can be difficult ti distinguish this entity from early MF. Phototherapy has been used to treat both hypopigmented MF and vitiligo, and can be used to remit the eruption and allow for its reevaluation should it recur.

Disorders of Pigmentation

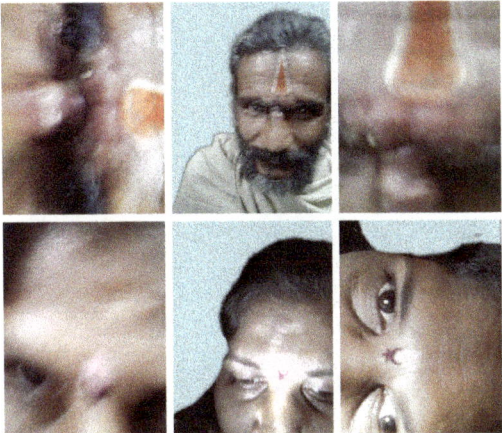

Fig. 13.48: Chemical dermatitis and depigmentation due to Tilak

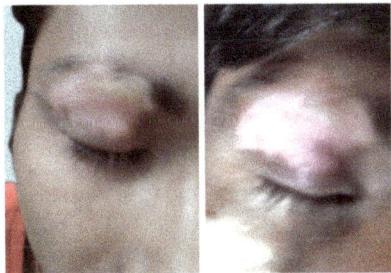

Fig. 13.49: Vitiligo on the upper eyelid

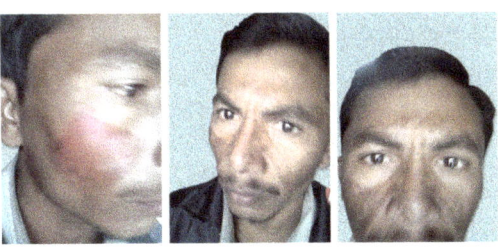

Fig. 13.50: Hyperpigmentation of the face due to application of some Ayurvedic creams

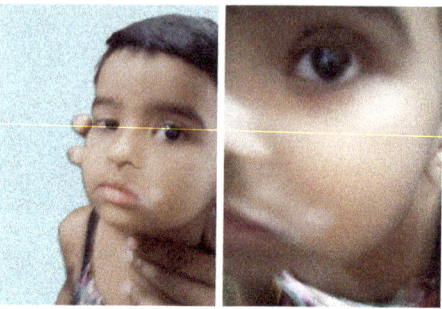

Fig. 13.51: Vitiligo near the angle of mouth

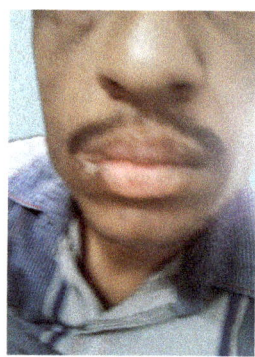

Fig. 13.52: Vitiligo of the lips

Hidradenitis Suppurativa

Clinical Presentation

Key points
- HS most typically occurs in the axillary, inguinal, perianal, perineal, mammary and inframammary regions
- The distribution pattern corresponds with the "milk line" distribution of apocrine-related mammary tissue in mammals
- The most commonly affected side is the axilla
- Perianal HS is associated with more debilitating outcomes.

CHAPTER 14

Drug Reactions

Drug eruptions, erythema, multiforme, Stevens-Johnson syndrome, etc.

COMMON ERUPTIONS DUE TO DRUGS

Fixed drug eruption	: NSAIDs, sulfonamides and tetranamides, phenolphthalein, dapsone
Maculopapular rash	: Ampicillin and other penicillins, NSAIDs, antiepileptics
Urticaria	: INH, glucocorticoids, androgens, iodides and bromides
Erythema multiforme	: Sulfonamides and penicillins, NSAIDs, rifampicin, antiepileptics, sulphones
Photosensitivity	: NSAIDs, tetracyclines and sulfonamides, phenothiazines, thiazides, sulfonylureas

Erythroderma	: Sulfonamides, penicillins, NSAIDs, antiepileptics
Lichen planus like eruption	: Chloroquine, gold, antituberculous drugs, antiepileptics, phenothiazines
Toxic epidermal necrolysis	: NSAIDs, antituberculous drugs, penicillins, antiepileptics, sulfonamides

Machanism Involved in Drug Reactions

1. Pharmacological. 2. Caused by overdosage or failure o excrete or metabolise. 3. Cumulative effects. 4. Altered skin ecology. 5. Allergic. 6. IgE-mediated. 7. Cytotoxic. 8. Immune complex-mediated. 9. Cell-mediated. 10. Idiosyncratic. 11. Exacerbation of pre-existing skin conditions.

Common Drugs that Cause Eruptions

Sulfonamides and cotrimoxazole (fixed drug eruption (FDE), erythema multiforme (EM) and Stevens-Johnson syndromes (SJS), aspirin and other NSAIDs (urticaria, maculopapular eruption, FDE, EM and SJS) and penicillins (urticaria and maculopapular eruption), tetracyclines (fixed drug eruption and photodermatitis), INH and systemic steroids (acneiform eruption), chloroquine, phenothiazines and sulfonylureas (lichenoid eruption and photodermatitis), barbiturates and phenytoin (acneiform eruption, lichenoid eruption and photodermatitis).

Therapy of Drug Eruptions

Withdrawal of the causative or suspected drug/drugs and application of topical steroids suffices for most of the eruptions. Patients with widespread eruptions (exfoliative dermatitis) or severe (blistering fixed drug eruption or erythema multiforme) eruptions frequently need a short course of systemic steroids for rapid resolution.

Stevens-Johnson syndrome and toxic epidermal necrolysis are medical emergencies and their therapy resembles that of extensive superficial burns. Admission to an acute care unit, warm surroundings, restoring water and electrolyte balance (input/output records and serum electrolytes to be monitored), parenteral nutrition are the supportive measures. Administration of parenteral dexamethasone 0.2 – 0.4 mg/kg/day and tapered rapidly within a week prevents progression and initiates healing.

Drug eruptions are uncommon in children. They appear usually within few days or hours of beginning a new drug. They are pruritic. Antibacterials, NSAIDs and antiepileptics are the most common causes of drug eruptions. Minor rashes subside on withdrawl of the concerned drug and applications of topical steroids. Severe (blistering) or extensive (exfoliative dermatitis) rashes need systemic steroids tapered over 1-2 weeks. Stevens-Johnson syndrome and toxic epidermal necrolysis are medical emergencies and the latter needs to be treated like 100% superficial burns.

FIXED DRUG ERUPTION

The peculiarity of this drug eruption is that it affects a particular body site repeatedly with every exposure to a particular drug, i.e. it is fixed to a particular site. This is a common drug eruption in India. Sulfonamides, NSAIDs, tetracyclines, phenolphthalein, barbiturates and phenytoin are common causes.

Fixed drug eruption recurs at the same site at every exposure to the offending drug. Sulfonamides, NSAIDs and phenolphthalein are common causes. Initial lesions are one or many dusky red, circular macules that soon turn bluish black in color. The pigmentation takes many months to fade and hence, patients may present with only pigmented macules or patches that represents inactive lesions. Acral and mucocutaneous junctional regions are commonly affected. Treatment is avoidance of the suspected drug and topical steroids, when lesions are active.

ERYTHEMA MULTIFORME

Erythema multiforme is a hypersensitivity reaction to herpetic, streptococcal, mycobacterial or mycoplasmal infections or to drugs like sulphonamides, NSAIDs, antibiotics, antituberculous agents and antiepileptics. Polymorphous rash includes the characteristic target lesions that comprise a dark center, surrounded by pale and bright red zones of edema and erythema respectively. Acral regions and mucocutaneous junctions are preferred sites. Therapy is symptomatic (other than identifying and treating the cause) except in severe cases when systemic steroids may be used.

STEVENS-JOHNSON SYNDROME

Stevens-Johnson syndrome is similar to erythema multiforme with the following differences. Etiology is similar to erythema multiforme, for the fact that drugs are more commonly implicated. Skin lesions are similar but target lesions are less common, bullae are more common and lesions tend to be concentrated over mucosae and mucocutaneous junctions leading to severe painful mucosal erosions and hemorrhagic crusting. Constitutional disturbance is severe and systemic complications are more common. A short course of high dose sytemic steroids along with supportive therapy in an acute care unit is needed.

TOXIC EPIDERMAL NECROLYSIS

Although etiopathologically related to erythema multiforme, toxic epidermal necrolysis is a life threatening disease due to necrosis of whole body epidermis and mucosal epithelia. Epidermis peels off in large sheets on a backgound of diffuse tender erythema and bullae all over the body. Mucosal lesions resemble Stevens-Johnson syndrome. Nikolsky's sign is positive. Systemic complications are fluid, electrolyte and temperature imbalance and propensity for developing infections. Therapy is similar to that of 100% superficial burns.

MISCELLANEOUS DRUG-INDUCED RASHES

Drug induced urticaria, maculopapular drug eruption, acneiform drug eruption, lichenoid drug eruption, drug induced photosensitivity.

Photosensitive Dermatoses

Photosensitivity (Photosensitive Dermatitis)

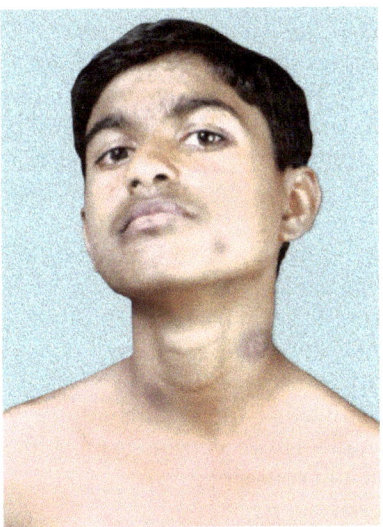

Fig. 14.1: Drug eruptions on the face and neck and around the lips

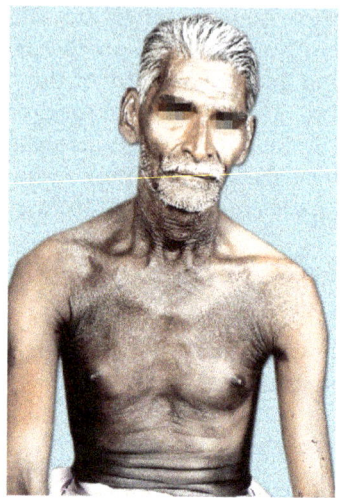

Fig. 14.2: Hyperpigmentation on the chest and abdomen

A state of heightened sensitivity of the skin to ultraviolet and, at times, visible spectrum of light is termed as photosensitivity. Such sensitivity may manifest as:
1. Phototoxicity, i.e. a predisposition to develop an eruption simulating sunburn.
2. Photoallergy, i.e. a delayed type of hypersensitivity (simulating 'eczema').
3. Photosensitivity may also occur as a component of multisystem diseases like:
    a. Pellagra (niacin deficiency)
    b. Systemic lupus erythematosus
    c. Porphyrias (except AIP).
4. Photosensitivity (tendency to sunburn) is a constant accompaniment of skin devoid of melanin as in:
    a. Oculocutaneous albinism
    b. Universal vitiligo
    c. White skin of caucasians
    d. Phenylketonuria.

5. Exacerbation of skin lesions with sunlight is known with:
   a. Rosacea
   b. Psoriasis
   c. Seborrheic dermatitis
   d. Pemphigus and other bullous disorder.
6. Photosensitivity due to unknown cause—polymorphous light eruption.

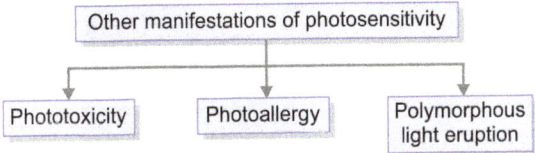

Photosensitive disorders include phototoxicity (induced by systemic or topical agents), photoallergy (systemic or topical agents), tendency to phototosensitivity due to reduced

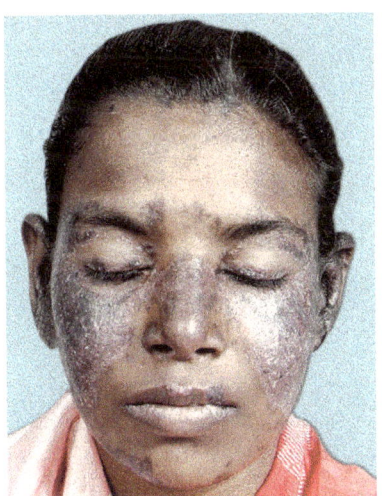

Fig. 14.3: Hyperpigmentation on the face—some drug recations after local applications (some creams)

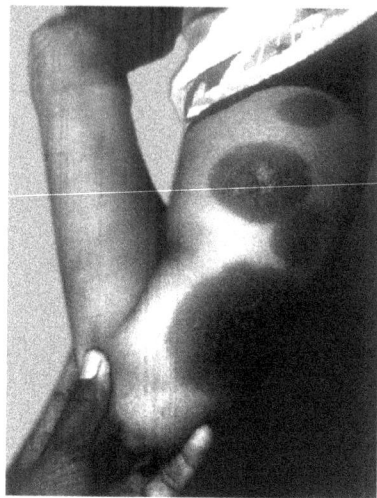

Fig. 14.4: Fixed drugs eruptions on the arm

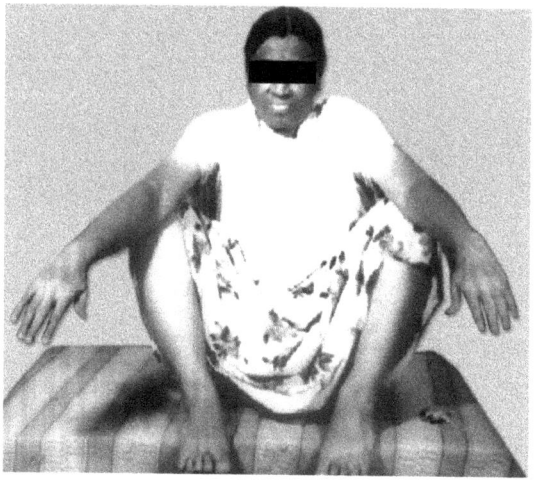

Fig. 14.5: Photosensitivity hyperpigmentation on face and arms

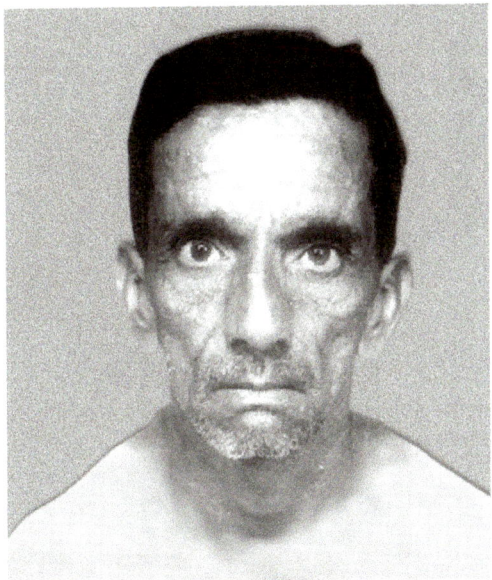

Fig. 14.6: Sun-exposure dermatitis hyperpigmentation on face, neck and chest

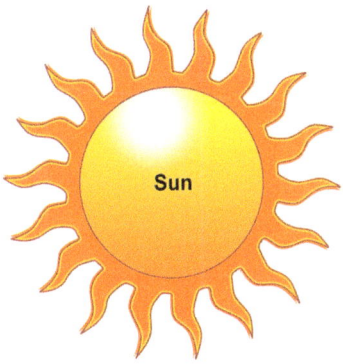

Fig. 14.7: The sun and the skin composition of the sunlight

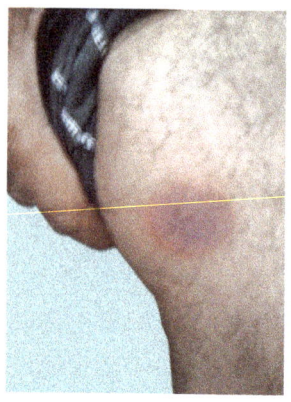 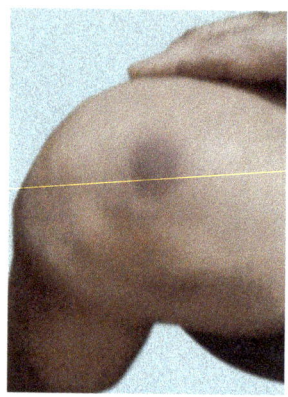

Fig. 14.8: Fixed drug eruption due to pain killers, brufen and combiflam

Fig. 14.9: Fixed drug eruption

Table 14.1

Y rays	X rays	UVC	UVB	UVA	Visible	Infrared
0.001/nm	200/nm	290/nm	320/nm	400/nm	1000/nm	

UV Blockers

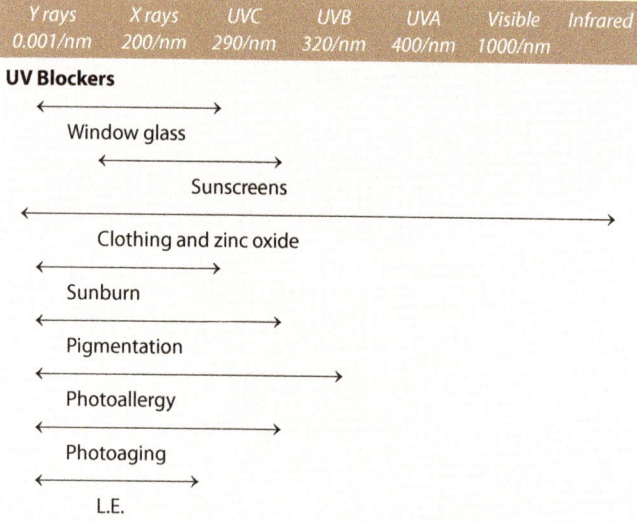

melanin (albinism, vitiligo) or to systemic disease (pellagra, SLE, porphyria) and photosensitivity of unknown cause (polymorphous light eruption).

Distribution of these diseases is restricted to sun-exposed parts of face, neck, chest, hands, forearms and feet. Phototoxicity is a sunburn-like response that occurs following local use of psoralens or certain perfumes. Photoallergy is an immunologically mediated eczematous response to topical (antibacterials, parthenium) or systemic (phenothiazines, sulfonylureas) agents. Polymorphous light eruption is diagnosed by exclusion of other photodermatoses.

Management of Photosensitive Disorders

Identifying an etiologic agent is tough but rewarding. Hence, all patients should be carefully questioned about possible contactants or ingestants. Topical steroids hasten healing. However, eliminating the cause and photoprotection are essential for lasting benefit.

Photoprotection

Topical steroids induce remission in mild cases, but identification and avoidance of a contactant or an ingestant responsible for the rash is crucial for cure. Avoiding sunlight, adequate photo-cover with umbrella, clothes or sunscreens (zinc cream, PABA and its esters) is essential. Moderate to severe cases of polymorphous light eruption need an extended course of chloroquine therapy (250 mg bd) with ophthalmic monitoring, sun screening agents.

CHAPTER 15

Disorders of Hair and Nails

ALOPECIA

Visible hair is the end product of cornification of cells of a skin appendage called the hair follicle. The stucture of a hair follicle is like a cup that gives rise to supports, and shapes the hair shaft. Ordinarily, there are about 1 lac hair on the scalp. Out of these, about 100 are lost every day. This is because the follicles continually pass through the 3 phase cycles of anagen (growth phase), catagen (phase of decay) and telogen (resting phase). When telogen ends, anagen begins, forming a new hair shaft that pushes the old resting shaft out of the follicle.

Classification, Clinical Features, and Management

Cicatricial

Acute Inflammations
Deep pyodermas, herpers zoster, tinea capitis.

Chronic Inflammations
Discoid LE, lichen planus, morphea.

Noncicatricial

Noninflammatory
Diffuse	Telogen effluvium, thyroid disorders, drugs
Patterned	Common baldness
Patchy	Alopecia areata, trichotillomania

Inflammatory — tinea capitis, superficial pyodermas

Scarring and Nonscaring Alopecia

Out of about 1 lac scalp hair, about 100 are lost every day. Hair are formed by hair follicles which continually pass through growth (anagen), catabolic (catagen) and rest (telogen) phases in a cyclical manner.

Loss of hair is termed alopecia. When follicles are destroyed (as judged by absence of follicular openings) the hair loss is said to be scarring and this is irreversible. Scarring alopecia occurs due to deep bacterial, viral or fungal infections, discoid lupus erythematosus and scleroderma. Nonscarring alopecia may be inflammatory (tinea capitis) or noninfammatory which can be localized (alopecia areata) or generalized (androgenetic alopecia, telogen effluvium).

Alopecia Areata

An autoimmune disorder, alopecia areata manifests as patchy loss of hair due to sudden precipitation of a group of contiguous hair follicles into telogen (resting phase). Alopecia areata is an autoimmune disease of hair follicles that affects young adults. It is occasionaly associated with atopy and other autoimmune diseases. Well-defined patches of non-scarring, non-inflammatory hair loss are characteristic. Any part of scalp or body (e.g. beard, moustache) may be affected. Affection of all scalp hair (alopecia totalis) and all body hair (alopecia universalis) carry bad prognosis. More than 50% cases regrow spontaneously. However, as most patients are worried about the condition, topical or intralesional steroid or topical minoxidil are the first line of therapy. Unresponsible cases can be managed with topical or systemic PUVA or topical DNCB. Systemic steroids are best avoided.

Androgenetic Alopecia (Common Baldness)

Therapy for androgenetic alopecia remains suboptimal. Topical minoxidil, 2% solution, to be applied twice a day, after hair washing, stops further hair fall and improves hair thickness. It gives cosmetically acceptable results only in patients who have a majority of hair of a thickness intermediate between vellus and terminal hair. The result takes 6–12 months and is maintained only if minoxidil is continued. Besides, minoxidil is expensive and requires monitoring of response and side effects by an expert.

Oral antiandrogens are contraindicated in men but may be used cyclically in females. Side effects should be explained to the patient and watched for, during the therapy. Surgical options for motivated men include hair transplant (which involves punch grafts of spared occipital hair to frontal and temporal regions) and scalp reduction.

This autosomal dominant trait needs androgens for its expression. The hair gradually become thinner and finally are lost. In males, it progresses in characteristics pattern (forehead – temples – vertex, gradually all regions coalescing till only a fringe of hair is left over the occiput and even this may be lost). In females, it presents as partial diffuse alopecia that rarely leads to bald patches. Topical minoxidil (2% solution) gives good results in selected patients but needs to be continued to maintain the improvement. Surgical options like hair transplant and scalp reduction are available for motivated patients. Biotin and finasteride are commonly used now.

Telogen Effluvium

Sudden precipitation of anagen follicles into telogen by major stresses (e.g. persistent high fever, difficult labor, major trauma) leads to loss of these telegen hair (10–20% of scalp hair) about 2–4 months after the stressful event. Hair grow back spontaneously.

Therapeutic Strategies

1. Gene therapy? (currently not available)
2. Modifiers of androgen metabolism: finasteride (available for men)

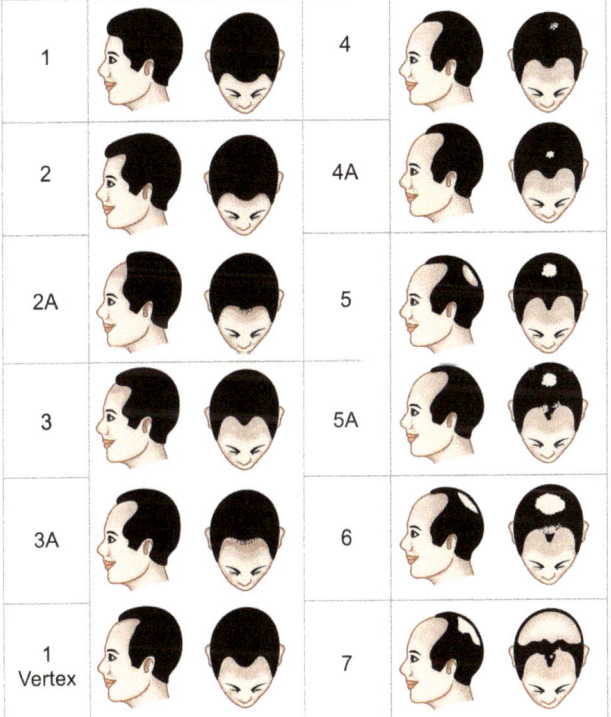

Fig. 15.1: Hamilton-Norwood scale of male pattern baldness

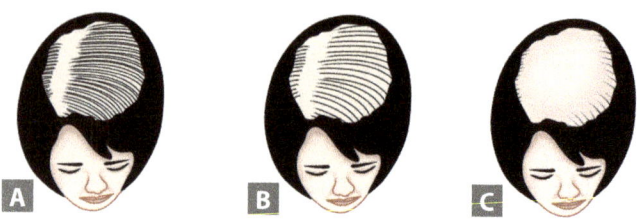

Fig. 15.2A to C: Ludwig classification for female pattern hair loss

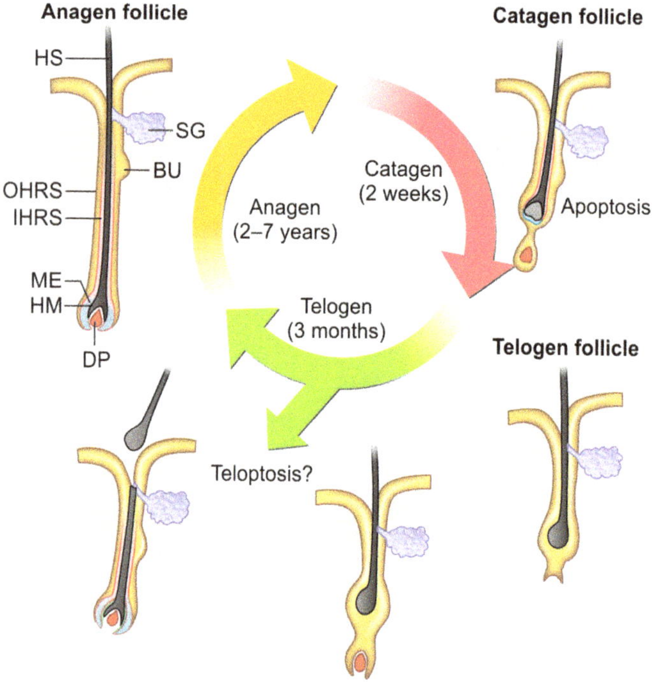

Fig. 15.3: Hair cycle

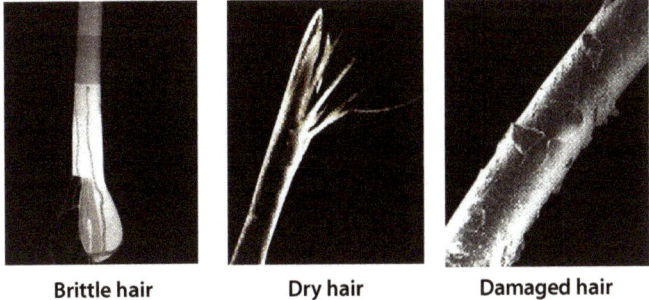

Brittle hair **Dry hair** **Damaged hair**

Fig. 15.4: Types of hair changes

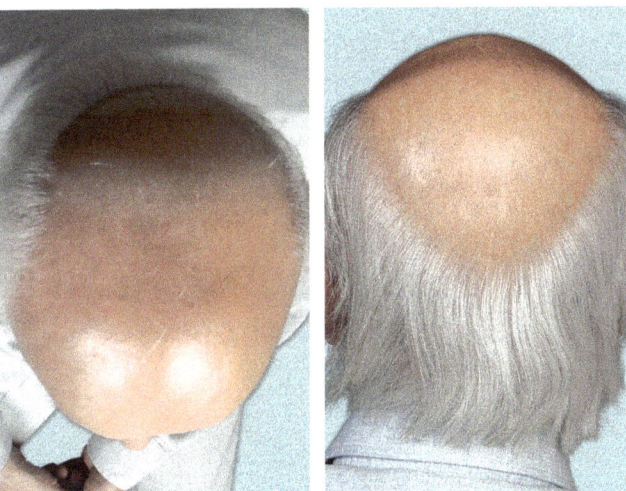

Fig. 15.5: Male pattern hair loss: front axial view

Fig. 15.6: Male pattern hair loss: back view

3. Antimicrobial shampoos?
4. Antiandrogens: cyproterone acetate (available for women).
5. Hair growth promoters: minoxidil (avaiable for men and for women).

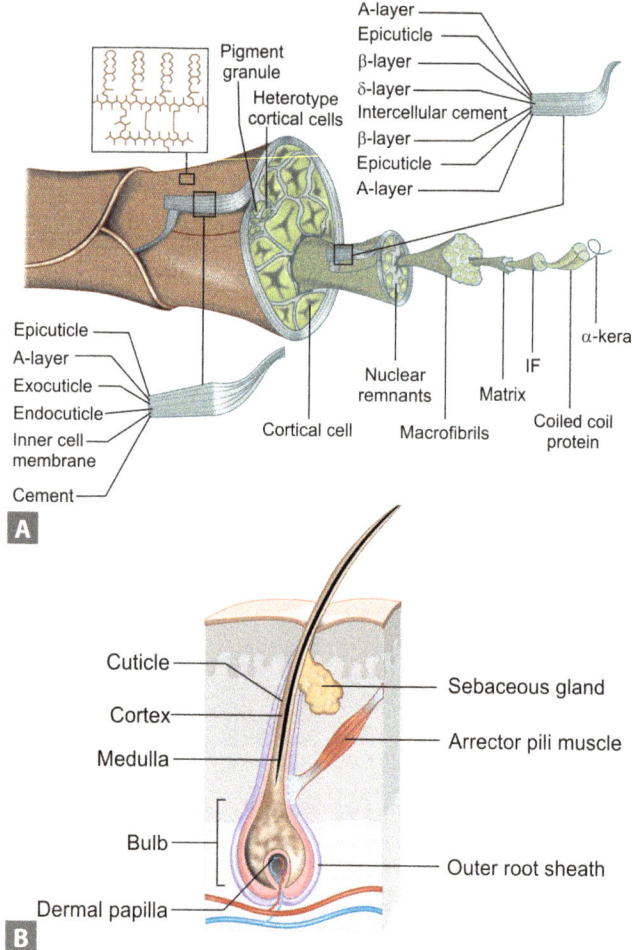

Figs 15.7A and B: Structure of human hair

6. Antiinflammatory agents?
7. Apoptosis modulating agents?

8. Hair transplantation (available), implantation of dermal papilla or cells of follicle dermal-sheath (impending)
9. Hair wigs.

Phototrichogram Analysis

Phototrichogram analysis of normal scalp hair characteristics in Asian populations is not well characterized. The mean hair density, hair thickness, and the white hair percentages were not significantly different between genders at any scalp site. The mean hair density and thickness may significantly different according to scalp sites. Hair density declined with age, especially at the peak between the top and back. Males and females showed different patterns of aging in hair density. Hair thickness changed little with age. Mean hair thickness generally tended to increase until the 20s, reach a plateau between the 20s and 50s, and decrease after the 50s. The mean white hair percentages were $1.84 \pm 4.24\%$ in males and $1.66 \pm 4.21\%$ in females. The mean white hair percentages were significantly increased in subjects over 40 years of age.

Hirsutism

Hirsutism is present in women of terminal hair in the distribution of a man.

Etiology of hirsutism

Racial　　Familial　　Hormonal　　Idiopathic

Ovarian causes
  Menopause
  Polycystic ovaries
  Arrhenoblastoma

Adrenal causes
  Cushing's syndrome
  Virilising tumors
  Adrenogenital syndrome

Flowchart 15.1: Androgenetic alopecia: pathogenic mechanisms

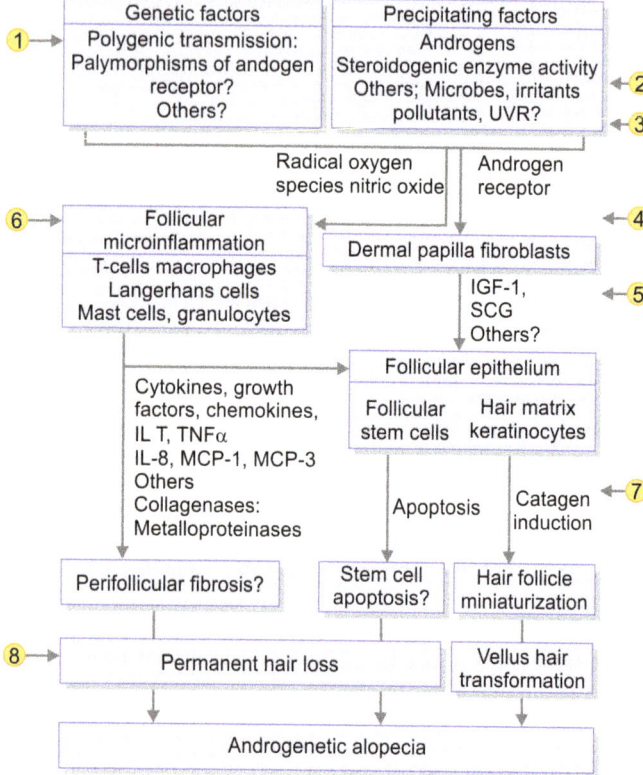

Pituitary causes
  Acromegaly
  Hyperprolactinemia

Iatrogenic
  Anabolic steroids
  Progesterones
  Adrenogenital syndrome.

Treatment

Underlying disorder must be treated.

HYPERTRICHOSIS

Hypertrichosis is an excessive growth of terminal hairs but once which does not follow an androgen-induced pattern.

Table 15.1: Causes of hypertrichosis

Localized	Generalized
Spina bifida	Hypertrichosis lanuginosa (congenital, acquired)
Melanocytic nevi	Drugs (minoxidil, corticosteroids, androgens, psoralens, phenytoin)
post-inflammatory	Hepatic porphyrias
	Some rare syndromes

NAILS

The common causes of nail disorders are as follows:
1. Congenital
2. Systemic diseases
3. Skin diseases
4. Occupation
5. Traumata
6. Vascular and neurogenic disorders
7. Infections
8. Nutritional
9. Psychogenic
10. Drugs
11. New growths

Chemical matricectomy for the treatment of ingrowing toenail

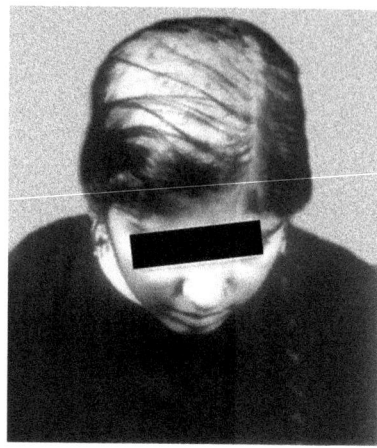

Fig. 15.8: Perifolliculitis decalvans—scarring alopecia with folliculitis

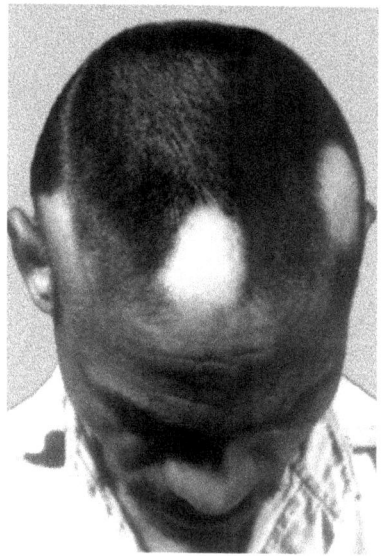

Fig. 15.9: Alopecia areata—rounded bald smooth patches over the scalp

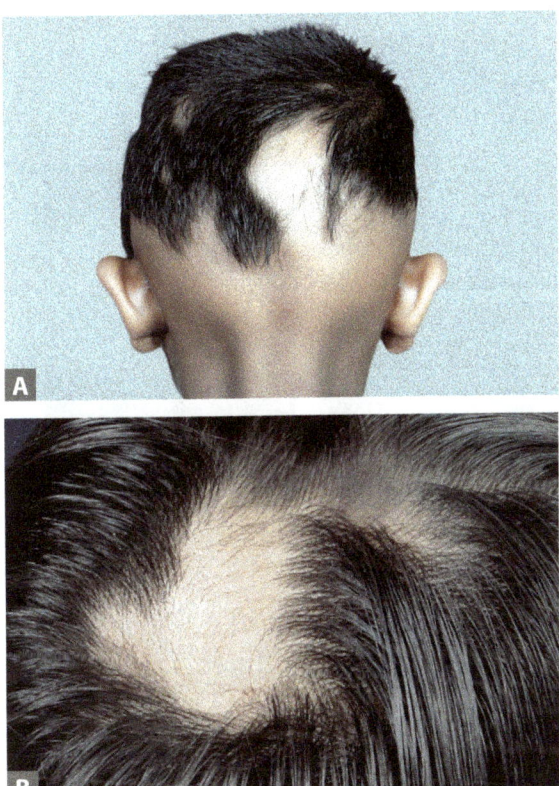

Figs 15.10A and B: Alopecia areata—see the presence of exclamation mark on back view

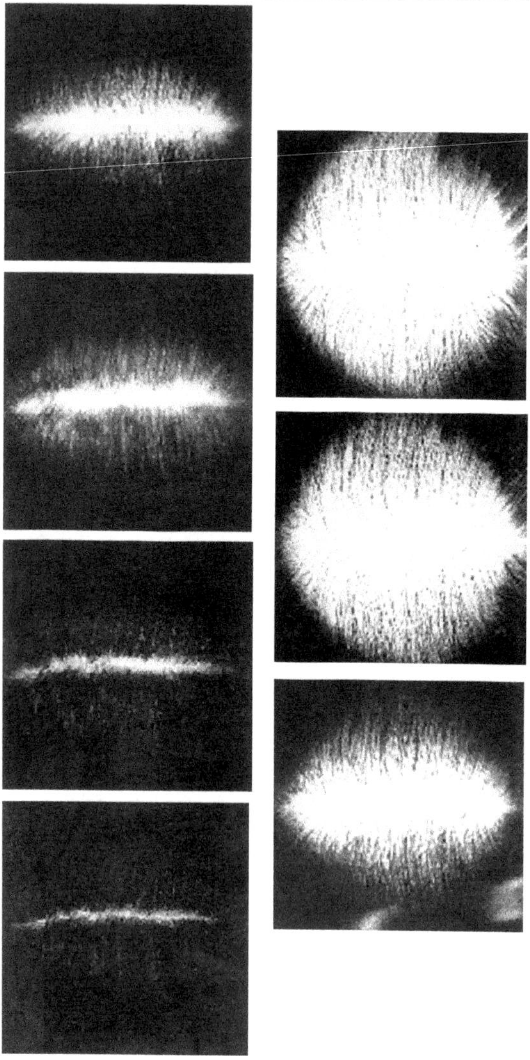

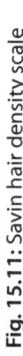

Fig. 15.11: Savin hair density scale

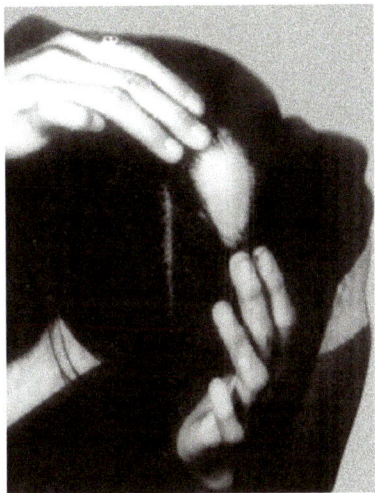

Fig. 15.12: Alopecia areata—see the sign of exclamation

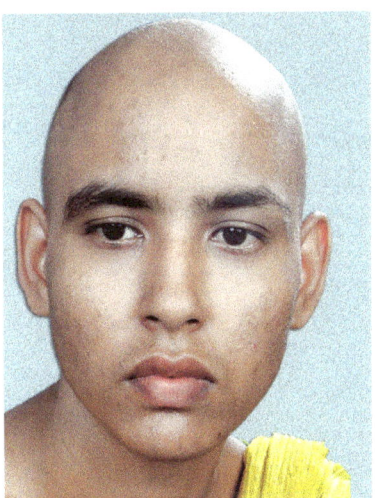

Fig. 15.13: Alopecia areata affecting scalp and face almost going for alopecia areata totalis

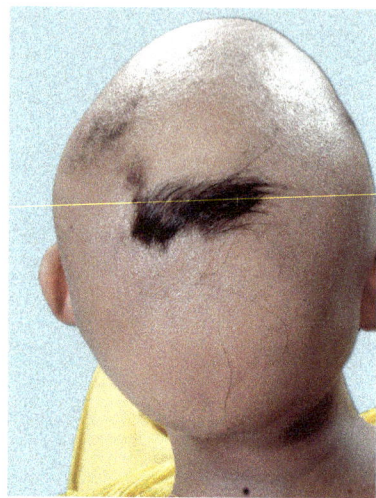

Fig. 15.14: Alopecia areata affecting scalp: back view—only a tuft of hair remaining

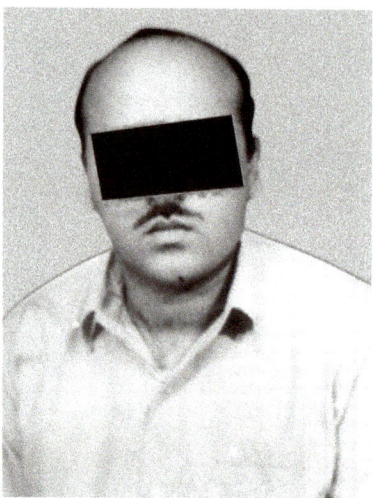

Fig. 15.15: Male pattern baldness see the "M" sign

Disorders of Hair and Nails

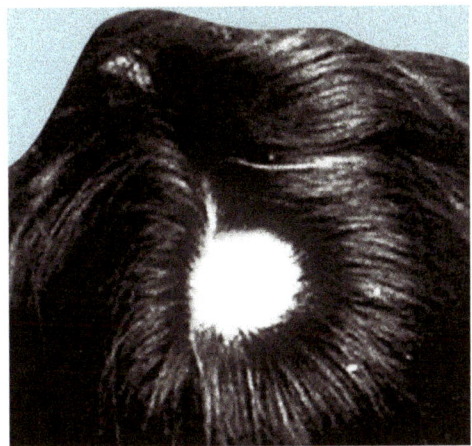

Fig. 15.16: Alopecia areata—see the round coin typed lesion, also see the scald and knits

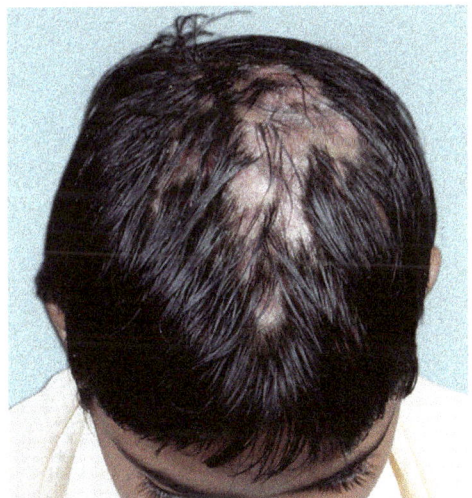

Fig. 15.17: Perifolliculitis decalvans—scarring alopecia with folliculitis

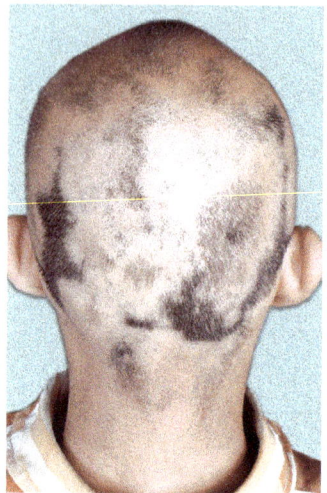

Fig. 15.18: Alopecia areata: back view

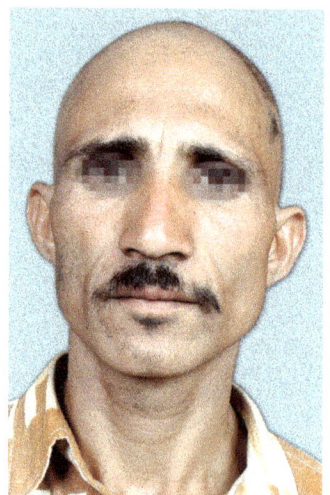

Fig. 15.19: Alopecia areata—scalp, beard and moustache: Patchy hair loss

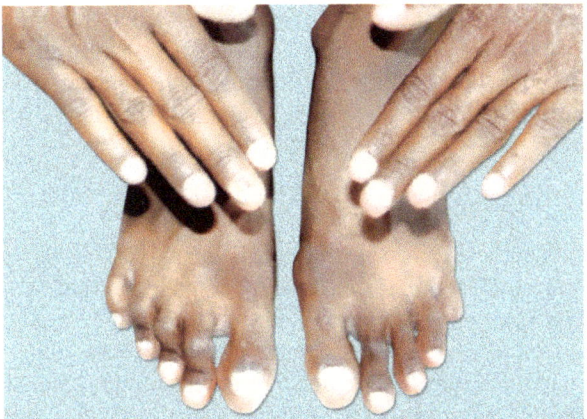

Fig. 15.20: Couping of nails in nutritional deficiency anemia

Most of these causes act on either of the following sites:
1. Posterior nailfold
2. Matrix.

Management of Chronic Paronychia

Chronic paronychia is an inflammatory disorder of the nail folds of a toe or finger presenting as redness, tenderness, and swelling. It is recalcitrant dermatoses seen commonly in housewives and housemaids. It is a multifactorial inflammatory reaction of the proximal nailfold to irritants and allergens. Repeated bouts of inflammation lead to fibrosis of proximal nail fold with poor generation of cuticle, which in turn exposes the nail further to irritants and allergens. Thus, general preventive measures form cornerstone of the therapy. Though previously antifungals were the mainstay of therapy, topical steroid creams have been found to be more effective in the treatment of chronic paronychia. In recalcitrant cases, surgical treatment may be resorted to, which includes en bloc excision of the proximal nailfold or an eponychial marsupialization, with or without nail plate removal. Newer therapies and surgical modalities are being employed in the management of chronic paronychia.

Etiology

It has a complex pathogenesis and is caused by multifactorial damage to the cuticle, thereby exposing the nailfold and the nail groove. Previously, it was believed that chronic paronychia is caused by *Candida*. However, recent data reveal that it is a form of hand dermatitis caused by environmental exposure. *Candida* is often isolated; however, in many cases, *Candida* disappears when the physiologic barrier is restored. Hence, the recent view holds that chronic paronychia is not a mycotic disease but an eczematous condition with a multifactorial etiology. For this reason, topical and systemic steroids may be used successfully, whereas systemic antifungals are of little value. Tosti et al. discovered that topical steroids were more effective than systemic antifungals in the treatment of chronic paronychia. Although *Candida* was frequently isolated from the PNF of their patients with chronic paronychia, *Candida* eradication was not associated with clinical cure in most patients.

In a study conducted by Rigopoulos D et al., tacrolimus 1% ointment and betamethasone 17-valerate cream was found to be more effective in patients of chronic paronychia than just emollient application, confirming allergens and irritants have indeed an important contribution to the pathogenesis of chronic paronychia.

Chronic paronychia commonly afflicts house and office cleaners, laundry workers, food handlers, cooks, dishwashers, bartenders, chefs, nurses, swimmers, diabetes, and patients on HIV-ART. Hypersensitivity to foodstuff is responsible for an increased incidence in food handlers.

There are many rare causes of chronic paronychia, which should always be kept in mind and some of which include the following:

- Infections (bacterial, mycobacterial, or viral)
- Raynaud's disease
- Metastatic cancer, subungual melanoma, squamous cell carcinoma. Benign and malignant neoplasms should always be excluded when chronic paronychia does not respond to conventional treatment
- Papulosquamous disorders like psoriasis, vesicobullous disorders-pemphigus
- Drug toxicity from medications such as retinoids, epidermal growth factor-receptor inhibitors (cetuximab), and protease inhibitors. Indinavir- induces retinoid-like effects and remains the most frequent cause of chronic paronychia in patients with HIV disease. Retinoids also induce chronic paronychia. The mechanism can be -nail fragility and minor trauma by small nail fragments.[10] Paronychia has also been reported in patients taking cetuximab (Erbitux), an antiepidermal growth factor-receptor (EGFR) antibody used in the treatment of solid tumors.

Differential Diagnosis

The differential diagnosis of chronic paronychia includes squamous cell carcinoma of the nail, malignant melanoma, metastases from malignant tumors. The clinician should consider the possibility of the carcinoma when a chronic inflammatory process is unresponsive to treatment. Any suspicion for the aforementioned entities should prompt biopsy.

Flowchart 15.2: Pathogenesis of chronic paronychia

```
┌─────────────────┐      ┌─────────────────┐      ┌─────────────────┐
│ Multifactorial  │      │    Loss of an   │      │    Infective    │
│    etiology     │      │     effective   │      │    organisms    │
│contact irritants/│─────▶│   seal leads to a│────▶│  and irritants  │
│ allergens are a │      │    persistent   │      │     within      │
│ common factor + │      │   retention of  │      │   the grooves,  │
│ physical trauma │      │     moisture    │      │ exacerbating the│
│  to the cuticle │      │                 │      │  acute flare-ups│
└────────┬────────┘      └─────────────────┘      └────────┬────────┘
         │                        ▲                        │
         ▼                        │                        ▼
┌─────────────────┐      ┌─────────────────┐      ┌─────────────────┐
│ Disrupt the seal│      │ Nailfolds round │      │   This vicious  │
│  between the    │      │ up and retract  │      │    cycle goes   │
│  nail plate and │      │ thereby exposing│      │  on compromising│
│ PNF allowing    │      │    the nail     │      │  the ability to │
│   substances/   │      │  grooves further│      │   regenerate the│
│   organisms to  │      │                 │      │     cuticle     │
│     cause       │      │                 │      │                 │
│  inflammations  │      │                 │      │                 │
└────────┬────────┘      └─────────────────┘      └────────┬────────┘
         │                        ▲                        │
         ▼                        │                        ▼
┌─────────────────┐      ┌─────────────────┐      ┌─────────────────┐
│   Secondary     │      │ Repeated bouts  │      │  The inflamed and│
│ colonization    │      │ of inflammation │      │   fibrosed PNF  │
│ with Candida    │─────▶│   leading of    │      │  progressively  │
│  albicans and/or│      │persistent edema,│      │    loses its    │
│ bacteria occurs;│      │    induration,  │      │  vascular supply│
│   episodes of   │      │   and fibrosis  │      │                 │
│  painful acute  │      │   of PNF, LNF   │      │                 │
│  inflammation   │      │                 │      │                 │
└─────────────────┘      └─────────────────┘      └─────────────────┘
```

Trichotillomania

Trichotillomania is characterized by the repeated urge to pull out hair, leading to noticeable hair loss, distress, and social or functional impairment. Most of the cases present initially to dermatologists with complaints of loss of hair and is often confused with other dermatological conditions like alopecia areata, tinea capitis, traction alopecia, and loose anagen syndrome. It is a chronic condition and difficult to treat.

Value of Trichoscopy Versus Trichogram for Diagnosis of Female Androgenetic Alopecia

Female androgenetic alopecia (FAGA) is a frequent cause of hair loss in women. Standard diagnostic methods are clinical inspection, pull test, and trichogram. It has been suggested that scalp dermoscopy (trichoscopy) revealing diversity of hair shaft diameter >20% is diagnostic of FAGA. Trichoscopy is a valuable and superior method to the trichogram for diagnosis of FAGA, especially in early cases, with the highest yield irrespective of the suggested cut-off of 20% diversity of hair shaft.

Phototrichogram Analysis of Normal Scalp Hair Characteristics with Aging

The mean white hair percentages were 1.84 ± 4.24% in males and 1.66 ± 4.21% in females. The mean white hair percentages were significantly increased in subjects over 40 years of age.

Increasing Hair loss and Scalp Disorders due to Pollution

There is a worldwide awareness on respiratory disease, sinus problem, allergies and lung cancers caused by air pollution. The skin and hair are exposed more directly to the surrounding environment forming the first barrier organ which responds to environmental damage. Though the gaseous contaminants and fine particles can enter the lung, all these plus the large particles, dust and heavy metals can affect the skin and hair.

The pollution levels also increase oxidative stress on the hair follicle cells, leading to increased hair shedding similar to the mechanism demonstrated by Philpott in persons suffering from the androgenic alopecia. The article is in press, to be published in the latest issue of Journal of Investigative Dermatology.

- Black woman's Hair loss Tied to braiding, Weaving.
- Therapeutic effect of Gelatin as a dietary supplement for female hair loss.
- Effect of arginine on human dermal papilla cells.
- Arginine could simulate the proliferation of DPC, wchich may be attribute to the effect of simulating the expressions of VEGF, FGF, and ER and inhibiting the expression of AR and SRD5A.
- Significant improvement of diffuse telogen effluvium with an oral fixed combination therapy- A meta-analysis.
- The treatment with a fixed oral combination containing medicinal yeast, l-cystine and pantothenic acid (Pantoger) has been investigated in several clinical studies.
- A fixed combination therapy of atleast 3 months with medical yeast, l-cystine and pantothenic acid can be recommended to patients with diffuse telogen effluvium
- The role of 5-hydroxytryptophan for chronic telogen effluvium treatment in women
- The significant reduction of hair loss observed by TrichoScan in patient who were taking 5-HTP, compared to women who use the placebo. The patient who took the 5-HTP reported mood improvement as well as significant reduction in anxiety.

A Descriptive Study of Alopecia Patterns and their Relation to Thyroid Dysfunction

It is well established fact that dysfunction of thyroid gland is associated with alopecia. Although there are many studies relating to thyroid and hair loss they are all based on a univariante analysis.

The most common was diffuse alopecia and thyroid dysfunction were urticaria (62.5%), vitiligo (50%), acanthosis nigricans (43%), premature graying (25%), hirsutism (27%), psoriasis (27%), seborrheic dermatitis (25%), ichthyosis (18%).

Hair and Scalp Evaluation by Trichoscopy in Female Patient with Thyroid Insufficiency

In patient with thyroid insufficiency the number of hairs per pilosebaceous unit was decreased but the most specific feature was presence of diffuse avascular areas.

Comparison of clinical efficiency between compound betamethasone injection (Diprospan) and triamcinolone acetonide injection in alopecia areata: A single center registry.

Compound betamethasone injection was efficacy and safety in treating alopecia areata, moreover it was suitable for mild and modrate patients.

The hair growth promotes effect of adiponectin *in vitro*.

The first is based on the hypothesis that spreading alopecia due to domino effect, i.e. affected follicles produce mediator(s), which then diffuse again to nearby follicles. The second is based on the idea that catagen-inducing mediator (s) can be produced everywhere within skin.

Senescence of Male Balding Dermal Papilla Cells is Associated with Oxidative Stress

Some researchers demonstrate that 2% O_2 appears to abrogate the negative effects of TGF-beta on cell growth, indicating a possible crosstalk between growth factors and celluar redox state. These data may therefore identify novel mechanisms by which hair follicle miniaturisation may occur in androgenetic alopecia.

Role of Estrogen Receptors in the Modulation of Hair Growth

ER signalling operate as a regulator of apoptosis in human anagen HFs, and further exploration of the mechanism if its action may result in potential application of selective

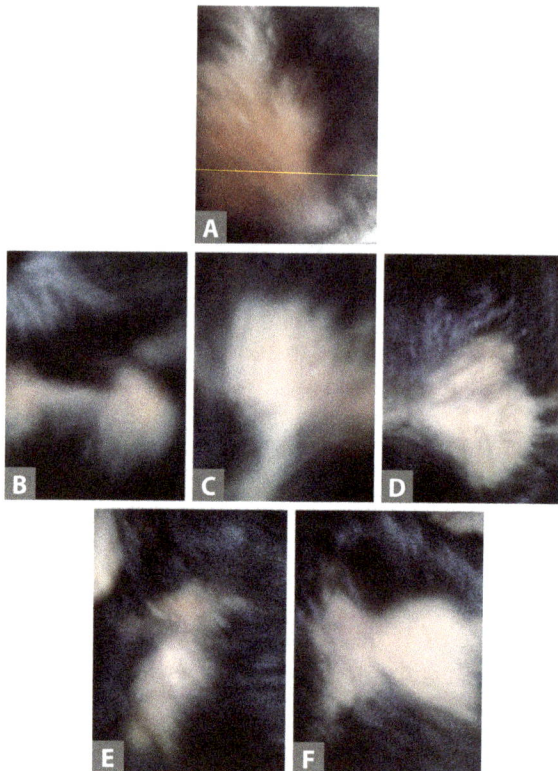

Figs 15.21A to F: Alopecia areata

estrogenists for the treatment of several hair growth abnormalities in clinical practice.

Optimization of Cell Construct Grafting Procedure for Hair Regeneration Therapy

Direct contact of epithelial and dermal components and better oxygenation (vascularity) are crucial for hair regeneration. HVS method is an effective transplantation method of a cultured DPC construct and easily applicable in the clinical setting due to its minimal invasiveness and no need of preparation of epithelial cells.

Modulation of Hair Growth Markers in Hair Follicle

Yeast extract included as increase in keratin 14 and 17 in the outer root sheath (ORS).CD34 staining around the blood vessels was increased whilst collagen IV staining of the basement membrane was more intense compared to the control. It is to be important for the strength and health of the hair fillcle. The corn extract causes an increase in beta-1 integrin, P63 and ki67 in the ORS of the treated human scalp skin grafts. Laminin-5(basement membrane) and fibronectin(dermal sheath) expression were also increase by the corn extract compared to the control. If the corn extract has stimulating effect on the hair growth, human scalp skin grafts were treated with PBS or corn extract(3%) daily for 21 days, Compared to PBS, Extract enhance hair shaft elongation after 14 and 17 days of treatment.

CHAPTER 16

Skin and Internal Disease

Skin manifestations of internal diseases—
Skin is said to be a mirror of health of the internal systems of the body.
1. Brain and spinal cord diseases
2. Cardiovascular system
3. Endocrine diseases
4. Gastrointestinal diseases

In addition to the various body systems like the cardiovascular, CNS, renal, hematologic, joints, gastro-intestinal systems, the skin examination provides valuable clues to the diagnosis of underlying malignancies, nutritional deficiencies, metabolic diseases, infections and autoimmune diseases like systemic lupus erythematosus.
A. Collagen vascular diseases
B. Vesiculobullous disorders of the skin
C. Nutritional deficiencies
D. Erythema nodosum, erythroderma.

SKIN MANIFESTATIONS OF COLLAGEN VASCULAR DISEASES

Collagen vascular diseases (sometimes referred to as collagen diseases or connective tissue diseases) are a group of multisystem autoimmune diseases that affect connective tissue, amongst other tissues. They include lupus erythematosus, scleroderma, dermatomyositis, rheumatoid arthritis, rheumatic fever and Sjogren's syndrome.

LUPUS ERYTHEMATOSUS (LE)

This may present as a multisystem disorder with affection of the skin and mucosa (systemic LE) or be restricted to the skin alone (chronic cutaneous LE). Please see section on systemic LE for details of skin lesions. In chronic cutaneous LE only discoid lesions occur over sunexposed regions of face, neck and scalp.

SCLERODERMA

Systemic sclerosis is seen as diffuse sclerosis of skin predominatly affecting the acral regions, i.e. hands, feet, fingers, toes and face. Other systemic affections include:
1. Raynaud's phenomenon
2. Pulmonary fibrosis
3. Gastrointestinal dysmotility
4. Glomerular sclerosis.

Calcinosis cutis, Raynaud's phenomenon, esophageal dysmotility, cutaneous sclerosis and skin telangiectasia occur together in the CREST syndome, which has better prognosis.

Localized scleroderma (morphea) presents as a rounded or linear indurated dyspigmented plaque with or without atrophy. Affected skin is sclerosed.
1. Dermatomyositis
2. Rhematoid arthritis
3. Rheumatic fever
4. Sjogren's syndrome.

Lupus erythematosus manifests on skin as discoid lesions, butterfly rash, oral ulcers, photosensitivity, alopecia and Raynaud's phenomenon. Localized scleroderma is seen as an indurated plaque with atrophy. Skin findings in sytemic sclerosis include diffuse or acral skin sclerosis, Raynaud's phenomenon, telangiectasia, dyspigmentation, cutaneous calcinosis and fignertip ulcers and scars. Violaceous lid edema and lichenoid papules on hands are manifestations of dermatomyositis. Subcutaneous nodules can be seen in rheumatoid arthritis as well as in rheumatic fever. Erythema marginaturm is a feature of rheumatic fever.

SKIN MANIFESTATIONS OF SYSTEMIC LUPUS ERYTHEMATOSUS (SLE)

1. *Discoid lesions (discoid lupus erythematosus):* They are seen as erythematous, indurated, rounded plaques with depigmented atrophic centers and hyperpigmented margins. Active lesions have a central adherent scale that has minute tacs on its undersurface (carpet tac sign). Malar regions, nose, ears, forehead, scalp and postauricular area affected commonly.
2. *Facial erythema (butterfly rash):* Bright red erythema involves the malar regions and nose symmetrically in a butterfly distribution. The rash has a tendency to wax and wane with disease activitiy.
3. *Photosensitivity:* Burning and itching on exposure to sunlight is followed by an erythematous maculopapular rash.
4. *Oral and nasopharyngeal ulceration:* Erosions and superficial ulceration of these mucosa (esp. hard palate) is common and keeps step with disease activity.
5. *Raynaud's phenomenon:* Exposure to cold elicits a vasospastic response, passing through the stages of pallor, cyanosis and rubor and is accompanied by pain.

Skin and Internal Disease

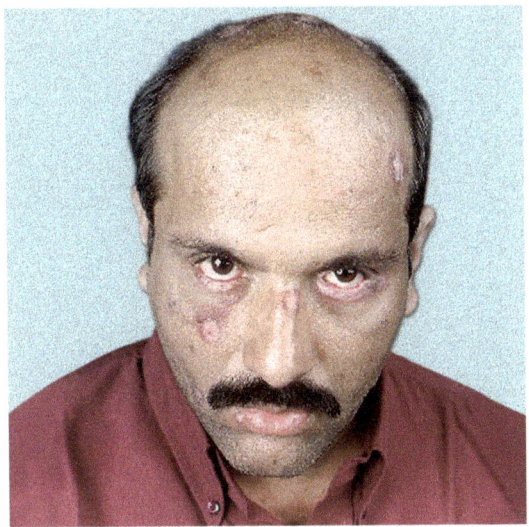

Fig. 16.1: Case of lupus erythematosus lesions around the nose and scalp, etc.

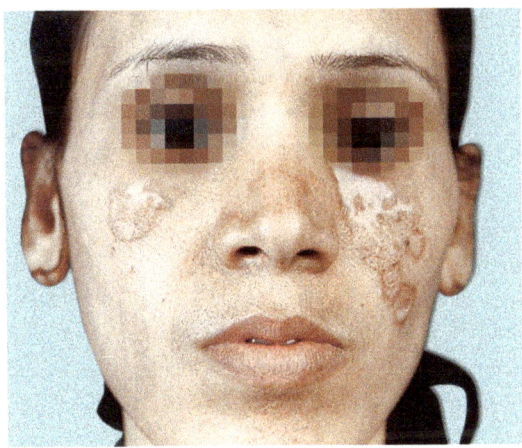

Fig. 16.2: Discoid lupus erythymatosus lesions on the cheeks and ears: Butterfly appreance on the face

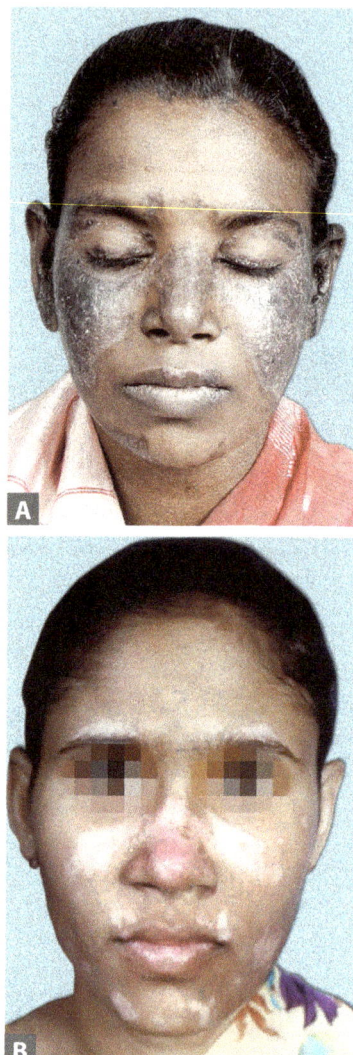

Figs 16.3A and B: Butterfly rash

6. *Alopecia:* Diffuse non-scarring alopecia that is in phase with disease activity is typical of SLE. Patchy scarring alopecia, related to discoid lesions, may occur in addition.
7. *Telangiectasia:* Punctate macular and papular telangiectasiae over face, exposed regions, palms and soles are typical of SLE. Linear telangiectasiae may be seen in addition, over the face and posterior nailfolds.
8. *Purpura:* This may be seen in SLE as a result of either thrombocytopenia or due to vasculitis.
9. Thrombophlebitis.
10. Peripheral gangrene and non-healing ulcers.

Cutaneous findings of systemic lupus erythematosus include specific skin lesions (seen only in lupus erythematosus) viz. discoid lesions and butterfly rash. Discoid lesions are erythematous plaques with central depigmentation, atrophy, follicular plugging and adherent scaling and affect the face. Butterfly rash is erythema that affects the malar regions. Nonspecific lesions include photosensitivity, oral ulceration, Raynaud's phenomenon, alopecia, and telangiectasia.

BUTTERFLY RASH

1. Physiological flushing
2. Actue contact dermatitis
3. Seborrheic dermatitis
4. Photosensitivity
5. Pellagra
6. Dermatomyositis.

Erythema involving butterfly region of face (cheeks and nasal bridge) suggests acute phase of systemic lupus erythematosus. Other findings of lupus erythematosus in the skin (discoid lesions, photosensitivity, oral ulcers, alopecia, Raynaud's phenomenon, etc.) and other systems (serositis, renal, CNS, hematologic, cardiac, hepatic, etc.) should be sought. Blood examination may show pancytopenia, ESR is elevated and there is proteinuria. ANA is positive. Other causes of facial erythema include other photodermatoses, flushing due to physiologic causes like fever, contact allergic dermatitis, and dermatomyositis.

CHAPTER 17

Vesicobullous Disorders

These are a group of autoimmune disorders that are characterized by formation of recurrent vesicles or bullae. They include pemphigus vulgaris, pemphigus foliaceus, bullous pemphigoid and dermatitis herpetiformis.
- Pemphigus vulgaris and foliaceus
- Bullous pemphigoid
- Dermatitis herpetiformis.

Chronic vesicobullous disorders are a group of immunological diseases that present as mucocutaneous blisters.

Table 17.1: Classification of bullous lesions based on the level of bulla

Subcorneal	Intraepidermal	Dermoepidermal
Bullous impetigo	Eczema	Pemphigoid
Staphylococcal	(allergic or irritant)	Dermatitis
Scalded skin	Viral infection	herpetiformis
syndrome		Toxic epidermal necrolyis
Miliaria (some forms)	Pemphigus	Epidermolysis bullosa
Subcorneal pustular dermatosis	Epidermolysis bullosa (some forms)	Bullous erythema multiforme

Common amongst these are pemphigus vulgaris, pemphigus foliaceus, bullous pemphigoid and dermatitis herpetiformis. Smear from bulla floor and skin biopsy for istopathology and immunofluorescence are useful for diagnosis. Systemic steroids are the treatment of choice except for dermatitis herpetiformis which responds to dapsone.

PEMPHIGUS

Pemphigus is a life-threatening bullous disorder characterized by severe mucocutaneous intraepidermal blisters. It is caused by the deposition of intercellular autoantibodies in the epidermis which cause acantholysis (separation of the epidermal cells from each other).

Etiology and Pathogenesis

Pemphigus is an autoimmune disorder in which IgG autoantibodies are produced against the complexes of polypeptides present in the inter cellular areas of the epidermis. The antibodies get deposited in the intercellular area and they induce the keratinocytes to release enzymes which dissolve the intercellular substance. The keratinocytes then separate from the adjoining cells. This process is called acantholysis.

Clinical Features

Epidemiology

Although rare in the West, pemphigus is the commonest cause of autoimmune blistering in India. It is mainly seen in the middle aged, but may occur in children as well.

Morphology

There are several forms of pemphigus. The commonest variety, pemphigus vulgaris is a blistering disease of mucosa and skin. The blisters in pemphigus vulgaris (though intraepidermal) are deeper. The hallmark is a flaccid bulla which appears on normal looking skin. On rupturning, the bulla leave behind erosions which have a tendency to spread, especially when tangential pressure is applied (bulla spread sign and Nickolsky's sign). These erosions take a very long time to heal. Pemphigus vulgaris is almost always associated with mucosal lesions, which manifest as painful erosions which extend peripherally with shedding of the epithelium. In almost half the patients, the disease begins with oral lesions and mucosal involvement is seen eventually in almost all patients.

A variant of pemphigus vulgaris is pemphigus vegetans. In this variety, the blistering is modified by heaped up

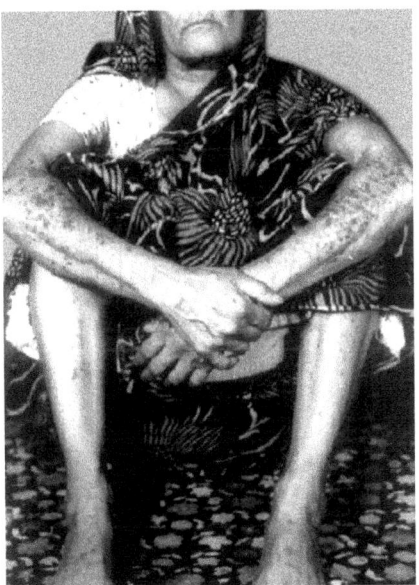

Fig. 17.1: A case of vesicobullous eruptions—pemphigus

cauliflower-like, exudative lesions in the groins and other body folds.

Apart from these two deeper types of pemphigus, there are two superficial varieties of pemphigus—pemphigus foliaceus and pemphigus erythematosus. In these, the blisters are superficial and rupture easily. Often the patient presents with extensive areas of scaling and crusting and no apparent blisters at all (Fig. 17.1). Oral lesions are infrequent. Pemphigus erythematosus is a less severe form of pemphigus foliaceus but is associated with dry, hyperkeratotic, scaly lesions on the face.

Associated Features

Lesions are frequently complicated by secondary infection.

Extensive lesions are often associated with dehydration and electrolyte imbalance especially if associated with oral lesions.

The disease runs a prolonged course even on therapy. Complications are inevitable, even with high doses of steroids.

Investigations

Histological and immunopathological changes are diagnostic in pemphigus.

Histology

Biopsy is best taken from the edge of the lesion. The bulla in pemphigus is intraepidermal, the split being suprabasal in pemphigus vulgaris and in the granular layer in pemphigus foliaceus. The presence of acantholytic cells is pathognomonic. These cells are rounded keratinocytes which float free in the blister cavity. The cytoplasm is condensed in the periphery and there appears a perinuclear halo.

Immunopathology

Every patient suspected of having pemphigus should be evaluated immunopathologically. Two types of tests need to be done in these patients. Direct immunofluorescence is done on skin lesions whereas indirect immunofluorescene is performed on patient's serum.

Direct immunofluorescence of normal skin shows intercellular deposits of IgG and C_3.

Indirect immunofluorescence, done on the serum, reveals autoantibodies. The titer of these antibodies correlates with the clinical activity and may be a useful guide to the dose of oral steroids needed.

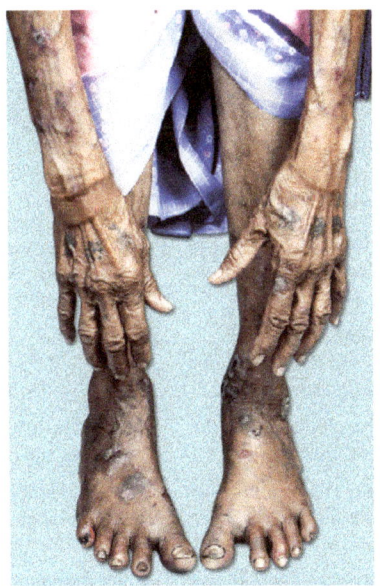

Fig. 17.2: Pemphigus foliaceus

Diagnosis

Diagnosis of pemphigus is based on:

Long history of vesiculobullous lesions.

Flaccid bullae which rupture to form nonhealing erosions; bullae may be transient in pemphigus foliaceus.

Positive Nickolsky's sign.

Painful oral erosions (in pemphigus vulgaris).

Histological and immunohistological confirmation.

Pemphigus needs to be distinguished from other bullous disorders like bullous pemphigoid.

After diagnosis of pemphigus is established, it is important to distinguish one variety of pemphigus from another. Table 17.2 shows the features of the two common varieties of pemphigus.

Table 17.2: Differences between pemphigus vulgaris and pemphigus foliaceus

	Pemphigus vulgaris	*Pemphigus foliaceus*
Morphology	Flaccid bullae which rupture to form superficial erosions	Blisters may not be obvious; extensive lesions with scales and crusts
Oral lesions	Universal	Infrequent
Distribution	Scalp, face, axillae; can be extensive	Initially seborrheic distribution; can become generalized
Course	More prolonged; greater morbidity and mortality	Lesser morbidity and mortality
Pathology	Suprabasal split with acantholysis	Subcorneal or granular layer split with acantholysis
Immunopathology	IgG and C_3 deposits in the intercellular spaces of epidermis	IgG and C_3 deposits in the intercellular spaces of epidermis
Treatment	High dose steroids and adjuvant therapy	Low dose steroids

Treatment

Many patient of pemphigus (especially pemp higus vulgaris) are gravely ill. Apart from specific therapy, supportive care and general measures are important.

General Measure
- Local and oral hygiene.
- Water and electrolyte balance.
- Treating secondary infection.

Specific Treatment

Specific treatment hinges on the use of immunosuppressive agents, (corticosteroids and cytotoxic drugs) since pemphigus is an autoimmune disorder.

Corticosteroids: They were initially used in high daily doses though, this was associated with decreased mortality, the side effects of corticosteroids resulted in increased morbidity. Many dermatologists continue to use high doses of oral steroids (80-160 mg prednosolone) to suppress the disease. The dose is gradually tapered off, when the patient improves. To circumvent the side effects of steroids, many dermatologists add immunosuppressive drugs.

Immunosuppressive drugs: These are used as adjuvants in patients, who either develop side effects to steroids or whose disease activity is not being controlled with steroid therapy alone. Immunosuppressives, which have been used, include cyclophosphamide, azathioprine and methotrexate.

Other therapies: Parenteral gold, plasmapheresis and extracorporeal photochemotherapy have been used with some success.

Combination therapy: A combination of steroid-cyclophosphamide has been used in monthly pulses in an attempt to reduce the side effects of conventional steroid therapy without compromising on efficacy. The regimen consists of giving 100 mg of dexamethasone in a dextrose drip (or betamethasone 100 mg orally) daily for 3 consecutive days with parenteral cyclophosphamide 500 mg monthly along with daily doses of cyclophos phamide (50–100 mg).

DERMOEPIDERMAL BULLAE

Bullous Pemphigoid

Etiology

This is an autoimmune disease mediated by IgG antibodies which bind to the bullous pemphigoid antigen in the lamina lucida at the dermo epidermal junction. Complement is activated and a dermoepidermal blister is formed by enzymes released from inflammatory cells attracted to the area by the chemotactic components of the complement cascade.

Clinical Features

Epidemiology: Bullous pemphigoid is a disease of the elderly.

Morphology: Itchy, tense bullae arise either on the normal skin or on large urticarial plaques. The bullae may be hemorrhagic (since they are dermoepidermal). The bulla spread sign and Nickolsky's sign are negative. Lesions heal with milia formation (these are intraepidermal cysts which appear as small pearly papules). Mucosal lesions are infrequent.

Distribution: The bullae may be seen all over the body, the most common sites being the lower abdomen, inner thighs, groins and the flexors of limbs (flexures and intertriginous areas).

Course: This is a self-limiting condition causing morbidity but is associated with very little mortality.

Complications: The disease is symptomatic (itching) and causes discomfort to the patient.

Association: Underlying malignancies should be ruled out.

Investigations

Biopsy shows a subepidermal blister.

Direct immunofluorescence shows a linear deposit of IgG and C_3 along the basement membrane zone.

About 70% of patients have IgG antibodies in their serum; this reacts with the basement membrane zone.

Bullous pemphigoid is characterized by:

Itchy, tense, hemorrhagic bullae, sometimes on erythematous base. Healing with milia formation. Infrequent oral lesions.

Dermoepidermal split on histology and a linear deposition of immunoglobulins on immuno fluorescence of skin biopsy.

Differential diagnosis: Bullous pemphigoid needs to be differentiated from other bullous disorders:

Pemphigus vulgaris: The bullae of pemphigus vulgaris are flaccid and rupture rapidly to leave erosions; oral erosions are present in all patients. Pemphigus occurs in a younger age group. Bullae of bullous pemphigoid are tense, hemorrhagic and oral lesions are seen only occasionally. It is a disease of elderly. Histology and immuno histology clinch the diagnosis.

Bullous erythema multiforme: An acute eruption chracterized by target lesions on the acral parts with history of antecedent herpes simplex infection or drug intake. Immunofluorescence findings are diagnostic of bullous pemphigoid.

Other disease like dermatitis herpetiformis, herpes gestationis, linear IgA bullous dermatosis may sometimes be confused with bullous pemphigoid.

Treatment

Though a chronic problem, the disease does not cause death, so the treatment need not be aggressive.

Mild-to-moderate disease: Safe drugs like dapsone (100–200 mg daily) and a combination of tetracycline (2 g daily) along with nicotinamide (1.5 g daily) have been found useful.

Severe disease: Steroids (prednisolone 40–60 mg daily equivalent) are the mainstay of treatment. Immunosuppressive agents may be added, if the steroids alone fail to control the disease.

Dermatitis Herpetiformis

Etiology

A gluten-sensitive enteropathy (though frequently asymptomatic) is always present. Absorption of gluten and other dietary antigens induces formation of circulating immune complexes which deposit in the dermal papillae, causing inflammation and a dermoepidermal split.

Clinical Features

Morphology: Extremely itchy, grouped papulovesicular lesions develop on normal or erythematous skin. Since the vesicles are extremely itchy, they are excoriated before they reach any size; such a patient shows only grouped excoriations. Repeated scratching may cause eczematous changes and secondary infection.

Associated Features and Complications

Gluten sensitive enteropathy (mild and patchy) is present in 100% of patients. Most patients, however, are asymptomatic. In a few patients it may be complicated by diarrhea, abdominal pain and malabsorption.

Rarely, small intestine lymphomas may complicate the enteropathy.

Distribution: The lesions are most frequently seen on the extensors: elbows, knees, buttocks and shoulders.

Investigations

Vesicles are generally not seen but when they can be biopsied, show a characteristic histology of a subepidermal blister with collection of polymorphs in the dermal papilla. Immunofluorescence studies of the skin show a granular deposit of IgA in the dermal papillae.

Diagnosis

Dermatitis herpetiformis is characterized by:

Grouped papulovesicular lesions, frequently manifesting as clustered excoriations on the extensors. Characteristic histology and immunofluorescence findings.

Differential diagnosis: Dermatitis herpetiformis has to be distinguished from scabies, nummular dermatitis and insect bites.

Treatment

A two-pronged approach brings about quick and lasting response.

Gluten-free diet which is slow to act on the skin lesions (several months) though the bowel changes revert to normal quickly. However, a gluten-free diet may be difficult to follow.

Dapsone (100–200 mg daily for adults) and sulfapyridine work dramatically. Response (within 48–72 hours) to dapsone has been used as a therapeutic test for diagnosis of dermatitis herpetiformis. Both these drugs can cause rashes, hemolytic anemia, thrombocytopenia, methemoglobinemia and peripheral neuropathy. Regular monitoring of blood counts is, therefore, essential.

ERYTHEMA NODOSUM

This is a pattern of hypersensitivity response of the skin to various infections or drugs. However, many a times, no etiologic factor can be identified.

Etiology

The different etilogic factors implicated are:
1. **Infections**

Bacterial	- Streptococcal (URTI), *Yersinia*, *Brucella* infections, *Tularemia*, cat scratch disease.
Mycobacterial	- Tuberculosis
Chlamydial	- Lymphogranuloma venereum
Spirochetal	- Leptospirosis
Fungal	- Histoplasmosis
Protozoan	- Toxoplasmosis

2. **Drugs** - Sulfonamides, estrogens, aspirin, iodides
3. **Internal Diseases** - Sarcoidosis, Behcet's disease, Crohn's disease.
4. **Malignancies** - Lymphoma, leukemia

Therapy

If an underlying cause is detected, treat it. If nose is found, therapy is only symptomatic since the disease is usually self-limiting. Ordinarily, it takes 3-6 weeks for the lesions to resolve by themselves. NSAIDs like ibuprofen are helpful in relieving pain in the nodules and joints.

Symmetrical, tender, erythematous nodules over shins of young women accompany fever and arthralgia. Tuberculosis, streptococcal infections and drugs are commonly implicated. Lesions subside over 3-6 weeks without ulceration. NSAIDs relieve the pain.

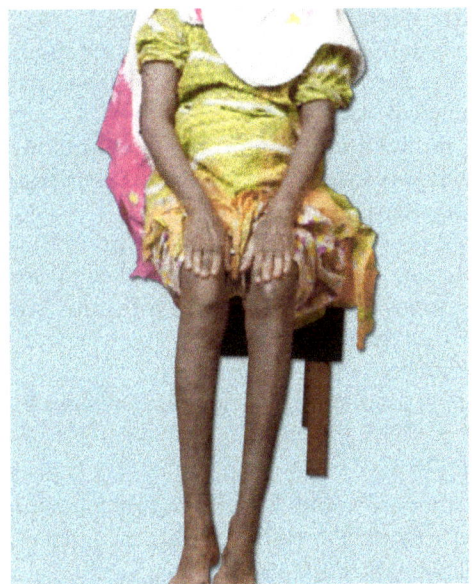

Fig. 17.3: Exfoliative dermatitis—see the erythema and scaling almost whole body affected

ERYTHRODERMA (EXFOLIATIVE DERMATITIS)

Erythema and scaling involving most of all of the body surface area is termed as exfoliative dermatitis or erythroderma. It develops either de novo (primary, idopathic or due to unknown cause) or as a progression of a preexisting skin disease (secondary erythroderma due to a known cause).

Etiology

Skin diseases that lead to secondary erythroderma by virtue of extension of skin lesions all over the body are as follows:

1. Psoriasis—acounts for about 40% cases.
2. Eczema/dermatitis group—accounts for about 20% and includes seborrheic dermatitis, allergic contact dermatitis and atopic dermatitis.
3. Drug induced erythroderma—accounts for 10-15% cases and is caused by sulfonamides, dapsone, NSAIDs, antiepileptic, penicillins, etc.
4. Miscellaneous—account for about 10% cases like ichthyoses, pemphigus, toxic epidermal necrolysis, staphylococcal scalded skin syndrome, Norwegian scabies and lymphoma.
5. Unidentified cause—
   In a small proportion, no cause may be found.

Management

Although therapy would differ according to the preexisting skin disease that led to erythroderma, the intial emergency care of all patients must ensure.
1. Omit and avoid suspected drugs.
2. Warm clothing and monitoring core temperature.
3. Monitor input/output, maintain fluid.
4. High protein diet.
5. Systemic steroids, oral or parenteral, equivalent of 1-2 mg/kg of prednisolone to be tapered gradually after 1-2 weeks.
6. Topical applications of soothing ointments like white soft paraffin soften and separate scales. Topical steroids, applied in limited quantities, releive pruritus and reduce erythema.
7. Investigations to monitor fluid and electrolyte balance, serum proteins and renal function are repeated at intervals till the skin lesions subside and other systems regain normalcy.

Erythroderma indicates erythema and scaling of the whole body surface. It may result from aggravation of a preexisting disease like psoriasis, contact allergic dermatitis or seborrheic dermatitis or may be induced by drugs like sulphonamides or NSAIDs. Features of the original skin condition may be identifiable clinically or on biopsy. Systemic problems due to persistent erythroderma include hypoproeinemia, cardiac failure, fluid, electrolyte and temperature imbalance and lymphadenopathy. Treatment is that of the cause. Supportive measures include high protein diet, warm clothing, maintaining fluid and electrolyte balance and topical application of soothing ointments. Systemic steroids are useful to expedite resoultion.

NUTRITIONAL DEFICIENCIES

Vitamin A Deficiency

Vitamine A deficiency leads to dry skin and phrynoderma.

Phrynoderma

This follicular papular eruption, seen usually in prepubertal children from developing countries, is thought to be due to a deficiency of vitamin A. However, another school of thought considers essential fatty acid deficiency as the cause. Ocular changes of vitamin A deficiency may be associted.

Phrynoderma is due to vitamin A/essential fatty acid deficiency. Grouped, keratotic, skin colored, conical, follicular papules over extensors of limbs are typical. Raising in take of Vitamin A containing foods (eggs, meat, carrots, beet, papaya, green leafy vegetabels) and oral supplementation (50,000 IU once a week or 5000 IU daily) improve lesions.

Vitamin B Complex

Many vitamin deficiencies from this group are commonly present in combination, thus some clinical features may overlap.
- Riboflavin deficiency
- Pyridoxine deficiency.

Actions of riboflavin and pyridoxine are closely related and interdependent. Hence, combined deficiency is a rule. Changes are early and prominent on face and include angular cheilitis, seborrheic dermatitis—like rash and a smooth magneta red tongue. Eggs, meat, liver, cereals and green vegetables are sources of riboflavin and pyridoxine. Oral therapeutic doses are 10–30 mg daily.

Pellagra (Niacin Deficiency)

Pellagra is due to niacin deficiency that affects NADP synthesis. Tryptophan is the dietary source of niacin and is present in eggs, meat, pulses, cereals and nuts. Alcoholism and a staple diet of jowar and maize predispose to pellagra. Sunbrun—like lesions involving face, 'V' of neck, dorsa of hands and forearms are characteristic. Tongue is smooth and dark red and other mucosae are inflamed. Diarrhea, behavioral changes, dementia And coma are the systemic changes that are serious but reversible with therapy. Nicotinamide 50 mg tid for many weeks and dietary correction are curative.

Vitamine deficiencies that rarely present with skin complaints:
- Thiamine
- Pantothenic acid
- Folic acid and cyanocobalamin

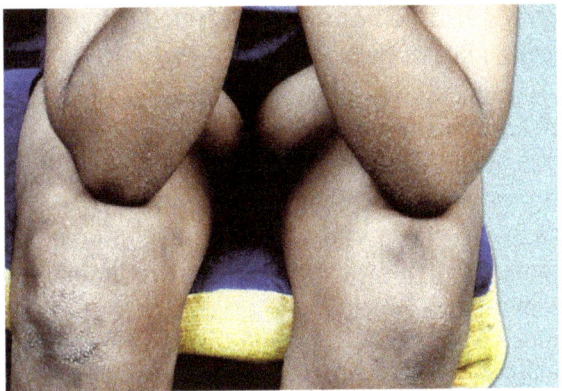

Fig. 17.4: Phrynoderma: Elbows and knees both sides

Vitamin C

Skin in infantile scurvy shows petechiae, ecchymoses and hematomas. Bleeding from gums is seen in older infants. Classic adult scurvy has petechial hemorrhages in perifollicular location with the central hair twisted like a corkscrew. Other evidences of mucocutaneous bleeding are common (esp. from gums). Therapeutic doses are 100 mg per day.

Vitamin E

Vitamin E deficiency is uncommon. Scaling, papular lesions and dryness are reported.

Vitamin K

Cutaneous hemorrhages can occur in severe vitamin K deficiency seen usually in premature babies.

Adjuvant Triamcinolone Acetonide Injections in Oropharyngeal Pemphigus Vulgaris

Enteric coated mycophenolate sodium in the treatment of refractory pemphigus.

Azathioprine is usually the first choice of adjuvant therapy but severe gastrointestinal symptoms are a drawback.

Stress and serum TNF-alpha level may predict disease outcome in patients with pemphigus: A preliminary study.

Emotional stress appears to be a significant factor affecting prognosis of the disease. Pretreatment assessment of serum TNF-alpha levels in case of patients with pemphigus may be a guide to the expected prognosis and selection of the proper treatment regimen.

CHAPTER 18

Skin Tumors

CUTANEOUS NEOPLASMS, BENIGN, PREMALIGNANT AND MALIGNANT TUMORS OF THE SKIN

Squamous Cell Carcinoma

This malignant neoplasm has the potential to lead to death by metastasis or local spread if left untreated. Affection of mucosae and mucocutaneous junctions is much more common in the brown skinned Indians than in the whites who develop these tumors on sun exposed skin.

Basal Cell Carcinoma (Rodent Ulcer)

This locally malignant neoplasm rarely metastasizes and thus leads to local destruction of tissues more commonly than death.

Therapy

Simple excision (with a margin of 5-10 mm) is the treatment of choice. Recurring lesions may need chemosurgery and inoperable lesions, radiotherapy.

Melanoma

This malignant tumor composed of melanocytes that may arise in the skin or other tissues harboring melanocytes, like the mucocutaneous juctions, mucosae including the conjunvtiva, iris, choroid and substantia nigra.

Melanoma is the malignant tumor of melanocytes. Sun-exposed regions are involved in whites whereas palms and soles are affected in Indians. It begins as a pigmented macule that grows slowly over months or years and then evolves into a papule or nodule on its surface indicating dermal involvement. Metastatic nodules signify poor prognosis. In the absence of metastasis, complete surgical excision, with a free magin of at least 1 cm, is curative.

Melanoma Epidemiology of Austria Reveals Gender-related Differences

Cutaneous melanoma shows gender-specific trends worldwide, with highest rates in older men. In Austria, women show greater knowledge about the early detection of skin cancer by screening. Our aim was to analyze national melanoma incidence and mortality rates with regard to gender to improve our prevention efforts.

Age-standardized incidence rates of melanoma increased for both genders from 4.9 in 1983 to 10.5 in 2008 ($P < 0.001$), for men more than women ($P < 0.005$). In 2006–2008 the lifetime risk of developing a melanoma was 1:123 (women: 1:128, men 1:117). In situ and local stages were more common in women, men presented with regional and distant disease. In 2008–2010 male mortality was 1.7 times higher than female ($P < 0.005$) and the lifetime risk of death from melanoma amounted to 1:570 (women 1:705, men 1:434; $P < 0.05$). Comparatively, men over 75 faced the highest risk of presenting with or dying from melanoma.

In Austria, melanoma epidemiology showed gender-specific differences. Efforts in early detection need to be increased in elderly men. As shown in the female population, a change in the melanoma-related epidemiology is feasible, most likely by means of secondary prevention.

BENIGN NEOPLASMS

Seborrheic Keratosis

Melanocytic nevi.

ACANTHOSIS NIGRICANS

This peculiar but benign condition of the skin is frequently a manifestation of an endocrine disorder. It implies papillomatous or verrucous hypertrophy of the skin combined with pigmentation occurring in streaks or patches in the axillae, groins, neck, submammary region and antecubital fossae. It may occur either in a mild or severe form; in the latter, there is accompanying dystrophy of the nails and hair, there being pigmentation of the other parts of the integument as well. There are two varieties of acanthosis nigricans:

1. *The juvenile type:* It is the benign type. It may be associated with endocrine, metabolic or digestive disorders.
2. *Adult type:* The prognosis is bad, since it is usually associated with abdominal cancer.

Third variety is known as pseudoacanthosis nigricans seen in obese individuals. Its course varies according to the weight of the body.

The treatment depends upon the primary cause which must be duly tackled. For local defects, salicylic acid ointment, retinoic acid, vitamins and thyroid may be tried.

CAROTINEMIA

It implies yellowish discoloration of the integument caused by the excessive consumption of carotin-rich foodstuffs, particularly carrots and oranges. The sites most commonly discolored are the palms of the hands, the soles of the feet and the nasolabial folds; later, other parts of the body may also be affected. The color varies from light-yellow to deep-orange. The pigmentations is only temporary, and when the cause is withdrawn from the diet, the color of the skin returns to normal.

CUTANEOUS HYPERPLASIAS

Keloid

Therapy

Therapy of keloids is not satisfactory. Intralesional injections of trimcinolone acetonide 10–20 mg/mL on several occasions may stop growth and soften the lesion. Persistent pressure with elastic bands has similar effect. Local cryotherapy or radiotherapy have a salutary effect on keloid growth. Surgical excision is fraught with the risk of recurrence. However, when surgery is followed up with intralesional steroid injection or pressure theraphy or radiotherapy of the excisiom scar the chances of recurrence are considerably reduced.

Palmoplantar Keratoderma

Marked thickening of the stratum corneum of palms and soles is seen in keratoderma. Keratoderma may be hereditary or may be due to an underlying condition like psoriasis, ichthyosis, long standing hand or foot eczema or tinea pedis.

Clavus (Corn)

Corns result from excessive concentration of perssure at one point.

Cutaneous Malformations

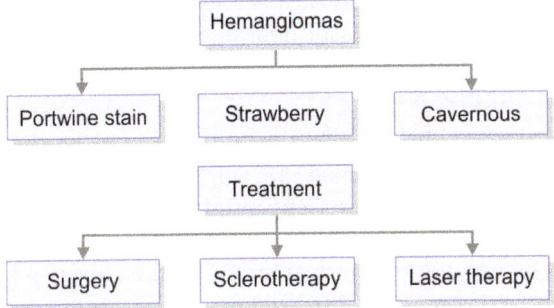

NEVI

The word nevus is derived from the Latin term meaning spot or blemish, originally used to describe the congenital lesions or birth mark (Mothers mark).

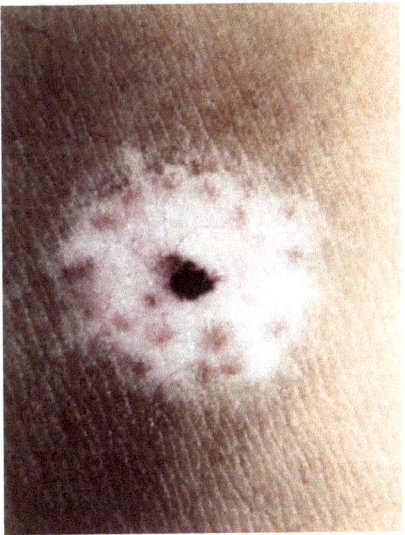

Fig. 18.1: Hollow nevus also known as Sutton's disease

The various types are keratinocyte nevi, follicular nevi, Sebaceous nevi, apocrine nevi, eccrine nevi, connective nevi, smooth muscle nevi, elastic neni, fat nevi, and vascular nevi.

Melanocytic Nevi

They are broadly classified into acquired or congenital. Acquired melanocytic naevi are subdivided into junctional, compound, and dermal. Congenital melanocytic nevi may be defined as melanocytic nevi present at birth.

A benign tumor, more common in the elderly people. Seborrheic keratosis (SK) occurs on any places, most frequently on the face and the upper trunk. Seborrheic

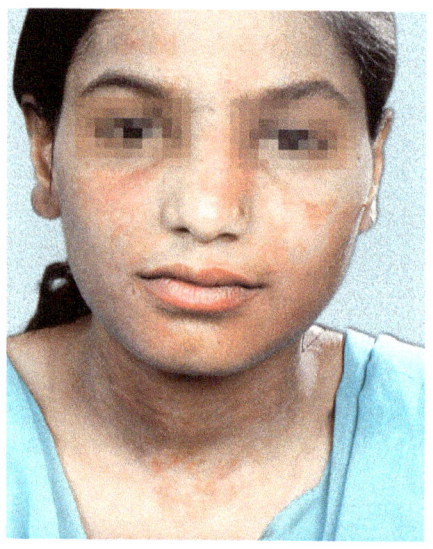

Fig. 18.2: Vascular nevus. See the red face extending up to neck signs at birth known as hemangioma

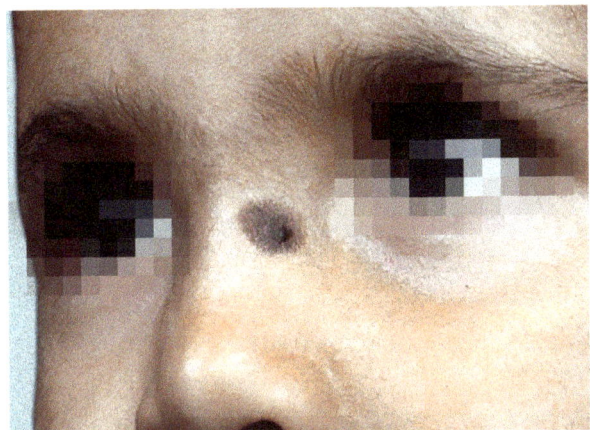

Fig. 18.3: Pigmented nevus or birth mark

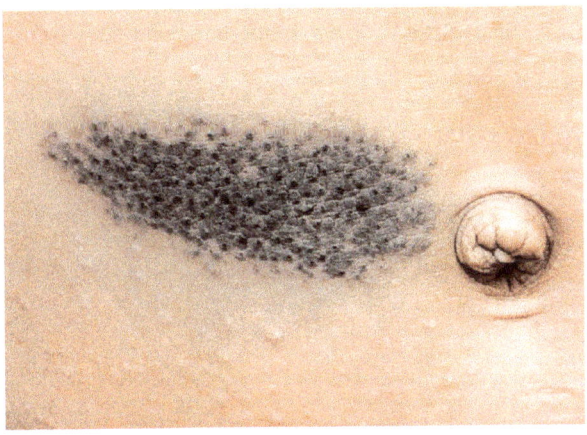

Fig. 18.4: Nevus on the abdomen

keratoses typically begin as flat sharply demarcated brown macules. Follicular prominence is one of the hallmarks of seborrheic keratoses. Later on, typical asymptomatic, slowly increasing, verrucous plaques develop and have a "stuck-on" appearance.

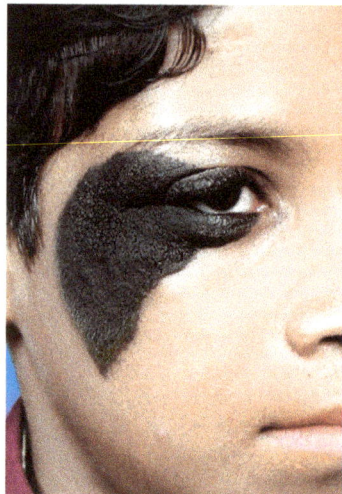

Fig. 18.5: Nevus on the cheeck and around the eye

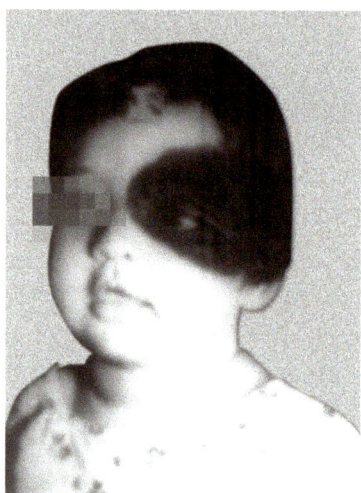

Fig. 18.6: Congenital melanocytic nevus with hairyness over the eye

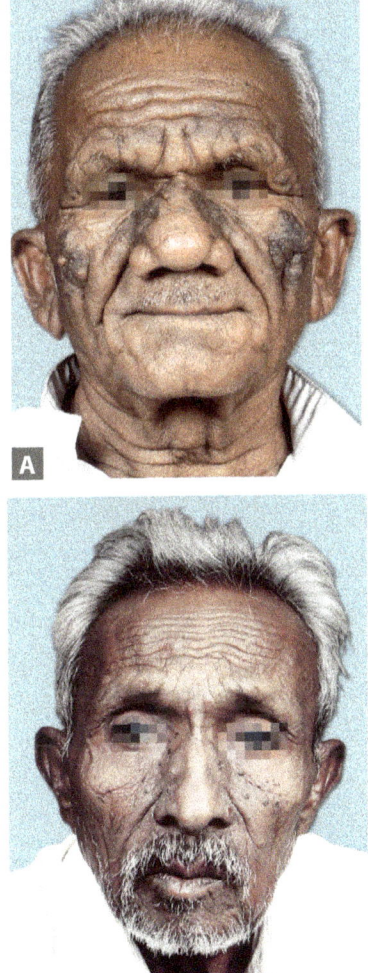

Figs 18.7A and B: Seborrheic keratosis

Treatment: Curettege, cryotherapy, or electrodesiccation.

A diagrammatic description of the antecedents, origin and growth of a malignant-melanoma are as follows:

The entire evolutionary process of a malignant melanoma must be considered in a evaluating patient's prognosis. The precancerous lesions is consistently cured by excision. Superficial malignant melanoma also has a good cure rate as compared to an advanced lesion with bulky overgrowth, arising precipitously. However, in order to give a fairly equivocal diagnosis it is necessary to make step sections of

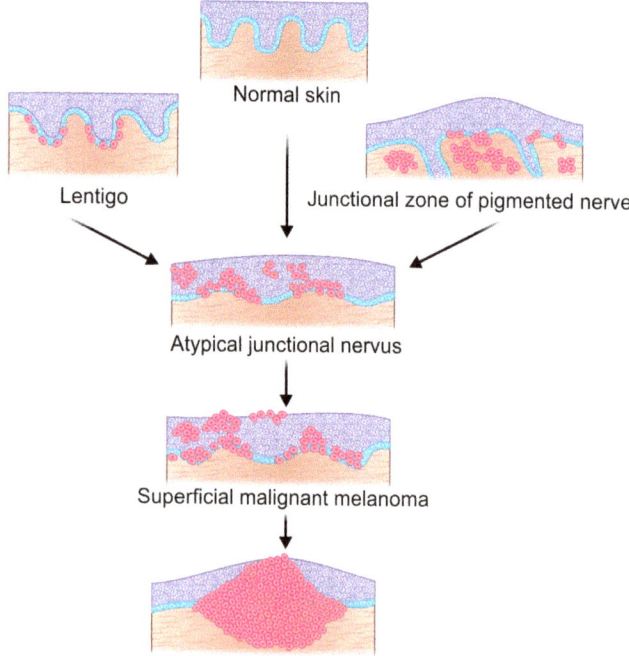

Fig. 18.8: Malignant melanoma with expansile growth

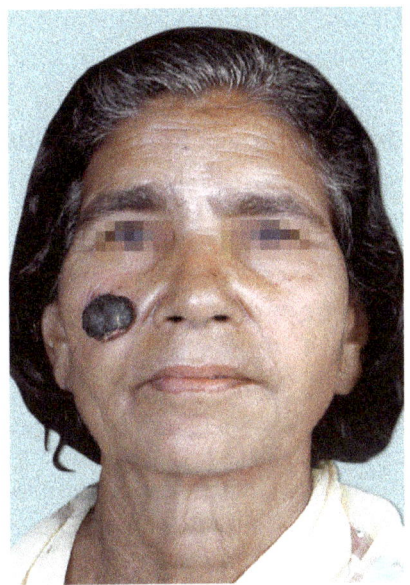

Fig. 18.9: Malignant melanoma: Small nevus growing into expansile mass and inflamation and pain surounded by redness

all tissues submitted, because the degree of alteration varies greatly in different sites. The importantce of determining the stage of development of the tumor is necessary for the prognosis of the case. In a series of cases studied by Hall et al. which were principally pigmentary alterations with little or no evidence of local growth (stage I) had an 82% five-year survival. Advanced local growth (stage II) reduced it to 45% five-year survial. If metastasis to the lymph nodes had occurred (stage III) only 11% survived for 5 years, and if the were present at the end of 5 years and if there were distant metastasis no survivors were present at the end of 5 years.

Photodynamic Therapy with Intradermal Administration of 5-Aminolevulinic Acid for Port-wine Stains

Photodynamic Therapy of Port-wine Stains

Nevus flammeus, or nevus telangiectasis, which occurs in 0.3–0.5% of newborns, is common congenital capillary malformation of the superficial layer of the cutis.

Melanoma Epidemiology of Austria Reveals Gender-related Differences

In Austria, melanoma epidemiology showed gender-specific differences. Efforts in early detection need to be increased in elderly men. As shown in the female population, a change in the melanoma-related epidemiology is feasible, most likely by means of secondary prevention.

Acquired Tufted Angioma in Pregnancy Showing Expression of Estrogen and Progesterone Receptors

Monosomy 18P is a chromosomal disorder resulting from the deletion of or all part of short arm of chromosome 18. The main clinical features are short stature, round face with short philtrum.

Pulpebral ptosis and protruding ears with detached pinnae. Monosomy 18p is very rarely concurrent with baldness. Thus, the baldness in monosomy18 has not been well addressed, not even as to whether it is hypotrichosis or alopecia.

Complete remission of extensive cutaneous metastatic melanoma on the scalp under topical monoimmunotherapy with diphenylcyclopropenone.

CHAPTER 19

Miscellaneous Disorders

SUBCUTANEOUS NODULES

Differential Diagnosis

Hypersensitivity Phenomena
- Erythema induratum (Bazin's disease)
- Erythema nodosum leprosum
- Erythema nodosum
- Periarteritis nodosa

Infections
- Furuncles
- Abscesses
- Cold abscess
- Nodulocystic acne

Granulomatous Disorders
- Rheumatoid nodules
- Rheumatic fever
- Sarcoidosis

Deposits

- Gouty tophi
- Amyloidosis

Tumors

- Neurofibroma
- Fibroma
- Lipoma
- Metastasis

Miscellaneous

- Hematoma
- Sebaceous cysts

Table 19.1: Different causes for the development of stretch marks

Different hypotheses on the development of stretch marks in the literature

Infection leading to the release of striatoxin that damages the tissues in a microbial toxic way

Mechanical effect of stretching, which is proposed to lead to rupture of the connective tissue framework (e.g. pregnancy, obesity, weight lifting)

Normal growth as seen in adolescence and the pubertal spurt that leads to increase in sizes of particular body regions

Increase in the levels of body steroid hormones; Cushing's syndrome, local or systemic steroid therapy that has a catabolic effect on fibroblasts

Genetic factors (absence of striae in pregnancy in people with Ehlers-Danlos syndrome and their presence as one of the minor diagnostic criteria for marfan syndrome suggest an important genetic element)

Immunosuppression states associated with pregnancy induced hypertension medication, human immunodeficiency virus or disease such as tuberculosis and typhoid

Associated with chronic liver disease

Table 19.2: Different topical products and their speculated modalities of action

Product	Indication	Suggested mode of action
Tretinoin	Therapeutic	Exact mechanism unclear, but recent studies suggest fibroblastic stimulation
Trofolastin	Therapeutic	Active ingredient (centella asiatica) stimulates fibroblasts and inhibits glucocorticoids
Verum	Preventive	Active ingredient hyaluronic acid is speculated to increase tensile resistance to mechanical forces
Alphastria	Preventive	Hyaluronic acid, the main ingredient, acts by increasing volume to oppose mechanical atrophy
Massage with oils	Preventive	Dual action of massage and hydrant action of oils.
Glycolic acid and trichloroacetic acid peels	Therapeutic	Glycolic acid is reported to stimulate collagen production by fibroblasts and to increase their proliferation in vivo and in vitro

Table 19.33: Summary of different laser and light source treatments for stretch marks

Type of laser	Effectiveness in striae distensae
Pulsed dye laser	Demonstrated to be effective only for the immature element of striae (striae rubrae), trageting the vascular element. Not effective in darker skin and associated with pregnancy induced hypertension. When combined with radio frequency, it showed a more promising response even on striae alba
Copper bromide laser	A 577-nm laser that showed a mild to moderate effect in one study on skin types II and III; no histological analysis was carried out. Needs much evaluation
1,450 nm diode laser	Not useful in skin of color (IV–VI) and associated with many complications

Contd...

Contd...

Type of laser	Effectiveness in striae distensae
1,064 neodymium-doped yttrium aluminium garnet laser	Targets immature striae and satisfactory results in the few studies so far
Excimer laser	A 308-nm xenon-chloride laser with a good safety profile, although only repigments temporarily and does not have an effect of atrophy
Intense pulsed light	A good alternative that was shown to be an effective tool in striae alba, although with a high incidence of pregnancy-induced hypertension
Fractional photothermolysis	Fewer studies conducted, although all reported efficacy in mature and immature striae and demonstrated an increase in the number of collagen and elastin fibers and a good safety profile

Erythema Nodosum

Erythema nodosum is the most frequent clinicopathologic variant of panniculitis. The disorder usually exhibits an acute onset and is clinically characterized by the sudden eruption of erythematous tender nodules and plaques located predominantly over the extensor aspects of the lower extremities. The lesions show spontaneous regression, without ulceration, scarring, or atrophy, and recurrent episodes are not uncommon. Erythema nodosum is a cutaneous reactive process that may be triggered by a wide variety of possible stimuli, being infections, sarcoidosis, rheumatologic diseases, inflammatory bowel diseases, medications, autoimmune disorders, pregnancy, and malignancies the most common associated conditions.

Clinical Features

Erythema nodosum can occur at any age, but most cases appear between the second and fourth decades of the life, with the peak of incidence being between 20 and 30 years of age, probably attributable to the high incidence of sarcoidosis at this age. Several studies have demonstrated that erythema nodosum occurs 3 to 6 times more frequently in women than in men, although the sex incidence before puberty is approximately equal. The typical eruption is quite characteristic and consists of a sudden onset of symmetrical, tender, erythematous, warm nodules and raised plaques usually located on the shins, ankles and knees. The nodules, which range from 1 to 5 cm or more in diameter, are usually bilaterally distributed.

Nodules may become confluent resulting in erythematous plaques. In rare instances, more extensive lesions may appear, involving the thighs, extensor aspects of the arms, neck, and even the face.

Treatment

Treatment of erythema nodosum should be directed to the underlying associated condition, if identified. Usually, nodules of erythema nodosum regress spontaneously within a few weeks, and bed rest is often sufficient treatment. Aspirin and nonsteroidal antiinflammatory drugs such as oxyphenbutazone, in a dosage of 400 mg per day, indomethacin, in a dosage of 100 to 150 mg per day, or naproxen, in a dosage of 500 mg per day, may be helpful to enhance analgesia and resolution. If the lesions persist longer, potassium iodide in a dosage of 400 to 900 mg daily or a saturated solution of potassium iodide, 2 to 10 drops in water or orange juice three times per day, has been reported to be useful.

Systemic corticosteroids are rarely indicated in erythema nodosum and before these drugs are administered an underlying infection should be ruled out. When administered, prednisone in a dosage of 40 mg per day has been followed by resolution of the nodules in few days. Intralesional injection of triamcinolone acetonide, in a dosage of 5 mg/mL, into the center of the nodules may cause them to resolve. Some patients may respond to a course of colchicine, 0.6 to 1.2 mg twice a day, and hydroxychloroquine 200 mg twice a day has been also reported to be useful in a recent report.

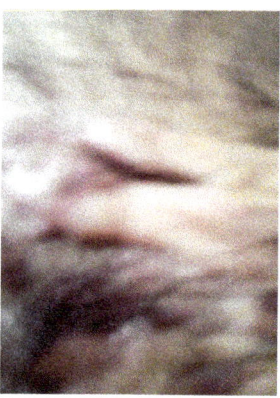

Fig. 19.1: Keloid—indurated and bifurcated

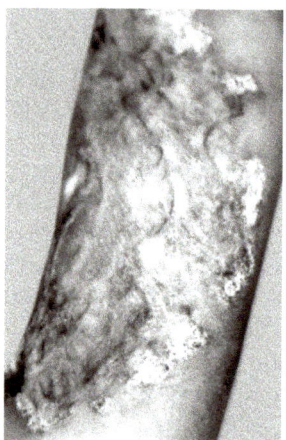

Fig. 19.2: Keloid—indurated skin lesion showing peripheral extensions

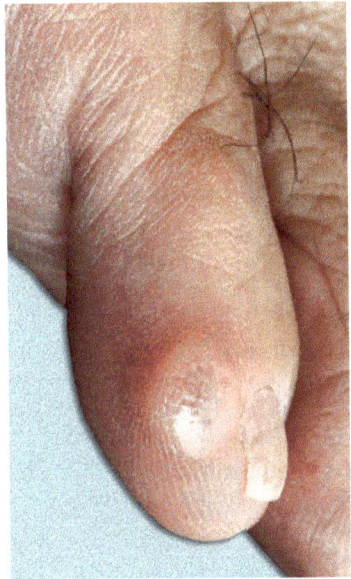

Fig. 19.3: Corns due to constant pressure of ill-fitted shoes

Subcutaneous nodules may result from hypersensitivity phenomena like erythema nodosum, infections like furuncles and abscesses, granulomatous disorders like rheumatoid nodules, deposits like gouty tophi or tumors like neurofibromas.

VESICULAR RASH
Differential Diagnosis
Infections
- Chickenpox
- Herpes simplex
- Herpes zoster
- Impetigo

Eczemas
- Atopic dermatitis
- Contact dermatitis
- Autosensitization eczema
- Id eruption.

Hypersensitivity Phenomena
- Erythema multiforme
- Stevens-Johnson syndrome.

Photosensitive Dermatoses
- Drug-induced photosensitivity
- Polymorphous light eruption.

Chronic Vesicobullous Dermatoses
- Dermatitis herpetiformis
- Pemphigus foliaceus.

Miscellaneous
- Miliaria crystallina
- Prurigo (insect bite reaction).

Differential diagnosis of vesicular rash includes infections caused by the herpes viruses and staphylococcal impetigo, eczematous dermatoses like contact allergic dermatitis and id eruption, hypersensitivity dermatoses like erythema multiforme and Stevens-Johnson syndrome, photosensitive dermatoses like polymorphous light eruption, chronic vesicobullous disorders like dermatitis herpetiformis and pemphigus foliaceus and miscellaneous conditions like miliaria crystallina and prurigo mitis.

RASH WITH FEVER
Differential Diagnosis
Viral Infections
- Chickenpox
- Measles

- Rubella
- Primary HIV infection
- Infectious mononucleosis
- Other viral exanthems.

Non-viral Infections

- Rickettsial infections
- Spirochetal infections
- Bacterial infections.

Hypersensitivity Phenomena

- Drug eruptions
- Erythema multiforme, Stevens-Johnson syndrome
- Toxic epidermal necrolysis
- Erythema nodosum.

Autoimmune Diseases

- Systemic lupus erythematosus
- Dermatomyositis
- Rheumatic fever
- Vasculitis of small or large vessels of varying causes
- Juvenile rheumatoid arthritis.

Miscellaneous

- Malignancies
- Disseminated intravascular coagulation
- Opportunistic infections.

Common conditions that presents with a combination of fever and skin rash are chickenpox, measles, rubella and other viral exanthems including primary HIV infection. Type II lepra reaction presents as fever with erythema nodosum leprosum. Occasionally, other infections like meningococcemia, syphilis, typhoid and leptospirosis may present as fever with rash. Drug eruptions, erythema multiforme, Stevens-Johnson syndrome and erythema nodosum are frequently associated with fever. Lupus erythematosus, dermatomyositis, rheumatic fever and vasculitis are some important autoimmune conditions presenting with this combination. Finally, malignancies and opportunistic infections in the HIV infected may also lead to fever and skin lesions.

HIRSUTISM

Growth of coarse hair in a male distribution, occurring in females is termed as hirsutism. Its causes include androgen excess due to tumors or hyperplasias, increased follicular sensitivity to androgens or drugs like anabolic steroids. Other features of virilization like clitoromegaly, husky voice and masculine body may be associated. Screening investigations include urinary 17-ketosteroids, serum testosterone and DHEA. Plucking, waxing, bleaching and electrolysis provide a choice of therapeutic procedures. Oral antiandrogens with

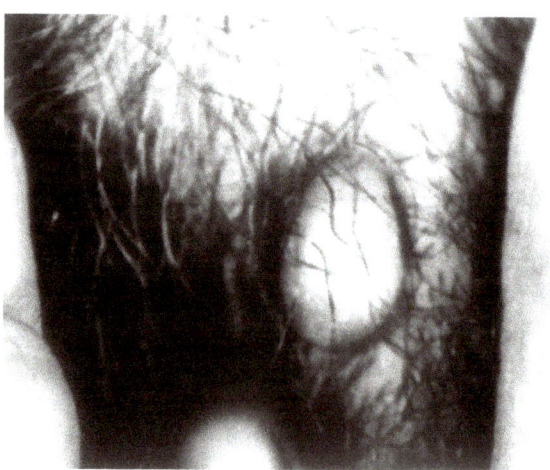

Fig. 19.4: Sebaceous cyst—round lobular, soft skin-colored growth

Miscellaneous Disorders

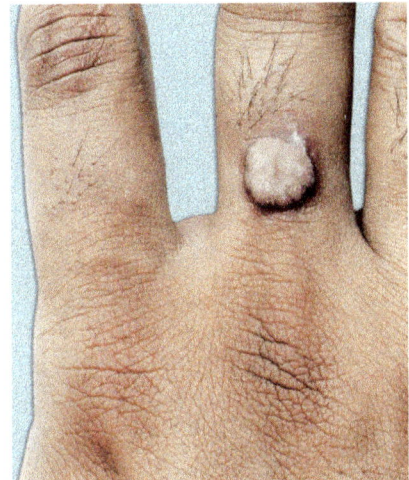

Fig. 19.5: Round nodule

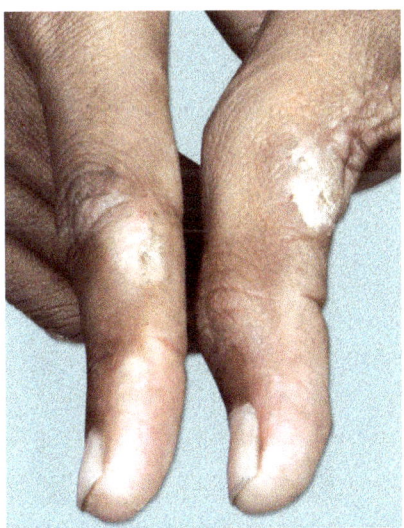

Fig. 19.6: Pressure corns and callosities on the both sides—identical lesions

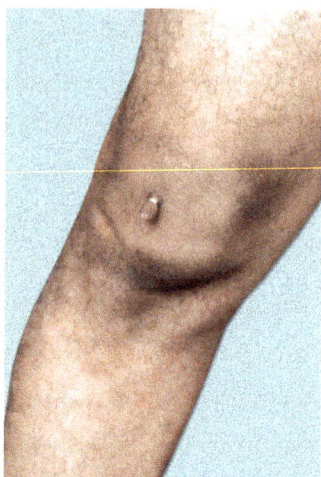

Fig. 19.7: Skin tags soft warts; acrochordons on the knee–see the hanging lesions

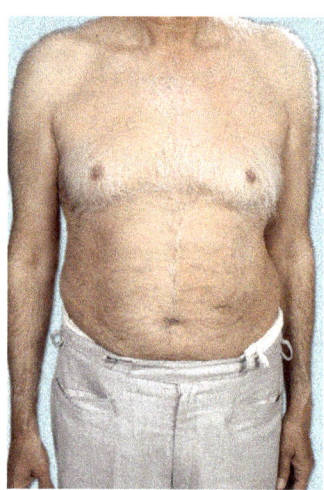

Fig. 19.8: Hypertrophic scar on the midsternum after bypass surgery—also see the racial excessive growth of hairs on the chest, shoulder and back and all over the arm

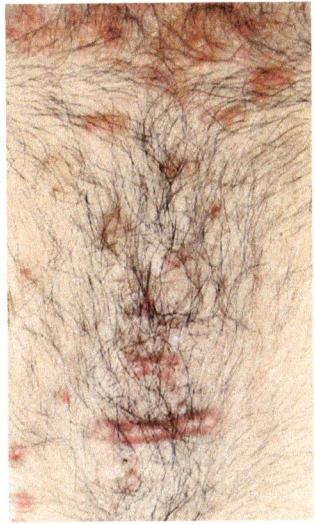

Fig. 19.9: Hypertrophic scar—see the horizontal scar

or without estrogens are used in cases with hyperplasias. Tumors must be removed.

PRURIGO MITIS

Prurigo mitis (prurigo simplex) an allergic response to bites of common insects like mosquitoes and fleas.

Vesicular and papulovesicular lesions on exposed parts (extremities and face) in children suggest this diagnosis. Treatment comprises topical steroids and avoidance of mosquito/flea bites.

APHTHOUS ULCER

Aphthae are a common causes of recurrent painful oral ulceration. Single or multiple, rounded ulcers with yellow slough over inner lips or cheeks characterize the disorder. Etiology being unknown and the condition being self limiting, the therapy is symptomatic.

MILIARIA (PRICKLY HEAT, HEAT RASH)
- Miliaria crystallina
- Miliaria rubra
- Miliaria pustulosa
- Miliaria profunda.

PRURITUS (ITCHING)

Pruritus is a sensation that evokes a desire to scratch. It may be due to skin diseases like miliaria, scabies, pediculosis, dermatophytosis, candidiasis, insect bite, allergy, urticaria, lichen planus, contact dermatitis, atopic dermatitis or seborrheic dermatitis. Systemic causes of pruritus include

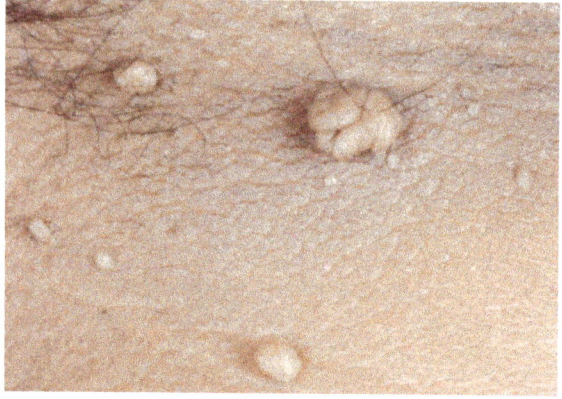

Fig. 19.10: Multiple round growths on the abdomen

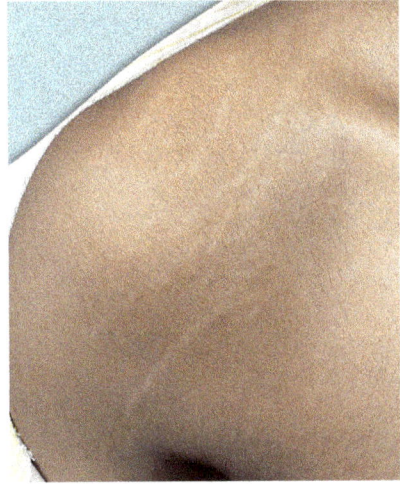

Fig. 19.11: Scratch marks—see the linear striae on the shoulder and back

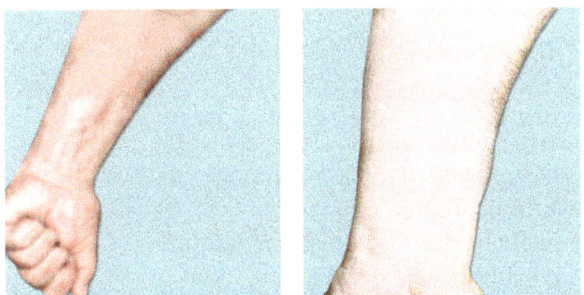

Fig. 19.12: Surgical scar after harvesting the radial artery for bypass surgery

hypothyroidism, diabetes mellitus, obstructive jaundice, lymphoma and renal failure. Oral antihistaminics (H_1 and H_2),

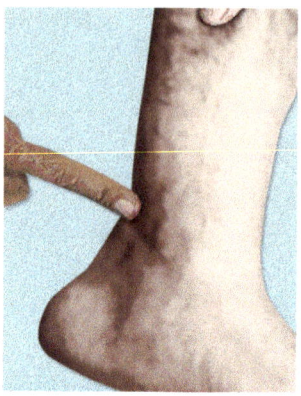

Fig. 19.13: Linear surgical scar after harvesting vein from the leg for by pass surgery

topical crotamiton and calamine lotion are useful in management which depends heavily on identification and treatment of underlying disorder.

Acquired

- Leprosy
- Drugs (clofazimine)
- Malignancies (lymphomas)
- Nutritional disorders
- Metabolic disorders (hypothyroidism)
- Systemic disease (sarcoidosis).

Ichthyosis

- Heterogeneous group of disorders (congenital and acquired)
- Fish-like scales, worse in winter.

URTICARIA, ANGIOEDEMA

Urticaria is a transient eruption characterized by circumscribed erythematous swelling in the skin. The lesions result from vasodilation of small venules and capillaries, and exudation of fluid into the superficial dermis. Angioedema is caused by a similar mechanism occurring in the deep dermis and subcutaneous tissues and is usually less pruritic and less well circumscribed. Urticaria (hives) usually occur on the trunk and proximal extremities while angioedema characteristically affects the face, hands, feet and genitalia. Involvement of the airways suggests C1 inhibitor-associated forms of angioedema. The most frequent type of acute urticaria and angioedema involve a period of less than 6 weeks in duration and occur commonly in children and young adults. In general, a younger and atopic populations is usually involved. Chronic urticaria, which lasts greater than 6 weeks in duration, peaks most commonly between the ages of 40 and 60, although children are also affected. Women are affected more commonly than men. In most studies, a specific cause is identified in less than 10% of cases.

Dermographism means 'skin waiting'. The most commonly encountered variants are immediatly simple dermographism and immediate symptomatic dermographism (factitious urticaria.

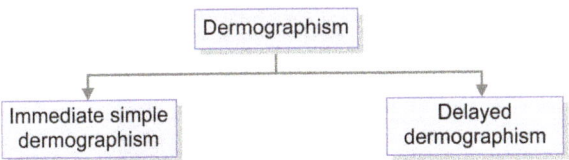

Treatment: Minimize heat and stress.
- Smoothing lotions
- Antihistaminics

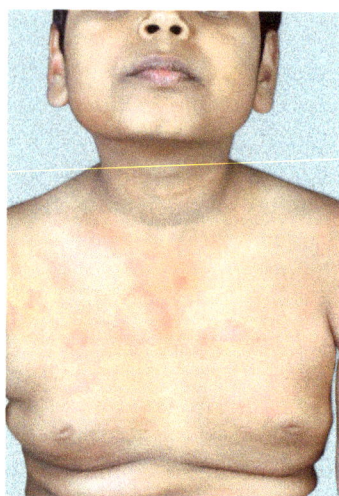

Fig. 19.14: Urticaria showing itchy erythematous wheals of various shapes and sizes—also see angioedema on the face

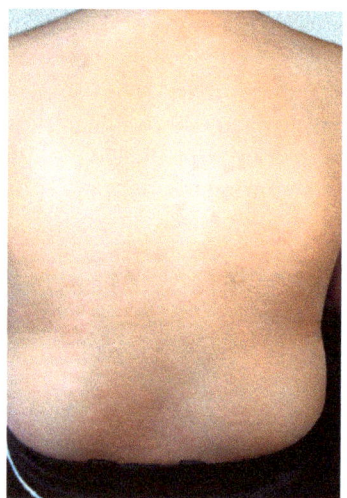

Fig. 19.15: Urticaria showing itchy erythematous wheals of various shapes and sizes on the back

Miscellaneous Disorders

Flowchart 19.1: Etiology, pathogensis and treatment of urticaria

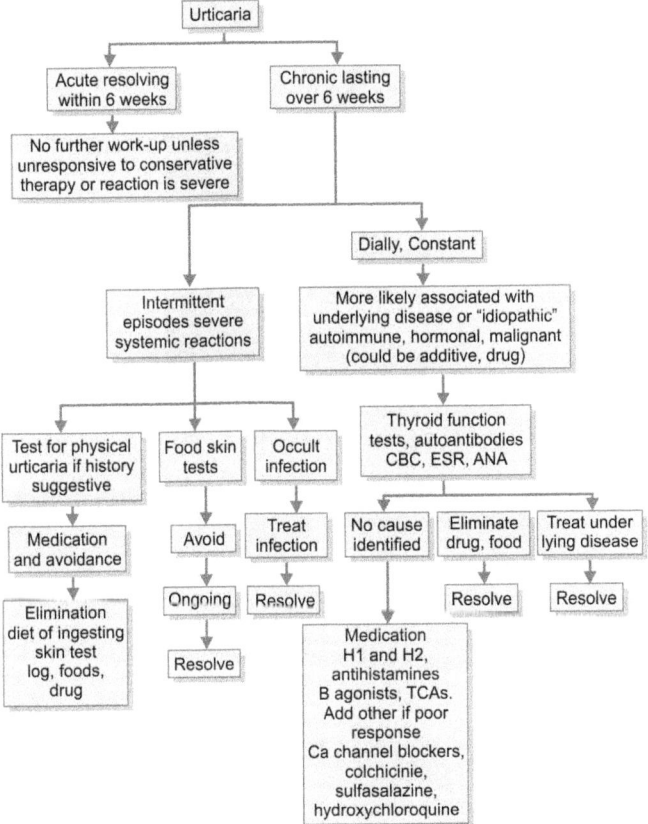

- H_1, H_2 antagonists
- Corticosteroids
- Adrenaline, in anaphylaxis.

Find out the cause and treat accordingly.

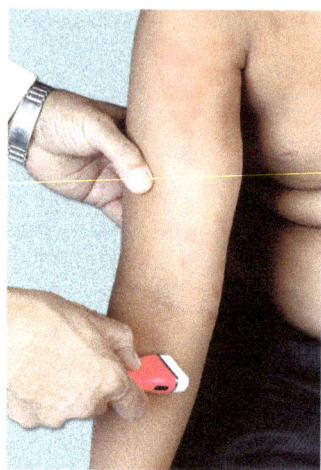

Fig. 19.16: Cold urticaria

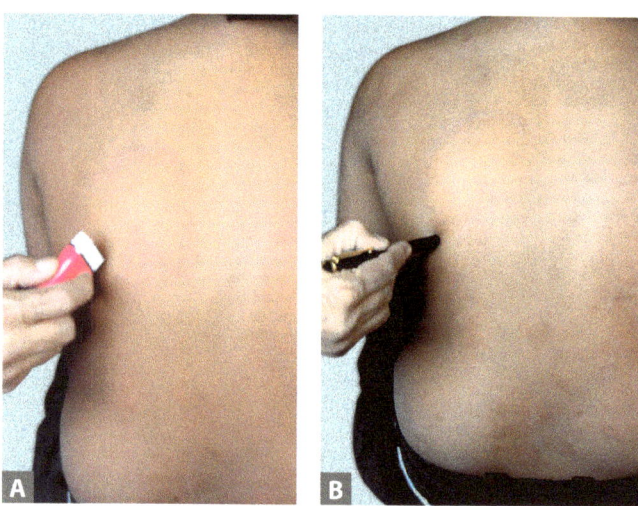

Figs 19.17A and B: Dermographism—stroking the skin with blunt metallic instrument results in an exaggerated triple response forming wheals along them

Table 19.4: Various etiological factors of acute urticaria

I. Infection	II. Drug	III. Food	IV. Food additives	V. Inhalants and contact allergens
Virus				
Hepatitis	Beta lactams	Eggs	Sodium benzoate	
Herpes	Aspirin	Peanut	Bisulfate	
Varicella-zoster	Lignocaine	Cow's milk		
Rubella	Amethocaine	Fish		
Measles	Insulin	Berries		
Mumps	Corticosteroids	Chocolates		
Epstein-Barr virus	Morphine	Mustard		
Cytomegalovirus	Quinine			
Influenza	Codeine			
Adenovirus	Curare			
Enterovirus infections	Radio contrast agents			

Flowchart 19.2: Classification of urticaria

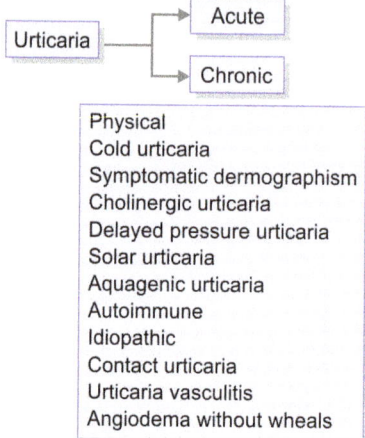

Current and Future Therapeutic Options for Management of Refractory Chronic Urticaria

Anti-inflammatory drugs

Dapsone	Studies have shown efficacy of dapsone(25–50) mg/day) in chronic urticaria/angioedema, including spontaneous CU
Sulfasalazine	Certain studies have shown efficacy and response of sulfasalazine(up to 2g/day)in CU
Hydroxychloroquine	Arandomized trail showed significant improvement in quality of life score in patients with CU treated with hydroxychloroquine, although urticaria activity scores change only marginally

	Biological
Omalizumab	Effective against different subsets of antihistamine—unresponsive CU angioedema of both autoimmune autoreactive and nonautoimmune autoreactive
Intravenous immunoglobulin	Possible therapeutic option in patients with chronic, unrimmiting urticaria with a positive autologus serum skin test and basophile histamine release assay who do not respond to other therapies
Rituximab	It destroys B cells thereby reducing antibody production including autoantibodies
Methotrexate	It is a steroid sharpening agent in recalcitrant chronic urticaria

SKIN CHANGES AND OLD AGE

Skin is effected by the general aging of the body. The basic molecular changes leading to skin aging and wrinkles are due to natural and secondary factors which lead to a breakdown of collagen, degradation of elastin polypeptides and break down in the lipidic matrix of the skin.

Formation of Wrinkles

Wrinkles is a furrow in the skin and is a natural process developed during aging. Premature wrinkles may be caused by deficiency of nutritional components in the different tissues, cellular destruction through excessive sun exposure, the effect of free radicals on the cellular membrane, and a deterioration in the genetic programming of the DNA. All this brings about the atrophy of the skin and, consequently, a general process of degeneration. Aging skin results from the passage of time, overexposure to the sun that destroys cellular ability to reproduce, lack of proper care while young, health problems and hormonal imbalances. When we express our emotions by smiling, frowning, squinting, our muscles

Flowchart 19.3: Factors affecting skin changes

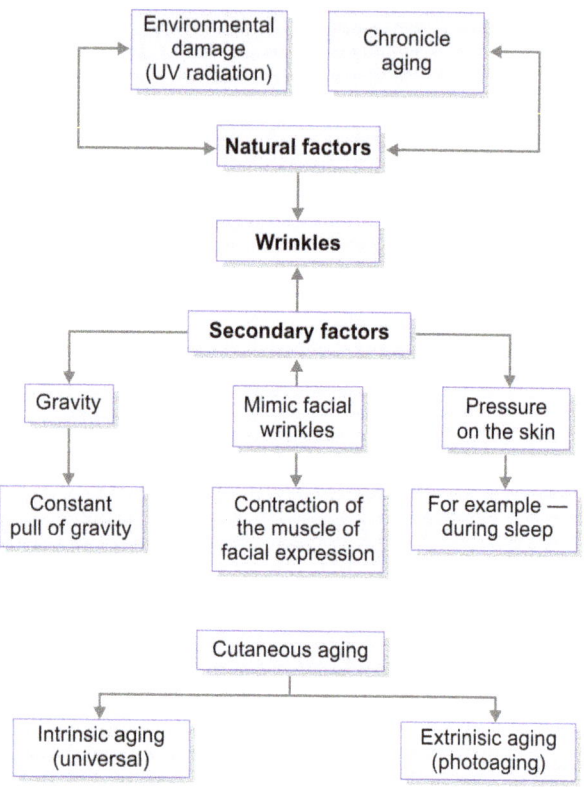

contract thousand of time every day. These movements exert tension forces to the dermis and results in formation of wrinkles around the mouth, forehead and eyes. One of the most striking signs of skin aging is the increased wrinkling of the face, neck and the area around the eyes. Wrinkles form due to the effect of constant pull of gravity over time, environment damage and continued facial expressions.

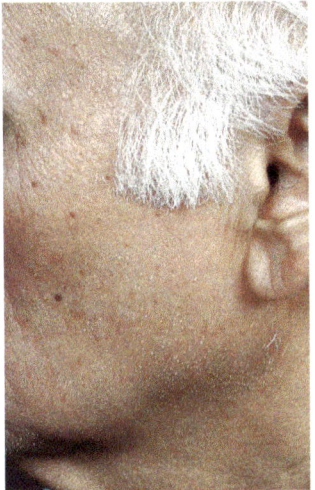 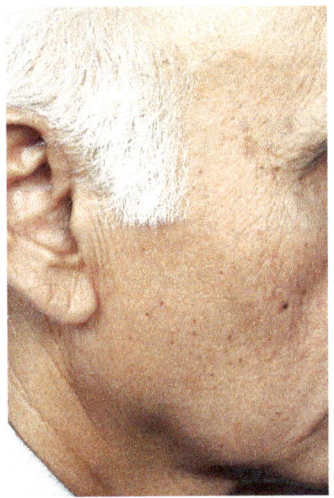

Fig. 19.18: See the aging process of the skin both external and internal signs of aging

Fig. 19.19: See the aging of the skin—sagging, hanging and wrinkles and photo marks

Treatment

1. Biorejuvenation is a common term to indicate mesotherapy for skin rejuvenation (also called biorevitalization or mesolift.

Drugs for Skin Rejuvenation

1. Hyaluronic acid alone (1.35%–3%)
2. Hyaluronic acid 0.2%, 1%, or 3%, plus other active ingredients.
3. Polynucleotide macromolecules.
4. Organic silicium.
5. Autologous cultured fibroblasts.
6. Growth factors.
7. Vitamins, amino acids, minerals, coenzymes, nucleic acids, β-glucan.

A. Injection Botox.
B. Cosmetic dermatosurgery.
C. Laser Resurfacing.
   a. High-energy, pulsed CO_2, laser.
   b. Erbium: Yttrium - aluminum - garnet (Er: YAG) laser.

HIDRADENITIS SUPPURATIVA

Table 19.5: Differential diagnosis of hidradenitis suppurativa

Early lesions	late lesions
Acne	Actinomycosis
Carbuncles	Anal fistula
Cellulitis	Cat scratch disease
Cutaneous blastomycosis	Crohn disease
Dermoid cyst	Granuloma inguinale
Erysipelas	Ischiorectal abscess
Furuncles	Lymphogranuloma venereum
Imflamed epidermoid cysts	Nocardia infection
Lymphadenopathy	Noduloulcerative syphilis
Periirectal abscess	Pilonidal disease
Pilonidal cyst	Tuberculous abscess
	Tularemia

Treatment

Key points

- There is no uniformly effective single therapy for HS; therefore, clinicians will likely have to try an array of different treatment modalities depending on the patient's disease
- For patients with extensive disease wide excision can dramatically improve the patient's quality of life
- Most of the listed therapies are ones that dermatologists possess intimate knowledge of and are thus in the best position to treat this debilitating disorder.

- **Antibiotics**
- **Retinoids**
- **Hormones**
- **Immunosuppressive and anti-inflammatory agents**
- **Neurotoxions**
- **Radiotherapy**
- **Light, radiofrequency, and other prodcedures**
- **Surgery**

Table 19.6: Treatment suggestion for hidradentis suppurativa based upon hurly stage or initial theapy

Hurly stage I disease or frist-line therapy	Stage II disease or second-line therapy	Stage III disease or third-line therapy
Antibiotics, either topic or systemic (A)	CO_2 laser ablation (A)	Radiation therapy (A)
Hormonal therapy (A)	Immunosuppressive therapies (A)	Wind excision
Retinoids (A)	Limited excisions (A)	Laying open of sinus tracts (C)
Zinc (A)	Radiation therapy (A)	
Cryotherapy (B)	Radiofrequency treatment (C)	
Botox (C)		
Radiofrequency treatment (C)		
Short-term corticosteroids		

Table 19.7: General treatment suggestion for all hidradenitis suppurativa patients regardless of hurly stage

Avoidance of tight-fitting clothing

Nonnarcotic analgesic

Reassurance

Smoking cessation

Stress management

Support group referral

Weight loss

- **Urticaria: it is rare forms**
- **Acquired angioedema [AAE]**
- **ACE inhibitor-induced angioedema**
  Episodic angioedema
- **Accompanied by eosinophilia [EAAE]**

Prophylactic use of topical silicone gel prevents prophylactic use scars and keloids.

Adams Oliver Syndrome: A Variant

A rare genetic disorder characterized by aplasia cutis congenital, variable limb defects and an associated spectrum of anomalies ranging from skin tag to lymphedema. A veriety of cranial and brain abnormalities can be described with AOS.

Extrinsic Skin Ageing Symptoms in Seafarers Subject to High Work-related Exposure to UV Radiation

The carcinogenic effect of UV radiation on the skin and eyes is well documented through experimental and epidermiological studies. While most available studies on adverse health effects of sun radiation have focus on development on skin carcinoma.

The development of photo-ageing is related to fair skin and history of long-term or intensive sun exposure. Due to repeated exposure to the sun, ability of skin to repair itself diminishes. Cigarette smoking is also known to cause biochemical change that accelerate ageing. Photogenitically, in photoageing, the repeated ultraviolet exposure breaks down collagens, induces inflammation and affect the synthesis of new collagen. Several studies have observed a significantly increased risk of photo-ageing out-door workers

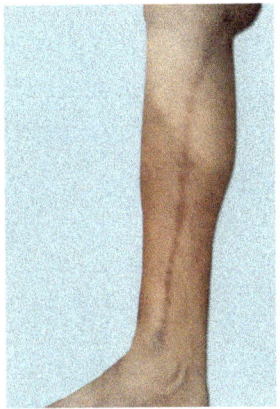

Fig. 19.20: Venous graft from leg for bypass surgery—linear scar

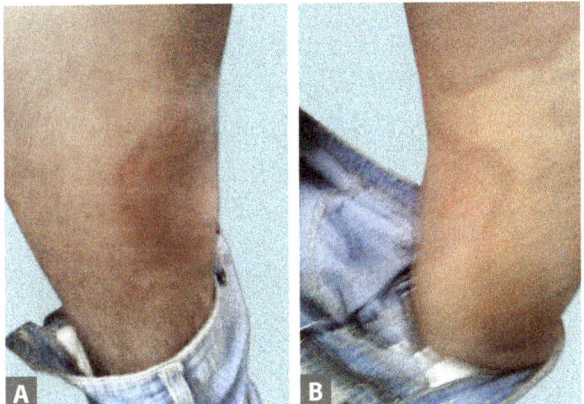

Figs 19.21A and B: Wheal thick-raised circular lesions of chronic idiopathic urticaria

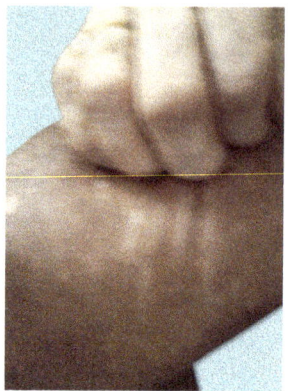

Fig. 19.22: Scratch marks

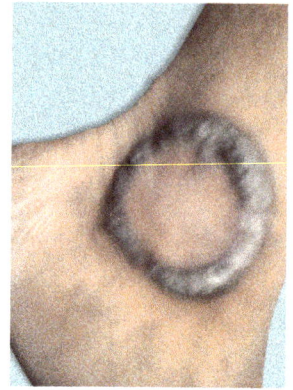

Fig. 19.23: Ringed region after artificial tattooing

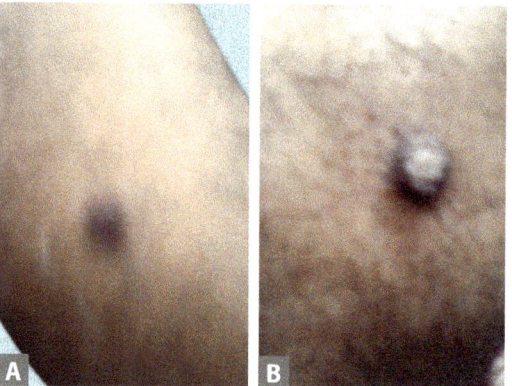

Figs 19.24A and B: Hanging growth innocent tumor

Miscellaneous Disorders

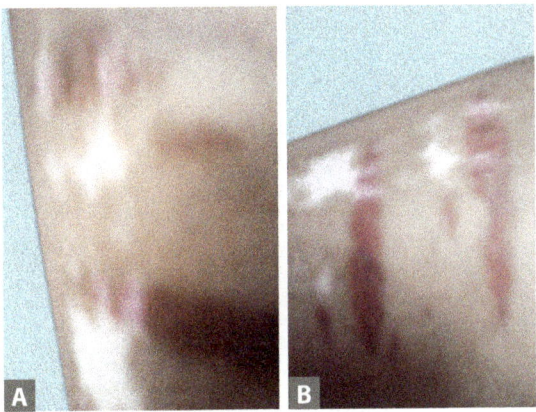

Figs 19.25A and B: Striae marks

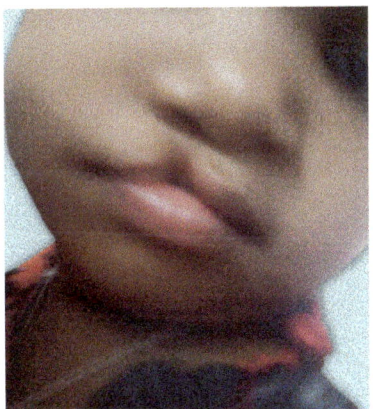

Fig. 19.26: Cleft lips

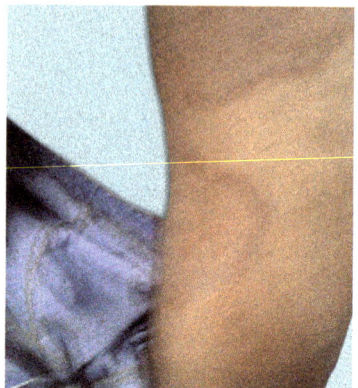

Fig. 19.27: Urticarial wheal

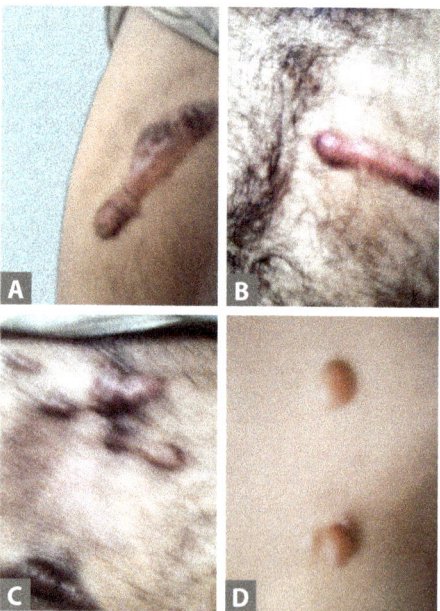

Figs 19.28A to D: Linear keloid

Miscellaneous Disorders

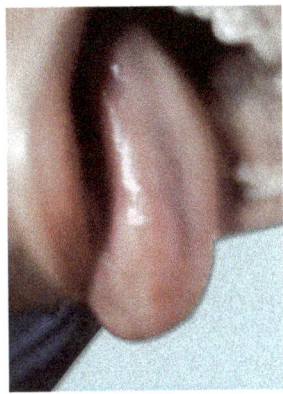

Fig. 19.29: Swelling of the lips

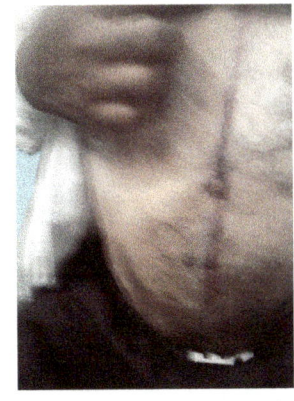

Fig. 19.30: Fungus infection of the axial. Chest showing linear mark of bypass surgery

compared to in-door workers and found a dose-effect relationship with increasing lifetime UV radiation exposure.

CHAPTER 20

Ichthyosis and Keratodermas

ICHTHYOSIS

Ichthyosis is derived from the Greek word for "fish". Ichthyosis, as dermatosis, is applied for skin disorders characterized by scaling in the absence of signs of inflammation. The ichthyotic disorders are generally inherited (and of several types) but can sometimes be acquired. These dermatoses generally worsen in winter.

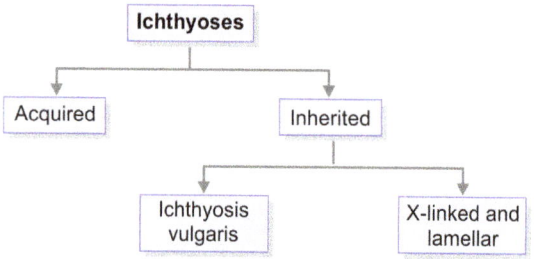

Acquired ichthyosis may result from:

(a) Infections : Leprosy, HIV infection
(b) Drugs : Cholesterol lowering agents, butyrophenones

(c) Metabolic causes : Malnutrition, essential fatty acid deficiency
(d) Systemic causes : Hypothyroidism, renal failure, anhidrosis due to neuropathies
(e) Malignancies : Hodgkin's lymphoma.

Table 20.1: Ichthyosis—causes and types

Congenital	Ichthyosis vulgaris
	X-linked ichthyosis
	Lamellar ichthyosis
	Non-bullous ichthyosiform erythroderma
	Epidermolytic hyperkeratosis
	Malignancies (lymphomas)
	Nutritional disorders
	Metabolic disorders (hypothyroidism)
	Systemic disease (sarcoidosis)

Points of focus: Ichthyosis.

Heterogeneous group of disorders (congenital and acquired).

Fish-like scales, worse in winter.

Ichthyosis Vulgaris

Etiology

A common disorder (incidence 4/1000), inherited as an autosomal dominant dermatosis.

Clinical Features

Morphology: The scales in ichthyosis vulgaris are small and branny and present on normal skin. The dryness is mild and the patients are either asymptomatic or have mild itching especially on the legs.

Distribution: The scaling is most prominent on the extensors of limbs. The major flexures are always spared.

Course: The scaling is not present at birth but usually begins during the first few years of life. Some patients may improve during adolescence, especially during the summer months and particularly if the patients moves to humid terrain.

Associated Features
- Hyperlinear palms and soles (accentuated skin creases).
- Keratosis pilaris.
- Atopic diathesis.

Complications
The dry skin chaps in winter and tolerates degreasing agents (soaps, detergents) poorly. Eczematization may complicate, especially in the presence of atopic diathesis.

Investigations
No needed.

Diagnosis
The diagnosis of ichthyosis vulgaris is based on the presence of:
- Fine branny scales.
- Characteristic distribution of scales.

Needs to be differentiated from X-linked ichthyosis on the basis of inheritance and the type and distribution of the scales (Table 20.2).

Table 20.2: Ichthyosis vulgaris and X-linked ichthyosis—how different?

	Ichthyosis vulgaris	*X-linked ichthyosis*
Sex	Both sexes	Males
Onset	First few years of life	Usually at birth
Course	May improve at adolescence	Persists
Scale	Small, branny	Larger, darker
Distribution	Extensors; flexural sparing	Generalized, encroaches flexures

Treatment

Many patients require treatment, particularly during winter months. The dryness (and the itching) is alleviated with the regular use of emollients. An array of these are available and the selection depends on individual preferences. Preparations containing urea and lactic acid are very helpful. Eczematized lesions may necessitate short courses of topical corticosteroid therapy.

Points of importance: Ichthyosis vulgaris
- Common, autosomal dominant dermatosis
- Asymptomatic (or mildly itchy) fine scaling
- Extensors of limbs, lower back. Flexures spared
- Topical emollients suffice.

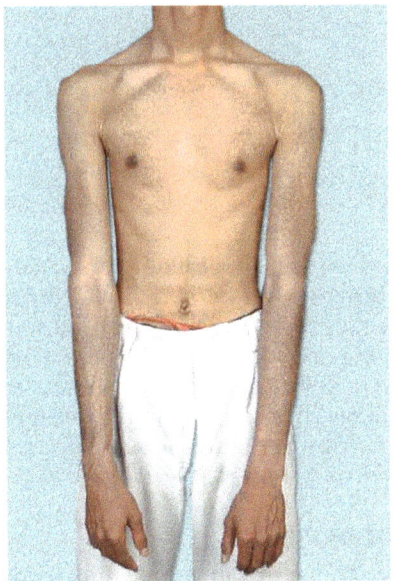

Fig. 20.1: Lamellar ichthyosis—brownish plate like scales over the trunk

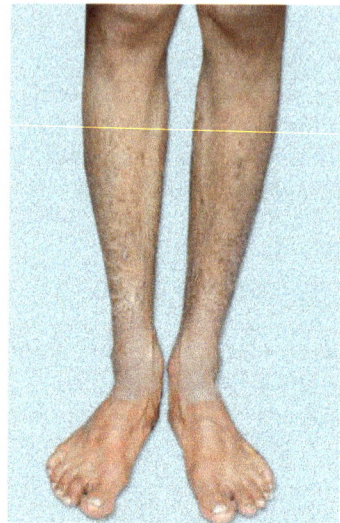

Fig. 20.2: Ichthyosis vulgaris—scaling limited to extensor aspects of limbs (skin)

X-linked Ichthyosis (Ichthyosis Nigra)

Etiology

Uncommon disorder, affecting one in 5,000 males. This variety of ichthyosis is inherited as an X-linked recessive disorder, the culprit gene being localized to the terminal part of the X-chromosome. The patients suffering from this disorder have a deficiency of the enzyme steroid sulfatase which hydrolyzes cholesterol sulfate. Since it is an X-linked disorder, in its complete form it only affects males; some female carriers may show mild scaling.

Clinical Features

Morphology: The scales in X-linked ichthyosis are large and brown, sometimes almost balck particularly in darker individuals—hence the name ichthyosis nigra.

Distribution: The involvement is generalized with no sparing of the body flexures.

Associated Features

No keratosis pilaris, hyperlinear palms, atopic diathesis. Corneal opacities may be seen.

Course: The scaling usually begins at birth and persists lifelong. The problem is generally more severe than ichthyosis vulgaris.

Investigations

None necessary; measurement of lowered steroid sulfatase in fibroblasts cultured from a skin biopsy can be done for research purposes.

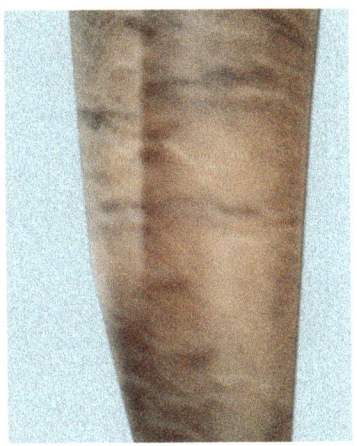

Fig. 20.3: Dry, ichthyososis and striated skin

Diagnosis

The diagnosis of X-linked ichthyosis is based on:
- Male patient
- Large, dark scales

- Involvement of extensors with encroachment of flexors
- Differentiate it form ichthyosis vulgaris.

Treatment

Topical therapeutic measures as for ichthyosis vulgaris usually suffice though they may need to be used more aggressively. Due to the benign nature of the disease and the side effects of oral retinoids, these are best avoided.

CHAPTER 21

Leprosy (Hansen's Disease)

"Leprosy work is not merely medical relief, it is transforming frustration in life into the joy of dedication, personal ambition into selfless service."

— **Rashtrapita Mahatma Gandhi**

Mycobacterium leprae, the causative organism of leprosy, in spite of being one of the earliest described (1872) pathogenic bacteria in humans, has not yet been grown in the laboratory. It can be grown in foot pads of mice, to a limited extent and can cause disseminated infection in 9-banded armadillos (South American Anteaters.)

M. leprae multiplies very slowly, doubling time being 14 days, compared to minutes or hour for most bacteria. The latter feature is responsible for the unusually long incubation period (2-10 years) and extremely slow evolution of the disease.

■ MODE OF TRANSMISSION

Contrary to popular belief, leprosy is not transmitted by skin to skin contact but by droplet infection. Nasal droplets of patients with lepromatous leprosy contain thousands of bacilli. However, most patients with leprosy have negative nasal smears and are therefore non-infectious.

INCUBATION PERIOD

Usually 3-5 years.

PREVALENCE

Of the total number of estimated leprosy cases in the world in 1994 (2.4 million), about 30% are in India. The prevalence of leprosy in India is between 1-2 per 1000 persons. The rate is higher (3-5/1000) in states like West Bengal, Orissa, Bihar; intermediate (1-2/1000) in Maharashtra, Tamil Nadu, Andhra Pradesh and low (0.1-1/1000) in punjab, Haryana, Rajasthan. Mumbai has a higher rate of about 3-5 per 1000.

CLASSIFICATION OF LEPROSY BASED ON CLINICAL, MICROBIOLOGIC, PATHOLOGIC AND IMMUNOLOGIC PARAMETERS

Indeterminate

Clinical

One or two, poorly defined, hypopigmented, slightly erythematous, macules or patches, generally smaller than 5 cm in diameter, with partial or no loss of sensation or sweating, usually over face or extremities of children are typical.

Bacteriology

Usually negative.

Histopathology

There is no granuloma; only sparse perivascular, periappendageal and peri and intraneural infiltrate of lymphocytes.

Immunology

Lepromin negative.

Tuberculoid (TT)

Clinical

One or two, well defined, hypopigmented or erythematous atrophic patches or plaques, smaller then 10 cm in diameter

Table 21.1: Classification of lepra reactions

Type I	Type II
Occurs in borderline leprosy.	Occurs in LL or leprosy.
Type IV	**Type III**
Hypersensitivity cell-mediated immunity.	Hypersensitivity immune complex disease (humoral immunity).
Change in pro-protective immunity either for better (upgrading from BL to BT) or for worse (downgrading from BT to BL)	No change in protective immunity. Patient's laprosy type does not change.
Common during first 6 months of beginning therapy when immunity is boosted with anti-leprosy treatment.	Common after first 6 months of initiating therapy when antigen relased from killed bacilli forms circulating immune complexes.
No or mild constitutional disturbance.	Severe constitutional symptoms and signs (fever, arthralgia, bodyache prostrataion) common.
Existing skin lesions change (lesions show erythema, edema hyperesthesia)	Existing lesions unaltered.
New lesions uncommon	New lesions (called erythema nodosum leprosum) occur as a rule and appear as crops of transient (last 3–10 days), red tender, dermal or subcutaneous nodules over face and extremities.

(commonly 3–5 cm), with a dry surface are noted over extremities or face. Sensations are totally lost or severely affected. Sweating is absent. A cutaneous nerve or a nerve trunk in the vicinity may be enlarged.

- **Borderline tuberculoid (BT)**
- **Mid-borderline (borderline borderline) BB**
- **Borderline lepromatus (BL)**
- **Lepromatus leprosy (LL)**

Neuritis is common to both types of reactions and manifests as pain, numbness, sensory loss, muscle weakness, deformity and tenderness in the region of affected nerve trunks.

Edema of hands/feet uncommon	Common
Other systems unaffected	Systemic affection commonly includes iritis, arthritis, periostitis, orchitis, glomerulonephritis and lymphadenitis.
Blood analysis normal	Raised (ESR, polymorphs) IgG, IgM, complement, circulating immune complexes.

Treatment of Lepra Reactions

Type I reaction: Sudden edema and erythema of existing lesions of leprosy with or without pain indicate type I reaction. Neuritis of the nerve trunk in the vicinity is common. Type I reaction signifies change in immune status for better (within 6 months of initiating therapy) or for worse (lack of treatment). Neuritis is an indication for systemic steroid treatment which avoids nerve damage.

Type II reaction: Reaction tends to begin 6 months after initiating therapy for leprosy and is due to immune complex deposition. Crops of symmetrical, tender, bright red nodules

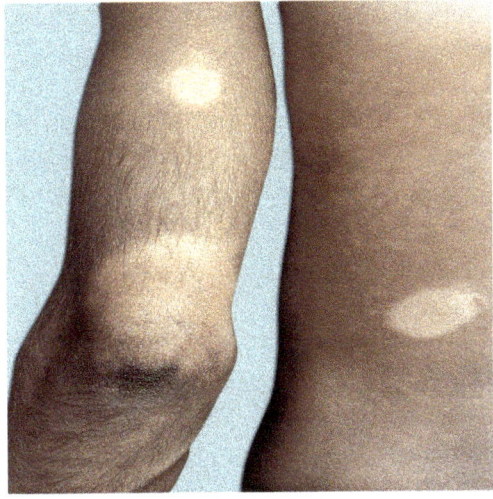

Fig. 21.1: Well-defined scaly and numb patches of paucibacillary leprosy

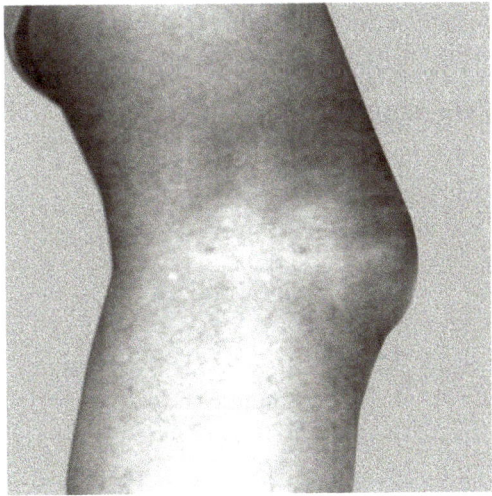

Fig. 21.2: A patch of maculo-anesthetic leprosy

and plaques occur over face and extremities (erythema nodosum leprosum). Lesions are transient lasting 2–10 days but new crops appear with severe constitutional disturbance. Neuritis may lend to nerve palsies. Iritis, orchitis, periostitis, myositis are common. High dose systemic steroids, instituted promptly and tapered gradually, avoid damage to nerves and organs.

Steps in disability prevention include:
(a) Identify patients at risk
(b) Give preventive advice
(c) Be alert to early warning signs
(d) Treat neuritis promptly
(e) Physical therapy during neuritis.

Correction of Deformities due to Leprosy

For the purpose of management, mobile deformities due to lepro can be divided into early deformities, mobile deformities and fixed deformities.

Treatment Regimes

- MDT regime

  ROM: Single dose of ROM—rifampicin 600 mg, ofloxacin 400 mg and minocycline 100 mg.
New regimes of short duration
1. RMM
2. U-MDT

Monthly administered ROM for MB and PB leprosy.

Quadruple Regime: Rifampicin (600 mg) + Ofloxacin (400 mg) + Clofazamine (100 mg) + minocycline (100 mg).

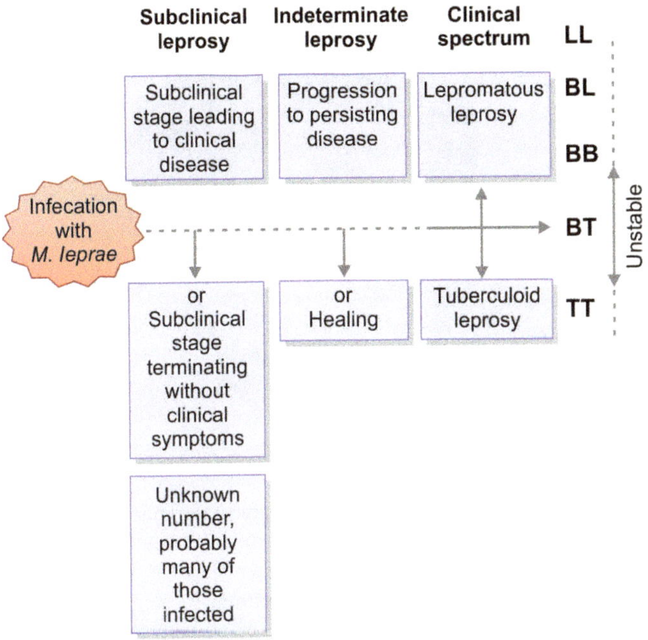

Leprosy (Hansen's Disease)

	Subclinical leprosy	Indeterminate leprosy	Clinical spectrum	
				LL
	Subclinical stage leading to clinical disease	Progression to persisting disease	Lepromatous leprosy	BL
				BB
Infecation with *M. leprae*				BT
	or Subclinical stage terminating without clinical symptoms	or Healing	Tuberculoid leprosy	TT
	Unknown number, probably many of those infected			

Fig. 21.3: The course after infection with *Mycobacterium leprae*

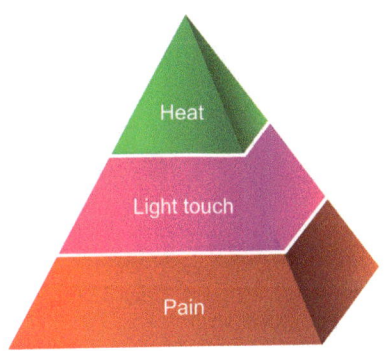

Fig. 21.4: The three cardinal diagnostic signs of leprosy

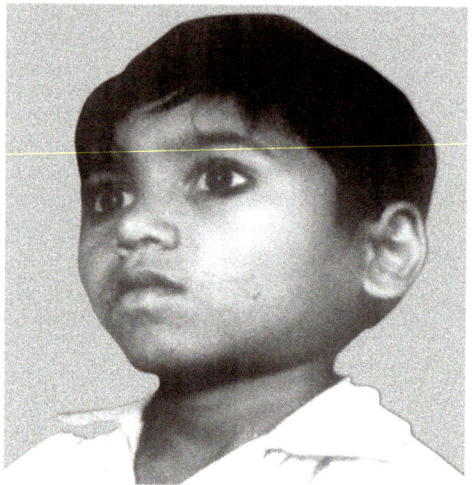

Fig. 21.5: Patch of paucibacillary on the cheeck

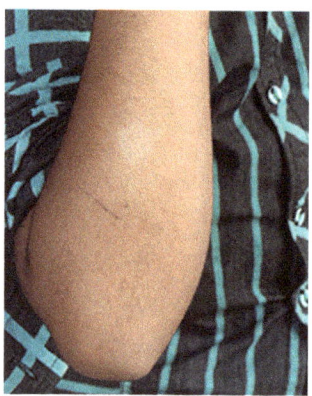

Fig. 21.6: Leprosy—single hypopigmented, anesthetic patch on arms

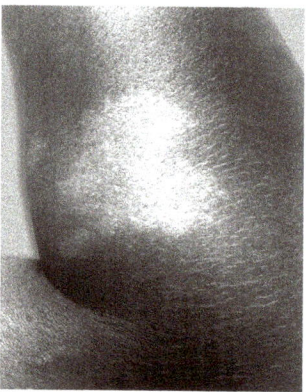

Fig. 21.7: Maculo-anesthetic patch on elbow

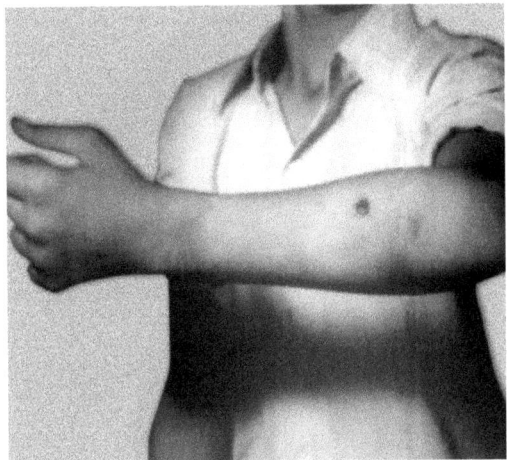

Fig. 21.8: Tuberculoid leprosy patch on the arm

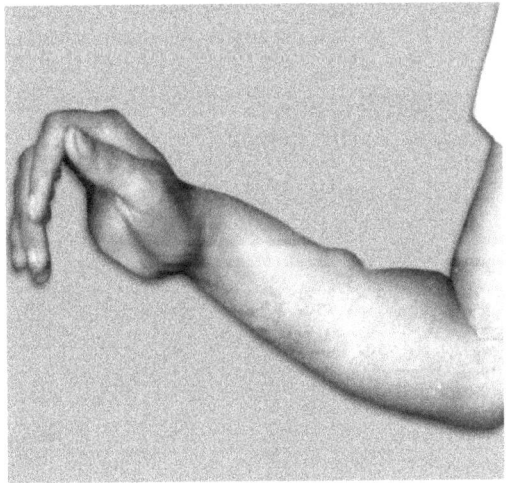

Fig. 21.9: Neuritic leprosy affecting ulnar

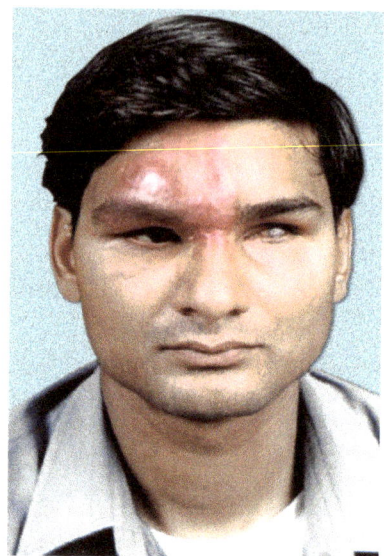

Fig. 21.10: Type 1 lepra reaction—the previously existing skin lesion over the face had become erythematous and edematous

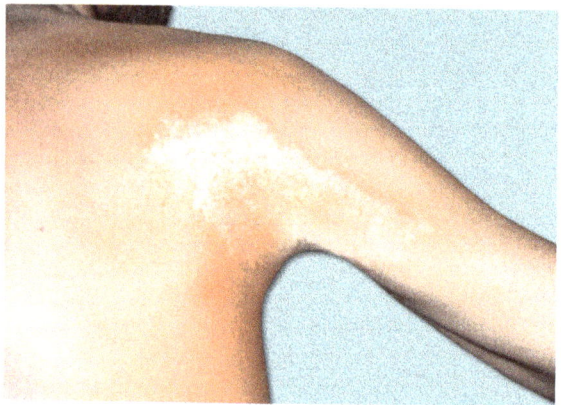

Fig. 21.11: Tuberculoid patch of leprosy on the back

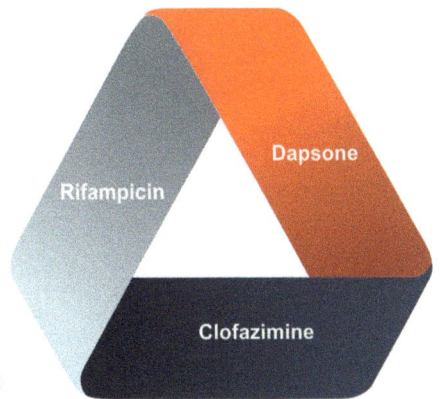

Fig. 21.12: Principal anti-leprosy drug

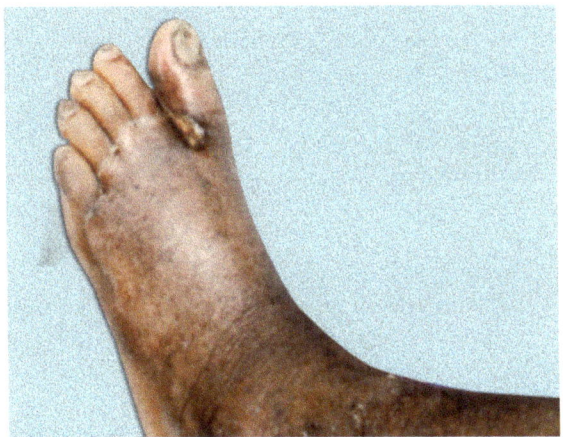

Fig. 21.13: Ulcer on the foot swelling and loss of sensation on the foot

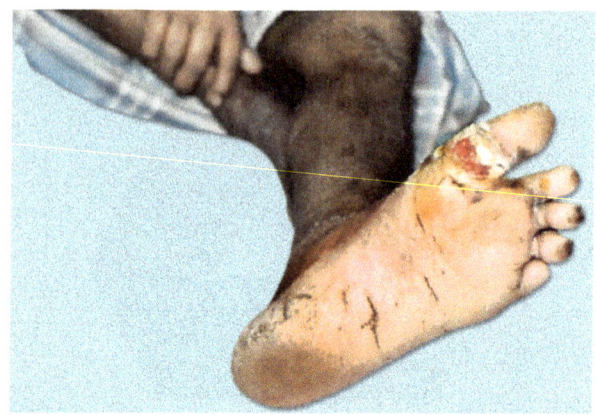

Fig. 21.14: Trophic ulcers on the sole and toes of the foot

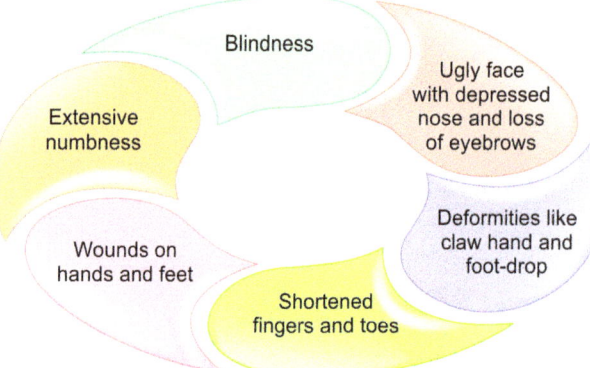

Fig. 21.15: Consequences of neglected and untreated leprosy

Leprosy (Hansen's Disease)

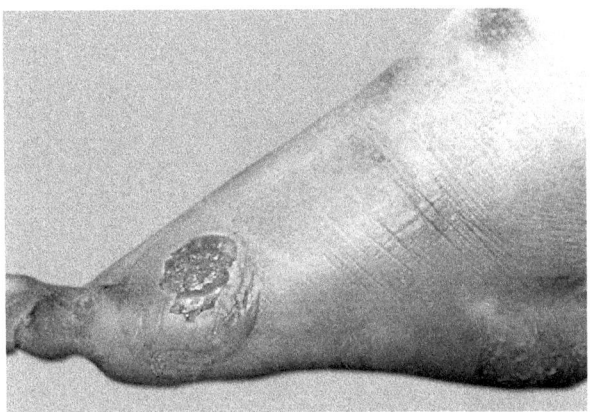

Fig. 21.16: Trophic ulcer and swelling on the foot due to leprosy

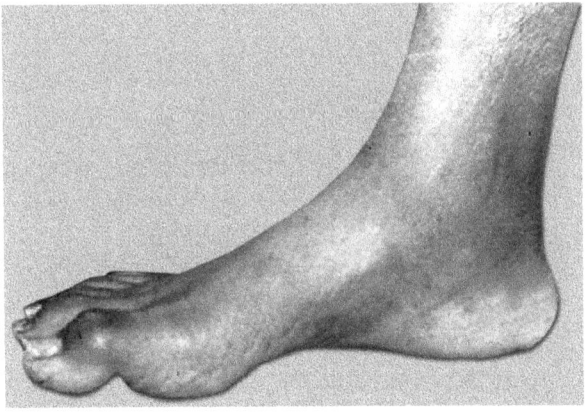

Fig. 21.17: Deformity on the foot due to leprosy

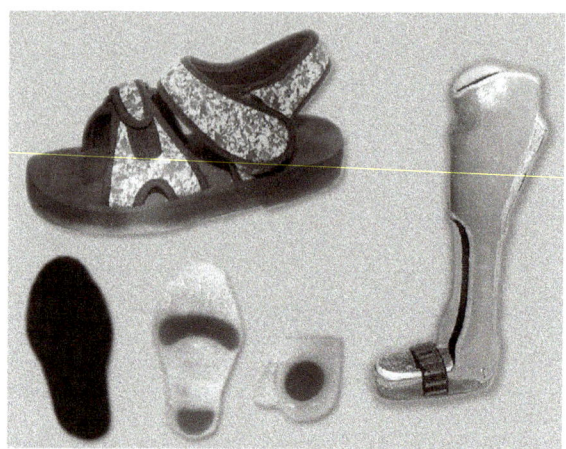

Fig. 21.18: Appliances use in leprosy deformities

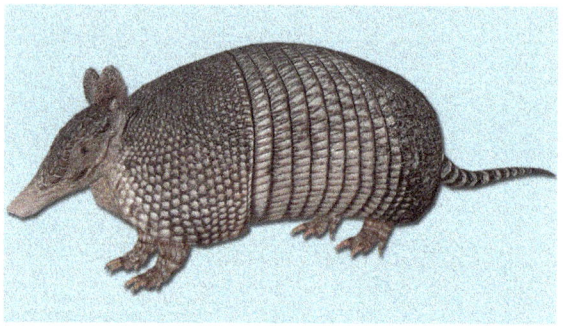

Fig. 21.19: 7-banded Armadillo, experimental animal used in leprosy research and leprosy vaccine

Prevention of Leprosy

1. Isolation
2. Chemoprophylaxis
3. Immunoprophylaxis
4. BCG
5. Armadillo-derived vaccine
6. Vaccines derived from cultivable mycobacteria.

Table 21.2: Recent advances in leprosy: Leprosy updates

New investigative techniques	New drugs and vaccines in leprosy
1. Chemical methods	1. Fluoroquinolones
2. Immunological methods	2. Minocycline (tetracyclines)
3. Molecular biological techniques	3. Clarithromycin (macrolides)
4. DNA targeting probes	4. Ansamycins
5. RNA targeting probes	5. Dihydrofolate reductase inhibitors
6. Gene amplification methods	6. Fusidic acid
7. Techniques to determine viability, drug susceptibility or resistance	7. Beta–lactam antibiotics
8. Bioluminescent techniques	*Immunotherapy and vaccines in leprosy*
9. Molecular methods for determination of viability and drug resistance	1. BCG vaccine
10. Techniques for eliciting strain differentiation for molecular epidemiology	2. *M. leprae* + BCG vaccine
11. Arbitrary primer amplification method	3. MW vaccine
12. Amplified—ribosomal DNA finger printing	4. ICRC vaccine
13. Strain specific probes	

Control of Leprosy

1. Case detection
2. Case holding, including treatment
3. Health education of the public and the patients
4. Implications of AIDS and HIV infections on leprosy control.

Rehabilitation in Leprosy

1. Prevention of deformity
2. Education of the community and the patient
3. Leprosy village and colonies
4. Capital intensive programs
5. Other rehabilitation program
6. Vocational training
7. Sheltered workshops
8. Crippled patients
9. Grip-aids.

CHAPTER 22

Sexually Transmitted Diseases

DEFINITION
Sexually transmitted diseases (STDs) are a group of contagious diseases transmitted through sexul contact.

The principal STDs include:
- Syphilis
- Gonorrhea
- Chancroid
- Donovanosis
- Lymphogranuloma venereum
- Herpes simplex
- Condyloma acuminata.

Genital infection due to:
- *Chlamydia*
- *Candida*
- *Trichomonas vaginalis*
- Hepatitis B
- HIV infection
- Public louse
- Scabies.

Prevention of STDs (Counseling for STD Patients)

This has assumed great importance in recent times with the emergence of HIV infection.

The various measures that can be advised include:
1. Abstinence from sex—impossible for most people.
2. Avoid sex with commercial sex workers because the chance of their being a carrier for STDs especially. HIV infection, is very high (60% of commercial sex workers in Mumbai are HIV Positive).
3. Restrict to one sexual partner. Avoid casual sex with someone whose antecedents are unknown.
4. If you must, then use a good quality condom every time. Learn how to use a condom in a proper way. Some of the spermicidal jellies (e.g. nonoxynol-9) are also active against bacteria and viruses.
5. After sex, pass urine after intercourse and wash genitalia as soon as possible with plenty of water and soap.
6. Prophylactic use of antibacterials like cotrimoxazole or tetracycline after an unprotected exposure is controversial. In any event, it is not useful for prevention against HIV.
7. Sex education forms an essential part of prevention of STDs. As it is only through such discussion that advice regarding condom usage, can be disseminated to the young.
8. Today, improving awareness about STDs in the community, with special reference to HIV infection, is a national priority. Prior knowledge of the far reaching medical and social consequences of HIV infection will go a long way in reducing risk taking behavior in the young.
9. *Pre-test counseling:* This refers to talking to persons with a history of activities with high risk for HIV infection (most commoly, unsafe sex) before doing a screening test (ELISA) for HIV infection. A little knowledge about

HIV infection with respect to its mode of transmission unique nature, virtual incurability and fatal outcome is necessary for all persons with a history of unsafe sex, even if they have never had any other STD. They must also be told about the fact the proper use of condom can prevent transmission of HIV infection. Without such information (and consent during the Elisa test) sceering test for HIV infection should not be performed.

Important sexually transmitted diseases include HIV infection, syphilis, gonorrhea, chancroid, donovanosis, lymphogranuloma venereum, herpes simplex, condyloma acuminata/non-gonococcal urethritis, hepatitis B, pediculosis pubis and scabies. Prevention of STDs is extremely important in the HIV era. Restricting to one sexual partner and, if this is impossible, use of condom during each and every unsafe intercourse are the two most important behavioral changes that need to be integrated into lifestyle in order to protect from HIV infection.

Vertical Transmission of STDs

- Syphilis
- Gonorrhea
- Herpes simplex
- Chlamydial infection
- HIV infection
- Condyloma acuminata

Vertical transmission of STDs refers to transmission from mother to her progeny either transplacentally, intrapartum or through breast milk. Most important STDs that are transmitted are syphilis (transplacental) herpes genitalis (intrapartum) and HIV infection (all 3 ways) vertical transmission of syphilis can cause abortion, stillbirth or congenital syphilis. That of HIV results in pediatric AIDS that is usually fatal in early childhood. Transmission of herpes genitalis induces disseminated neonatal herpes infection that has high morbidity and mortality.

SYPHILIS

Acquired Syphilis

Acquired syphilis is sexually transmitted. After an incubation period of about 2-4 weeks, if untreated, it passes through primary, secondary stages and may later go into the tertiary stage. The first two years of infection are termed early syphilis (infectious) and the later part called late syphilis (non-infectious).

Primary Syphilis

A primary sore (hard chancre) and regional lymphadenopathy are the clinical components. Signs and symptoms regress spontaneously in 2-6 weeks even without therapy.

Primary syphilis consists of a chancre and regional lymphadenopathy. The hard chancre is seen as a single, painless rounded, indurated ulcer, with pale granulation and serosanguinous discharge in the floor and which does not bleed on manipulation. Smear for dark ground microscopy demonstrates treponemes. Serum VDRL is positive later in the course of the ulcer. Therapy is that of early syphilis.

Secondary Syphilis

Secondary syphilis presents with mucocutaneous lesions, generalized nontender, shotty lymphadenopathy, arthralgia and fever. The lesions are nonpruritic, symmetric, widespread and dull red in color. Deep dermal tenderness is positive over the skin lesions which may be macular papular, papulosquamous, pustular, acne form or annular. Condyloma lata mucous patches are the moist lesions that occur over genitalia, flexures, mucocutaneous junctions and mucosae.

Dark ground illumination for treponemes from the moist lesions and positive serology (VDRL test or a specific test like TPHA) establish the diagnosis. Procaine penicillin (fortified) 8 lac IU IM OD for 10 days is curative. For HIV positive persons the dose is 24 lac IU IM OD for 14 days. Tetracycline or erythromycin can be given (500 mg QDS for 30 days) in case of penicillin hypersensitivity.

Latent Syphilis

Infection with *T. pallidum* may persist without causing any signs or symptoms and may be detected during accidental screening. According to whether the infection is acquired during the first two years of infection or later, it is termed as early latent or late latent syphilis.

Benign tertiary syphilis of the skin and mucoase presents as painless, indolent single or few, indurated plaques or noduloulcerative lesions with annular or serpiginous outline. Spontaneous healing leads to tissue paper scarring face, head, nasal and oropharyngeal mucosae are frequently affected. Diagnosis can be confirmed with serologic tests and skin biopsy. Therapy is that of late syphilis.

Cardiovascular and Neurosyphilis (Quaternary Syphilis)

Diagnosis of syphilis depends on demonstraton of either the organisms (by dark ground illumination from smears of moist lesions) or the antibodies to it. VDRL test is the commonest used screening test for syphilis. However, it can give false positive results and hence sometimes its results may need to be confirmed with specific tests like TPHA and FTA-ABS test. A VDRL titer of 1:8 usually indicates infection, if the clinical findings coincide. After therapy, VDRL titer falls gradually and this is useful for monitoring the response. Skin biopsy is rarely needed for diagnosis. It shows a lymphoplasmocytic and histiocytic infiltrate. CSF studies may be done in cases of late syphilis.

Therapy of Syphilis

Penicillin injections, after test dose, is the treatment of choice for syphilis. While a single injection of benzathine penicillin, 2.4 MU IM ATD can be used for early syphilis in HIV negative, it should be avoided in others. Procaine penicillin, 8 lac IU IM OD ATD for HIV negative and 24 lac IU for HIV positive for 10-14 days is the preferred therapy. For persons with late syphilis, unless CFS studies rule out asymptomatic neurosyphilis. For persons with penicillin hypersensitivity, oral erythromycin or tetracyline, 500 mg QDS for 30 days can be used, After treatment, patients need to be followed up every 3 months with a serum VDRL to ensure a cure.

Congenital Syphilis

Treponemes cross the placenta from an infected mother to the fetus after the first trimester. Routine antenatal screening of mothers with a serum VDRL test is advised to prevent this dangerous possibility.
1. Clinical implication
2. Early congenital syphilis
3. Late congenital syphilis
4. Stigmata of congenital syphilis

Clinical Implication

Therapy of syphilis during pregnancy : Prompt institution of therapy is important. Avoid drugs other than penicillin because they are either contraindicatd (e.g. tetracyclines) or have poor penetration across the placenta (e.g. erythromycin). Avoid benzathine penicillin because it does not cross placenta very well. If any of these are used, it is mandatory to treat the body at birth.

Severity of this transplacental infection varies according to the duration of infection in the mother. Older the infection, milder the affection. Thus, this may cause abortion or stillbirth (in severest infections) or present as congenital syphilis at birth or later in infancy or childhood (in mildest infections).

Early Congenital Syphilis

During the first two years of life, the infection is termed as early congenital syphilis (infectious). Most common age of presentation is between 2–6 months and the complaints: low birth weight, failure to thrive, weak or hoarse cry, persistent rhinitis with or without epistaxis, generalized lymphadenopathy, hepatosplenomegaly, fever, pseudoparalysis due to metaphysitis and a mucocutaneous eruption similar to secondary syphilis in adults. Syphilitic dactylitis, choroiditis and meningoencephalitis are uncommon. Diagnosis can be confirmed by a smear for treponemes obtained from wet

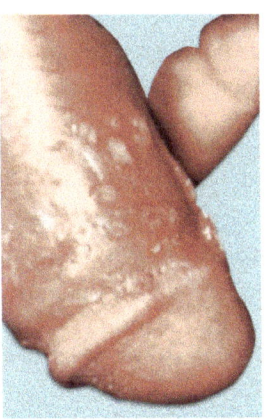

Fig. 22.1: Syphilis—painless indurated clean ulcers on the glans penis

mucosal lesions. A high titer of VDRL test (especially when this is compared to mother's VDRL titer) is usual. Specific tests like TPHA are also positive. X-ray of painful long bones (esp. tibia) may show metaphysitis. Therapy comprises procaine penicillin 50000 IU per kg body weight IM OD after test dose for 10 days. Benzathine penicillin 50000 IU IM single dose (half in each buttock) can also be used but is not preferred due to improper absorption and poor penetration into CSF.

Late Congenital Syphilis

This is now rare. After the first two years of life, the infection is called late congenital syphilis (non-infectious). Mucocutaneous lesions resemble those of late acquired syphilis. Interstitial keratitis occurs after 6 years of age and if not treated with steroids, may lead to blindness. Clutton's joints represent an arthritis with joint effusion that does not revert after antisyphilitic therapy. Persistent periosteitis leads to periosteal thickening (sabre tibia). Neurolabyrinthitis results in eighth nerve deafness, vertigo and tinnitus. Interstitial keratitis, eighth nerve deafness and Hutchinson's teeth are collectively termed as Hutchinson's triad that is diagnostic of late congenital syphilis.

Diagnosis depends on clinical features, through obstetric history, examination and investigation of mother and father and a positive serum VDRL or TPHA. Therapy is similar to acquired late syphilis.

Stigmata of Congenital Syphilis

These are residual of the post-inflammatory processes due to congenital syphilis and hence may be seen in untreated and treated patients for the rest of their lives. Some popular stigmate include Hutchinson's teeth (peg shaped incisors), mulberry molars, depressed bridge of nose, frontal bossing and rhagades.

Transplacental transmission of syphilis leads to with decreasing severity of infection, either abortion, stillbirth, congenital syphilis at birth or later. Most cases are daignosed during the first two years of life (early congenital syphilis). This manifests as low birth weight, failure to thrive, rhinitis, hoarse cry, hepatosplenomegaly, skin rash resembling secondary syphilis and painful limbs due to metaphysitis. Diagnosis depends on clinical features and demonstration of treponemes and a positive serology. Treatment consists of procaine penicillin 50000 IU/kg body weight IM OD ATD for 10 days.

URETHRITIS

Gonococcal urethritis is still the commonest cause of urethritis in India. Other organisms that may cause urethritis (non-gonococcal urethritis) include chlamydia, mycoplasma, trichomonas and candida. Uncommonly when urethritis is not due to any specific infectious cause it is termed as non-specific urethritis. Due to the longer length and type of cells lining the male urethra, urethritis is much more common and symptomatic in the males.

Proctitis, pharyngitis following anal or oral sex and disseminated gonococcal infection can occur in both sexes. Disseminated infection may present in the septicemic phase or the later, arthritic phase.

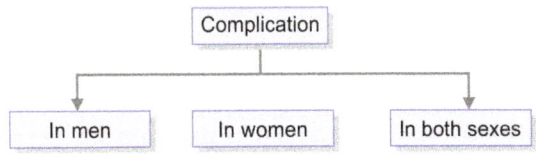

Gonorrhea presents most commonly as an acute uncomplicated urethritis in males. A promiscuous young adult complains of burning while passing urine and purulent discharge per urethra. Examination reveals thick, profuse, purulent urethral discharge. In women, it present as gonococcal cervicitis with or without asymptomatic urethritis. Diagnosis can be confirmed with smear and culture of urethral or endocervical discharge. Complications in women, bartholinitis, salpingitis, pelvic inflammatory disease and infertility are common complications.

Treatment of Gonorrhea

Uncomplicated gonorrhea in men responds well to either single dose norfloxacin 800 mg or to ciprofloxacin 500 mg/day for 3 days. Other drugs like kanamycin 2 g IM or ceftriaxone 500 mg IM also work well in a single dose. For women, although single dose therapy may be nearly as effective multiple dose regimes are preferred because of chances of serious complications norfloxacin, ciprofloxacin or clavulanate potentiated amoxicillin, all for 5 days duration, are effective in females.

Diagnosis of Urethritis

Urethritis is symptomatic in males and a frequently silent in females. Clinically, profuse purulent urethral discharge and a short incubation period favors gonorrhea whereas its absence indicates other organisms. More than 5 pus cell per hpf in early morning urine indicates urethritis. Smear and culture of material (urethral discharge or scraping in males and endocervical discharge in females) is required to establish the diagnosis of gonorrhea (Gram stain, Thayer Martin medium), chlamydial (Giemsa stain, tissue culture) or mycoplasmal (Gram stain, tissue culture) infections.

- Non-gonococcal urethritis
- Chlamydial urethritis
- Mycoplasmal urethritis

NON-GONOCOCCAL URETHRITIS

Any urethritis that is not caused by gonococci is included under this title. Common causes of non-gonococcal urethritis are *Chlamydia trachomatis* and *Mycoplasma* (ureaplasma urealyticum). Other organisms like herpes simplex, gram negative bacilli (*E. coli, Proteus, Klebsiella*), *Trichomonas, Candida* and condyloma acuminata (human papilloma virus) occasionally cause urethritis.

Chlamydia Urethritis

This is the most common cause of non-gonococcal urethritis and is important because it can cause female genital infections and all its accompanying complications (including sterility and ectopic pregnancy) similar to gonorrhea.

Mycoplasma Urethritis

Although the pathogenic status of these organisms was doubted for many years, now with increasing reports of this

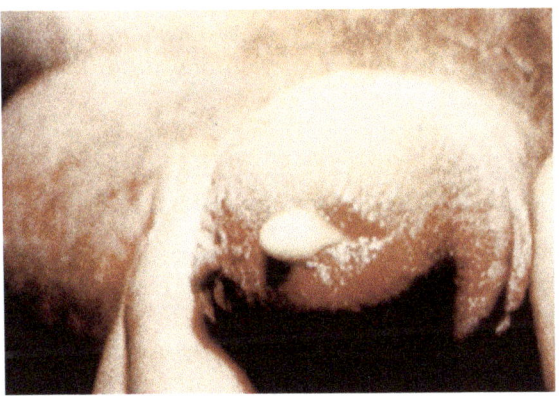

Fig. 22.2: Gonorrhea

infection in males and females (with resultant complications) it is an established condition.

Please see 'Diagnosis of Urethritis' for further details on clinical features and investigations in non-gonococcal urethritis.

Therapy

Erythromycin 500 mg QDS for 10 days or doxycycline 100 mg BD for 7-10 days are effective against both these common non-gonococcal pathogens. Alternatively tetracycline 500 mg QDS for 10-14 days can also be given. Co-trimoxazole (2 tabs BD for 10 days) is effective against *Chlamydia* but not against *Mycoplasma*.

Urethrtis due to non-gonococcal causes is termed as non-gonococcal urethritis. Common causes are *Chlamydia trachomatis* and *Mycoplasma*. Unusual causes include herpes genitalis, candidiasis, trichomoniasis and secondary to upper urinary tract infection. Diagnosis is suspected when a male presents with burning micturition, but with scanty mucoid or mucopurulent discharge per urethra. Urine shows increased pus cells. Urethral smear and culture is negative for gonococci but positive for *Chlamydia* or *Mycoplasma*. Treatment consists of oral erythromycin or tetracycline 500 mg QDS.

GENITAL ULCERATIVE DISEASE (INCLUDING DD OF GENITAL ULCERS)

The term genital ulcerative disease is used to denote genital ulcers caused by STDs as against non-STD causes like Behcet's syndrome or traumatic ulcers. Their effective management is important as they can significantly increase the risk of transmission of HIV between sex partners. STD causes of genital ulcers include chancroid, syphilis, donovanosis herpes simplex, lymphogranuloma venereum.

CHANCROID (SOFT CHANCRE)

Chancroid is a common STD caused by *Haemophilus ducreyi*. It presents as multiple, painful ulcers over inner or other prepuce in males or labia in females. The ulcers are tender, nonindurated and bleed on touch. They are covered with slough and have ragged undermined edges. A tender, suppurative, inguinal lymphadenopathy (bubo) occurs in 30% and if untreated, rupture of the nodes leads to an ulcer. Phagedena and balanoposthitis are other common complications.

Diagnosis is clinical but can be confirmed with smear and culture. Ruling out syphilis and HIV infection by a VDRL and an ELISA, is a must frequent washes with a mild antiseptic solution for the ulcer and aspiration for the bubo are needed. Oral cotrimoxazole, erythromycin or tetracycline give good results. Streptomycin 1g IM OD is added in cases with inguinal buboes. Balanoposthitis and phagedena need crystalline penicillin and metronidazole to control the anerobic infection.

Donovanosis

Donovanosis is a STD caused by *Calymmatobacterium granulomatis*. It induces a relatively painless ulcer with elevated beefy red granulation in the base that bleeds on touch. The edges are rolled out and a smear of the granulation reveals dumbbell shaped coccobacillary organisms within macrophages. Complications include pseudobubo, scarring, lymph stasis and carcinoma. Treatment consists of streptomycin 1 g IM OD for 2–3 weeks. Co-trimoxazole, tetracycline or erythromycin are also effective.

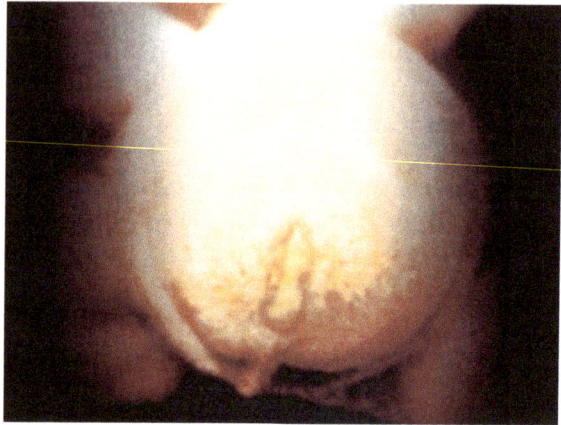

Fig. 22.3: Non-gonococcal urethritis

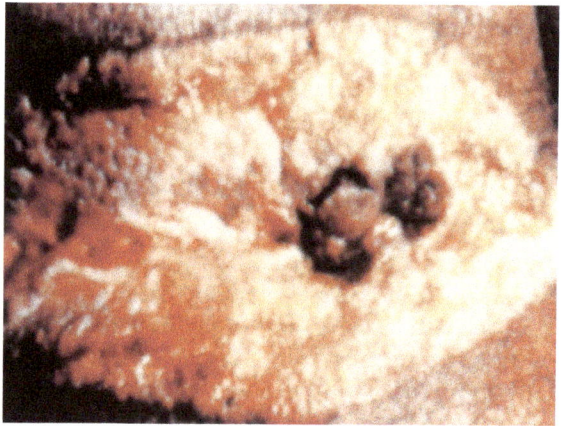

Fig. 22.4: Granuloma inguinale

Table 22.1: Differential diagnosis of ulcer on genitalia

	Chancroid	Donovanosis	Primary syphilis	Herpes genitalis
1. Causative organism	Haemophilus ducreyi	Calymmatobacterium granulomatis	Treponema pallidum	Herpes simplex virus type 2
2. Incubation period	3 to 5 days	8 to 80 days	9 to 90 days	3 to 6 days
3. Symptoms	Painful	Variable	Nil	Painful
4. Onset	Acute	Insidious	Insidious	Acute
5. Lesions preceding ulcer	Vesiculopustule	Papule	Papule	Grouped vesicles
6. No. of ulcers	Multiple	Single/multiple	Single	Multiple
7. Size of ulcers	0.5 to 2 cm	2 to 10 cms	1 to 2 cm	2 to 3 mm
8. Base	Soft	Variable	Indurated	Soft
9. Tenderness	+	+	–	+
10. Bleeding	+	++	–	–
11. Floor of ulcer	Slough	Dark red granulation tissue	Pale granulation	Slough
Slough	++	+/–	–	–/+
Depth	Deep	Deep	Variable	Superficial

Contd...

Contd...

	Chancroid	Donovanosis	Primary syphilis	Herpes genitalis
Raised above the surface	+/–	++	+/–	–
12. Edge of ulcer	Undermined	Rolled out, variable	Variable sometimes punched out	Sloping
13. Discharge	Purulent, profuse	Serosanguinous profuse, variable	Serosanguinous scanty	Serosanguinous, variable
14. Surrounding skin	red	variable	normal	variable
15. Progress	Fast	Slow	Slow, self healing	Fast, self healing
16. Smear	Gram's stain- Gram negative bacilli in parallel chains	Wright's stain- coccobacilli within macrophage	Dark ground illumination - T. pallidum	Wright's stain- multinucleated epithelial giant cells
17. Standard therapy	Co-trimoxazole Erythromycin	Streptomycin Co-trimoxazole Erythromycin	Injectable penicillin	symptomatic

STDs

- Herpes simplex
- HIV infection
- Secondary septic lymphadenitis due to other STDs
- Non-STDs

FILARIASIS

The differential diagnosis of the common causes of inguinal lymphadenopathy is presented in Table 22.1. Other than these, herpes simplex, HIV infection and scabies amongst the STDs and filariasis amongst the non-STDs also cause inguinal lymphadenopathy.

LYMPHOGRANULOMA VENEREUM (LGV)

Lymphogranuloma venereum is a STD, caused by *Chlamydia trachomatis*, that affects promiscuous adult males. Primary lesion is a self healing genital sore. After a few weeks, regional lymph nodes become enlarged, matted and form an inguinal bubo situated on both sides of the inguinal ligament. The bubo is multilocular, pointing and bursting through many openings. The chronicity of the secondary lymphadenopathic stage leads to lymphedema, distortion of genitalia (ram's horn penis and esthiomene), urethral, vaginal and rectal strictures and fistulae. Infection responds to co-trimoxazole, tetracycline or erythromycin. Complications need surgical correction.

PRACTICAL MANAGEMENT OF STDs (SYNDROMIC MANAGEMENT OF STDs)

In the HIV era, efficient management of STDs has become a national priority because
1. HIV and other STDs commonly affect the same person as their mode of transmission is similar.

2. Presence of an ulcerative STD increases the chances of HIV transmission 10 fold and that of an inflammatory STD (e.g. urethritis, cervicitis, vaginitis) increases it by 4 fold.
3. STDs when associated within the same patient are more servere and frequenty unresponsive to conventional treatment.

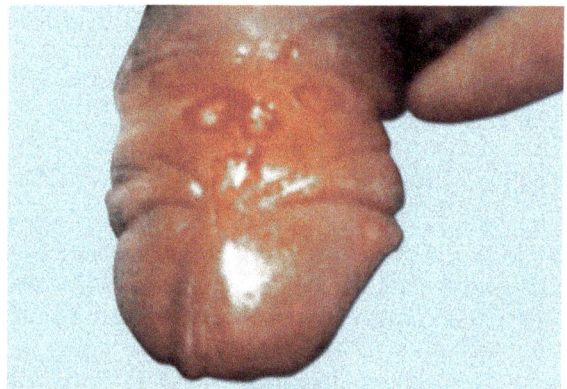

Fig. 22.5: Chancroid

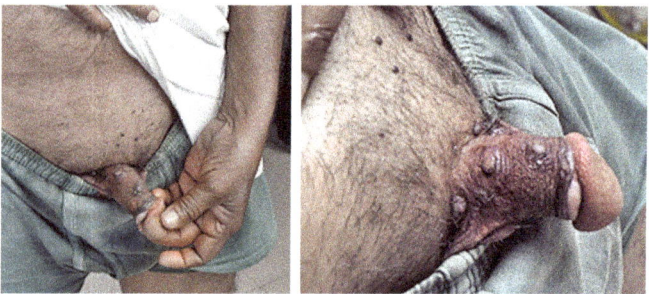

Figs 22.6A and B: Patient of STD showing multiple venereal warts and painless indurated clean ulcers in a HIV positive

Hence, correct and promt treatment of STDs should be administered by the primary care physician by following a standard protocol even in the absence of facilitis for establishing the correct diagnosis. Such an approach is based on identifying the correct syndrome in a patient and treating accordingly. This is called the syndromal approach to STD management.

All common STDs can be divided into the following well defined syndromes that can be identified without any facilities.
1. Genital ulcer
2. Urethral discharge
3. Inguinal bubo
4. Vaginal discharge.

Genital Ulcer: In both Males and Females

Treat with injection benzathine penicillin 2.4 MU IM after test dose (1/2 in each buttock, preferably treat the spouse as well, if possible after a VDRL of both) in addition to erythromycin 500 mg QDS or tetracycline 500 mg QDS or co-trimoxazole 2 tabs BD for 14 days.

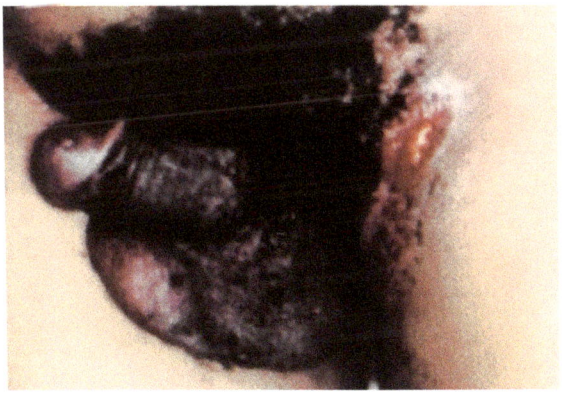

Fig. 22.7: Lymphogranuloma venereum (LGV)

Urethral Discharge in Males

Treat with oral norfloxacin 800 mg single dose followed by doxycycline 100 mg BD for 10 days.

Inguinal Bubo

In both sexes—with or without genital ulcer. If suppurative—treat with injection streptomycin 1 g IM OD for 10 days with oral erythromycin 500 mg QDS for 14 days. If non-suppurative injection benzathine penicillin 2.4 MU IM after test dose (preferable after a VDRL).

Vaginal Discharge

Treat with oral norfloxacin 80 mg OD for 3 days with doxycycline 100 mg BD for 10 days and metronidazole 200 mg TDs for 7 days along with vaginal tablets of clotrimazole 100 mg OD for 7 days. This takes care of gonococcal and chlamydial genital infections and trichomonal and candidal vaginitis.

For all theses patients, it is mandatory to explain about prevention of HIV and STDs use of condoms (including where they are avail.

CHAPTER 23

HIV and AIDS

The impact of HIV infection on modern medicine as well as human life during the last decade stands unmatched. The HIV epidemic soon turned into a pandemic and this infection has now become endemic in many countries including India. Knowledge regarding HIV infection is in a state of flux and is gradually evolving as more and more experience is gained. The information presented here is in tune with the current experience but it may need modification at a latar date.

HUMAN IMMUNODEFICIENCY VIRUS

It was initially identified as the underlying cause for the epidemic of *Pneumocystis carinii* pneumonia and Kaposi's sarcoma affecting homosexuals in the USA during the year 1984. It is a retrovirus with an affinity for CD4 receptor bearing cells in the body. Hence it selectively infects, replicates within and destroys T4 helper/inducer lymphocytes that are the key cells in mounting an effective cellular immune response. Loss of this effector arm of immune function results in a plethora of infections and malignancies.

HIV belongs to the family of retroviruses that need the enzyme reverse transcriptase for multiplication. The virus has an envelope made of glycoproteins that are crucial to the pathogenicity of the virus. Antibodies against them are of diagnostic importance. The central core has the RNA fragment and the enzymes. A core antigen p24 is important for early diagnosis. HIV 1 subtype is the agent causing HIV has affinity for the CD4 receptors and thus selectively kills the T helper lymphocytes. Loss of T cell function leads to infections and malignancies.

IMMUNOPATHOGENESIS OF HIV INFECTION

With its affinity for CD4 receptors, HIV selectively targets T helper cells. During T cells release hundreds of virions further infect. Early in the infection, the virus is neutralized by CD8 positive cells in the blood and is therefore confined to the lymph nodes. This results in peristent generalized lymphadenopathy which last for a few years. Polyclonal B cell activation occurs in some patients. With disease progression, immune system gets exhausted and the virus appears in the blood. This tends to reduce CD4 cell count by destroying them. Loss of this effector arm of immunity leads to a variety of infections and malignancies.

EPIDEMIOLOGY AND TRANSMISSION OF HIV INFECTION

More than 4 million persons are estimated to be infected with the HIV in India. In the city of Mumbai more than 2 lakh people are estimated to be infected. HIV prevalence rates in many parts of India exceed one percent of the population. Women and children are increasingly (25% of total and 40% of newly detected cases) infected. The major route of HIV transmission is heterosexual (80%). Perinatal transmission (5%), blood transfusions and intravenuos drug abuse (5%) and homosexual intercourse (5%) account for other cases.

NATURAL HISTORY OF HIV INFECTION

Within 6-12 weeks of the infection about 50% may show a flu like self-healing illness. After a variable asymptomatic phase (average 3-5 years but can vary from 1-10 years) minor infections like herpes zoster or molluscum contagiosum may occur. Lymphadenopathy may be seen during this stage. Within 1-2 years this progresses to more internal infections that may be initially typical and later atypical. They include

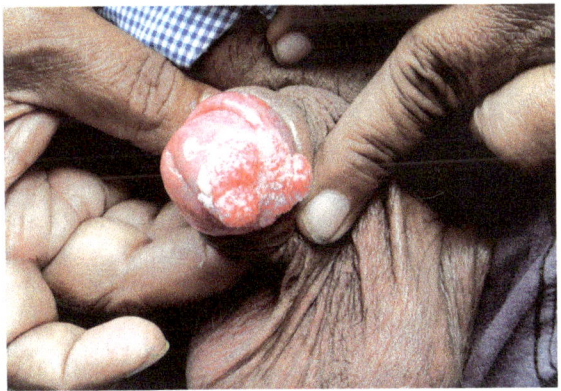

Fig. 23.1: Multiple venereal warts in a HIV positive patient

bacterial, mycobacterial, fungal and parasitic infections and infestations with associated weight loss, fever and diarrhea. This phase lasts 1-3 years. Serious infections (e.g. cryptococcosis, toxoplasmosis, systemic candidiasis, and cytomegalovirus) soon supervene and death results from one of these within the next 1 year. Malignancies like squamous cell carcinoma, lymphomas and Kaposi's sarcoma occur during the last stage.

CLINICAL FEATURES AND STAGES OF HIV INFECTION

Primay Infection Illness (Seroconversion)

About 50% of infected persons develop a flu like illness 6-12 weeks after the infection. Constitutional signs and symptoms, like rhinitis, pharyngitis, lymphadenopathy and rash lasting 1-3 weeks are common. The plasma viral load is very high during this period at the end of which serum ELISA turns positive.

Early HIV Disease (Latent HIV Infection/Asymptomatic HIV Infection)

Usual duration of this phase in Indians is 2-5 years. Persistent generalized lymphadenopathy (PGL) is the only sign of this relatively asymptomatic phase. Lymph nodes are 1-3 cm sized, non-tender, firm and discrete. Recurrent minor fungal and bacterial infections (including STDs) of the skin occur. Molluscum contagiosum, typical herpes zoster or unresponsive seborrheic dermatitis could serve as clinical markers of this phase in adults. Plasma viral load is low and CD4 count is normal.

HIV and AIDS

Table 23.1: Mucocutaneous manifestations of HIV infection

Sexually transmitted diseases

Unusually florid or non-responsive
- Syphilis
- Chancroid
- Donovanosis
- Herpes genitalis
- Condyloma acuminata
- Molluscum contagiosum

Other infections

Viral:
- Herpes zoster
- Warts
- Oral hairy leukoplakia (EBV)

Bacterial:
- Unusually extensive or florid pyoderma
- Bacillary angiomatosis

Mycobacterial:
- Scrofuloderma
- Orificial tuberculosis
- Atypical mycobacterial infections

Fungal:
- Candidiasis
- Dermatophytosis
- Cryptococcosis
- Penicilliosis
- Histoplasmosis

Parasitic:
- Crusted scabies
- Demodicidosis

Malignancies
- Squamous cell carcinoma
- Lymphoma
- Kaposi's sarcoma

Autoimmune diseases
- Thrombocytopenic purpura
- Vasculitis
- Reiter's disease

Drug eruptions
- Stevens-Johnson syndrome
- Toxic epidermal necrolysis

Other inflammatory skin disorders
- Seborrheic dermatitis
- Psoriasis Papular eruption of HIV
- Eosinophilic folliculitis

Miscellaneous changes
- Hyperpigmentation
- Ichthyosis
- Xerosis
- Premature graying of hair

Oral cavity lesions
- Aphthous ulcers
- Candidiasis
- Oral hairy leukoplakia
- Herpes labialis/stomatitis
- Mucous patches of syphilis
- Periodontitis
- Addisonian pigmentation
- Warts
- Kaposi's sarcoma
- Squamous cell carcinoma

Intermediate Stage HIV Disease (AIDS-related Complex/Symptomatic HIV Infection without AIDS)

The intermediate symptomatic phase of HIV infection lasts 1-2 years. Typical systemic infections like pulmonary tuberculosis or scrofuloderma occur commonly. Others include recurrent upper and lower respiratory tract bacterial infections, unresponsive or severe STDs, herpes zoster or oral candidiasis, CD4 counts fall steadily and plasma viral load rises gradually during this phase. Mild to moderate constitutional symptoms and signs, i.e. fever, anorexia, weight loss and night sweats are usual.

Late Stage HIV Disease (AIDS)

Serious opportunistic infections occur in this phase including:
- Disseminated or multiple attacks of pulmonary or extrapulmonary tuberculosis,
- Cryptococcosis (CNS, skin, lungs)
- Candidiasis (visceral—esophageal and disseminated)

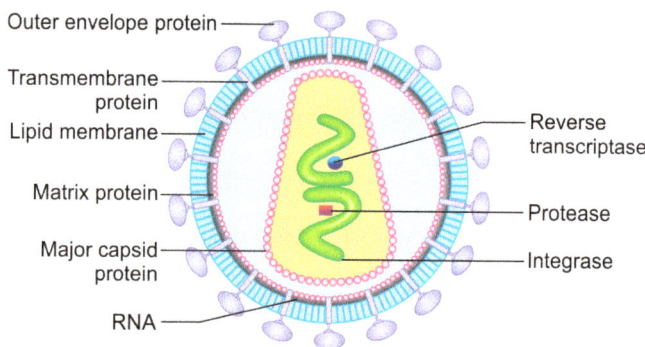

Fig. 23.2: Human immunodeficiency virus

- Toxoplasmosis (CNS, eye lungs)
- Herpes simplex and zoster—(encephalitis, radiculitis)
- *Pneumocystis carinii* (lungs)
- Atypical mycobacterial infections (lungs), diarrhea due to unusual organisms like *Cryptosporidium* or *Isospora*,
- JC polyomavirus (PML, progressive multifocal leuko-encephalopathy)
- Please see Tables 23.1 and 23.5 for details of systemic affection in HIV disease.

Malignant Tumors like

- Non-Hodgkin's lymphoma
- Cervical and anorectal carcinomas and
- Kaposi's sarcoma occur.

Direct Effect of HIV Infection like

- Malabsorption due to persistent diarrhea, wasting or slim disease, resulting from severe weight loss
- HIV encephalopathy
- Retinopathy
- Peripheral neuritis manifest in this stage.

Serious internal opportunistic infections like disseminated tuberculosis, cryptococcal meningitis, cerebral toxoplasmosis, cryptosporidial diarrhea are common causes of death during late stage HIV infection in Indian patients. Herpes encephalitis, *Pneumocystis carinii* pneumonia or cytomegalovirus infections, may also occur and may lead to death. In Indian HIV patients, malignancies like squamous cell carinoma and lymphoma are more frequent when compared to Kaposi's sarcoma. Later, severe weight loss follows. HIV encephalopathy or peripheral neuropathy or HIV enterooathy are some late effects due to long-standing HIV infection.

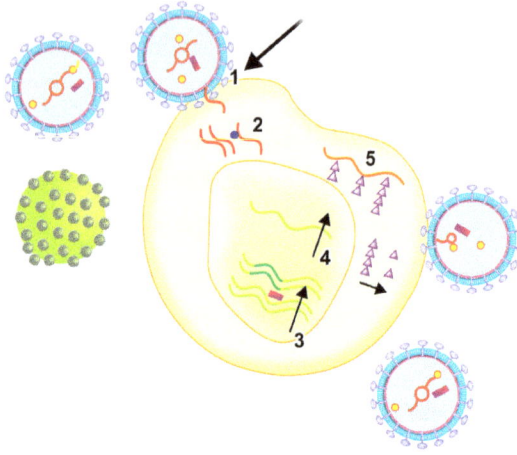

1. Entry can be blocked by entry inhibitors
2. Reverse transcription can be blocked by nucleoside reverse transcriptase inhibitors (NRTIs) and non-nucleoside reverse transcriptase inhibitors (NNRTIS)
3. Integration
4. Transcription
5. Translation
6. Viral assembly can be blocked by protease inhibitors (PIs)

Fig. 23.3: HIV replication and sites of drug action

Classification of antiretrovirals update–

Nucleoside reverse transcriptase inhibotors (NRTIs)	Non-nucleoside reverse transcriptase inhibitors (NNRTIs)	Protease inhibitors (PIs)
Zidovudine	Nevirapine	Indinavir
Stavudine	Efavirenz	Nelfinavir
Lamivudine	Delavirdine	Ritonavir
Didanosine		Saquinavir
Zalcitabine		Atazanavir
Emtricitabine		Amprenavir
Abacavir		Lopinavir

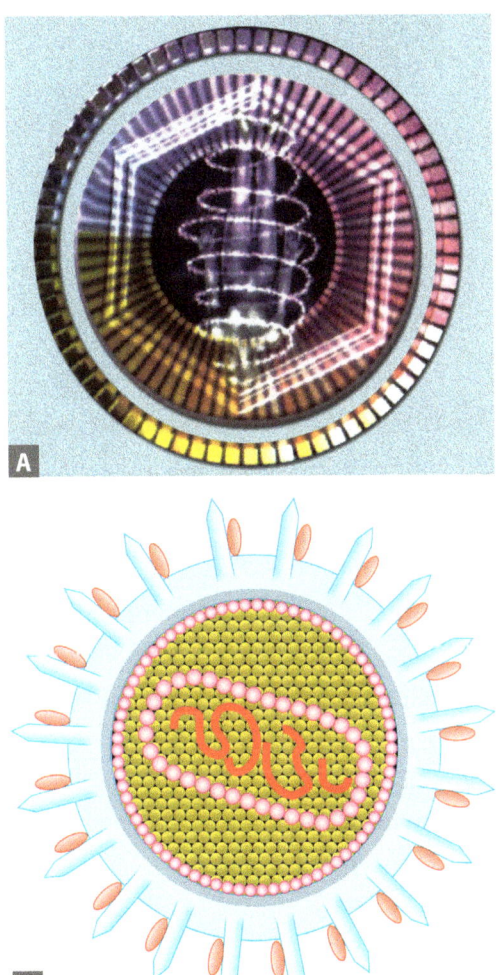

Figs 23.4A and B: HIV virus

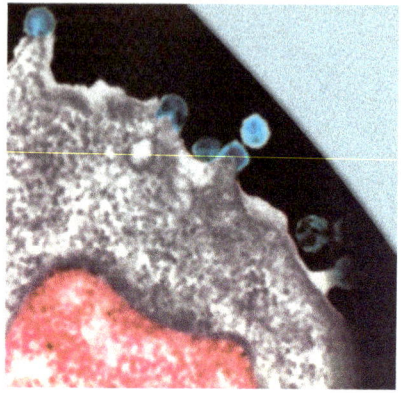

Fig. 23.5: HIV virus—under the electron microscope

New Drugs

Nucleotide analogue	Tenofovir
Entry inhibitor	Enfuvirtide
Protease inhibitor	Fosamprenavir

HIV and Pregnancy

Management of pregnancy in HIV infection.

Women and HIV

Pediatric HIV infections
Homosexuality and AIDS

Prevention of AIDS/HIV Infection

(a) Health promotion
(b) Specific protection
    (i) General population
    (ii) Health workers

Protection in the work place.

HIV Vaccines

A cure has not yet been found for HIV infection. In such a scenario, an effective vaccine would have been an ideal way to arrest the march of HIV infection. Approaches to vaccine development have included targeting the viral envelope and making it dysfunctional or producing antibodies to it. Use of viral peptides or viral particles to stimulate immunity against the virus has also been tried. Combining these viral proteins with other benign viruses (vector controlled vaccines) can improve their performance. Composite DNA vaccines comprise several viral proteins and hence are stronger immune stimulators.

The main hurdle to vaccine development has been the ability of HIV to mutate rapidly and form newer viral strains with a different genetic make-up. This makes vaccines against earlier strains ineffective. Till now none of the vaccines have reached final stage of clinical evaluation although some are

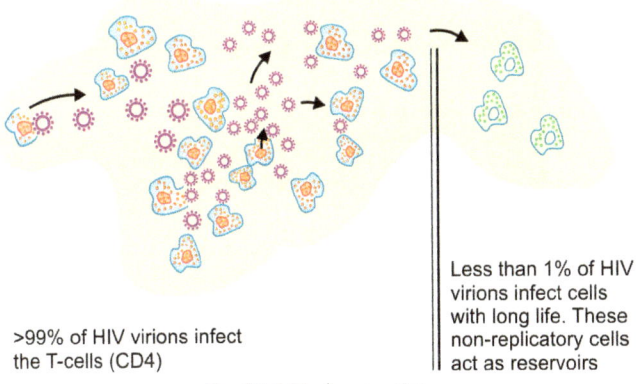

Fig. 23.6: Viral reservoirs

Table 23.2: Tests for diagnosis of HIV infection

	Early disease	Intermediate disease	Late disease	Advantages	Disadvantage
ELISA	+ve	+ve	+ve	Inexpensive	False-positive or negative occurs in 1–3%
WB	±	+ve	+ve	Diagnostic if positive	False-negative common in early infections
P24	±	-ve	+ve	Becomes +ve earlier than ELISA	False-negative common in intermediate and early stage
Qualitative PCR	+	+	+	Diagnostic and relatively inexpensive	Gives no information about severity of viremia
Viral load	++	+	+++	Quantitative, used for prognosis or for monitorning therapy	Very expensive
Viral culture	+	+	+	Positive early, used for prognosis	Very expensive, not easily available. False-negative common

Table 23.3: Antiretroviral drugs

Drugs	Doses	Side effects	Comments
AZT	200 mg tds orally as parts of MDT; 2 mg/kg QDS in children as part of MDT; 1000 mg/day as monotherapy (post-exposure); 500 mg/day in pregnancy from 14–34 weeks up to delivery; 2 mg/kg QDS orally for 6 weeks for prevention of transmission in neonates; 20 mg/m^2/h infusion for HIV encephalopathy	Intolerance, Granulocytopenia, anemia, hepatitis, myositis	Anchor drug for MDT; can be used as monotherapy in special situations. NSAIDs, co-trimoxazole, fluconazole and acyclovir increase chances of toxicity
3TC (Lamivudine) (NRTI)	150 mg BD as part of MDT; 4 mg/kg BD in children; 2 mg/kg BD in neonates	Intolerance, hepatitis, pancreatitis, granulocytopenia	Drug with better tolerance and compliances. Co-trimoxazole increases blood levels
Didanosine (ddC) (NRTI)	125 mg BD as part of MDT; 2–3 mg/kg BD in children; for better absorption, take on empty stomach	Intolerance, neuropathy pancreatitis, hepatitis	Poor tolerance. Interferes with ddC action. Hence, never given together with ddC

Contd...

Contd...

Drugs	Doses	Side effects	Comments
Zalcitabine (ddC) (NRTI)	750 µg TDS as part of MDT; 10 µg/kg TDS in children	Intolerance, neuropathy, pancreatitis, hepatitis, skin rash, stomatitis, granulocytopenia	Poor tolerance. Interferes with ddI action. Hence, never given together with ddI
d4T (Stavudine) (NRTI)	30 mg BD as part of MDT; 1 mg/kg BD in children (up to a maximim of 30 mg BD)	Nausea, vomiting, diarrhea	Anchor drug; used as alternative to AZT in patients with poor bone marrow function. Lower dose in patients with renal failure
Nevirapine (NNRTI)	200 mg BD as part of MDT; 3–4 mg/kg BD in children	Intolerance, skin rash (Stevens Johnson syndrome)	Better tolerated. Can be used during pregnancy. Induces hepatic cytochrome p 450. Hence, increases metabolism of all drugs (including protease inhibitors) metabolized by p 450
Saquinavir (PI)	600 mg TDS as part of MDT; used in children	Intolerance, induction of diabetes mellitus, skin: photoallergy	Do not use with rifampicin or nevirapine. Compared to other PI, it is absorbed poorly from the GI tract

Contd...

Contd...

Drugs	Doses	Side effects	Comments
Indinavir	800 mg TDS as part of MDT; 10 mg/kg TDS in children	Intolerance, diabetes, hepatitis nephrolithiasis	Do not use with rifampicin (Finish AKT first then start ART) or nevirapine. Take ddI at least 2 hours apart

NRTI: Nucleoside reverse transcriptase inhibitor; **PI**: Protease inhibitor; **NNRTI**: Non-nucleoside reverse transcriptase inhibitor.

MDT: Multidrug therapy; **AKT**: Anti-Kochs therapy; **ART** Anti- retroviral therapy

Note: Intolerance includes headache, abdominal pain, diarrhea, anorexia, nausea, vomiting. Intolerance of variable severity, is common to most of the antiretroviral drugs and its severity/persistence determines if the drug can be continued or needs to be omitted /replaced. 2 mg/kg QDS in children as part of summary: Currently antiretroviral therapy is so expensive that it is out the reach of most (99%) HIV infected patients in India. Useful antireteroviral drugs include reverse transcriptase inhibitors like AZT (azidothymidine) or 3 TC (lamivudine) or ddI (didanosine) and protease inhibitors like indinavir or ritonavir. Monotherapy with AZT is contraindicated because of the likelihood of resistance to the drug. Monotherapy with AZT is indicated for post-exposure prophylaxis of HIV infection and in prevention of HIV transmission from mother to child. A combination of AZT, 3TC and indinavir (HEART, Highly effective antiretroviral therapy) is recommended for affording patients. Such therapy is shown to reduce the incidence of opportunistic infections and improve life expectancy. The efficacy of such therapy can be monitored by doing plasma viral load.

Table 23.4: Skin care guideline for patients with HIV infection

Sl. no.	Conditions	Drugs of choice	Alternative therapy	Comments
	Bacterial			
A.	Syphilis, without central nervous system (CNS) involvement	Benzathine penicillin — 2.4 million U for 3 weeks 1 per week	NA	In patients who are penicillin sensitive and coinfected with HIV and syphilis, both the AHCPR and the CDC recommend consultation with a specialist for desensitization and penicillin treatment
B.	Syphilis, with CNS involvement	2 million to 4 million U aqueous penicillin IV every 4 hours for 10 to 14 days	NA	—
C.	*Staphylococcus aureus* Superficial infection	Penicillinase resistant penicillin/first generation cephalosporin	NA	Antibacterial soaps/antihistaminic used as adjunctive
D.	*Staphylococcus aureus* Chronic condition	Minocycline 100 mg	NA	Long-term therapy
E.	*Staphylococcus aureus* Deep infection			
F.	*Staphylococcus aureus* Recurrence			
G.	*Pseudomonas*			

expected to reach that stage in the next few years. A more practical use of the vaccines is in immunotherapy of an HIV infected mother to reduce the risk of transmission to her fetus or for immunotherapy of a newborn of an HIV infected mother.

Latency: In spite of rapid and powerful viral suppression, HAART is a lifelong therapy. Initial speculation that, with 3 years duration of treatment, HIV can be eradicated, proved to be to optimistics. Scientists have observed a rebound of viral load after discontinuation of any powerful HAART therapy. They explain that there are some segments of body, infact macrophages and memory T-cells that get infected and harbor them for a very long time. The HIV virus cannot multiply on its own but is dependent on the replicatory stages of the host cell. The virus waits for the host cell to replicate (latency).

Post-exposure Prophylaxis (PEP)

Occupational exposure to HIV.

CDC guidelines for post-exposure prophylaxis (PEP)
1. Immediate measures to treat the exposure site
2. Evaluating the risk of HIV transmission
3. Initiating post-exposure prophylaxis (PEP)
4. Regimens for PEP
   Basic regimen (28 days)
   Duovir   or   lamivir - S
   Expanded regimen (28 days)
   Duovir   or   lamivir - S
                +
   Indivan   or   efavir
5. Follow-up.

Table 23.5: Treatment of opportunistic infections

Pathogen/disease	Site of infection	Treatment
Aspergillus	Lungs, sinuses, disseminated	IV amphotericin B itraconazole
Bacterial	Lungs, sinuses, disseminated	Standard antibiotics IV immunoglobulin
Candidiasis	Mucous membranes, skin, lungs	Ketoconazole, fluconazole
Cytomegalovirus	Retina, GIT, lungs, brain, heart, kidneys, adrenals	IV ganciclovir IV foscarnet
Coccidioidomycosis	Lungs, lymph, nodes, spleen	IV amphotericin B
Cryptococcus	Brain, lungs, disseminated	Fluconazole; IV amphotericin
Cryptosporidium	GIT, lungs	Paromomycin; azithromycin
Hairy leukoplakia	Tongue, buccal mucosa	Topical podophyllin; acyclovir
Herpes simplex	Mouth, lips, genitals	Acyclovir
Herpes zoster	Trunk, face, extremities	Acyclovir; foscarnet
Histoplasmosis	Lungs, skin, GIT	IV amphotericin B; itraconazole
HPV	Genitalia, anus	Cryotherapy, alpha-interferon Topical 5-fluorouracil
Isospora	Intestines	Co-trimoxazole
Kaposi's disease	Skin, lymph nodes, GIT, lungs	IV vincristine; IV doxorubicin IV amphotericin B
M. avium complex	Lungs, disseminated	Rifampin, ethambutol and ciprofloxacin Rifampin, ethambutol, ciprofloxacin and clofazimine Clarithromycin

Contd...

Contd...

Pathogen/disease	Site of infection	Treatment
Microsporidium	GIT	None; try albendazole
Molluscum contagiosum	Skin	Cryotherapy
Pneumocystis carinii Pneumonia	Lungs, lymph nodes, spleen liver	Co-trimoxazole and IV pentamidine
Salmonellosis	GIT, disseminated	Ciprofloxacin; co-trimoxazole Ampicillin
Neurosyphilis	CNS	IV crystalline penicillin
Thrombocytopenia	Megakaryocytes	IV immunoglobulin IV vincristine ; steroids
Toxoplasmosis	Brain	Sulfadiazine + Pyrimethamine Clindamycin + Pyrimethamine Azithromycin + Pyrimethamine Atovaquone
Tuberculosis	Lungs, lymphatic system, CNS	INH + rifampicin + pyrazinamide + ethambutol For 2 months; then Rifampicin + INH for 7 months

How can Patients Live Longer and Healthier after HIV Infection?

Whether a patient is a candidate for antiretroviral therapy or not, some general measures should be followed to improve overall health status and prevent opportunistic infections.

Persons who are HIV-infected have a higher rate of infection caused by intestinal pathogens such as *Salmonella*,

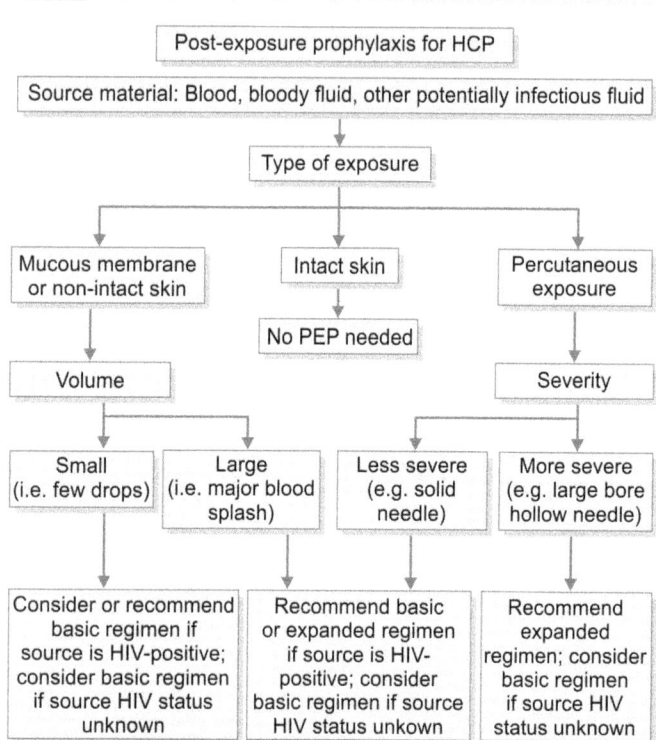

Fig. 23.7: Post-exposure prophylaxis for healthcare personnel (HCP)

Shigella and *Campylobacter*. HIV-infected persons should therefore avoid uncooked food (such as raw eggs) and unpasteurised dairy products and should also thoroughly wash cutting surfaces and implements used with raw food. Limiting exposure to cryptosporidial infection can be achieved by using filtered water. Other important measures include eating a well-balanced diet, exercising regularly, maintaining good personal hygiene and avoiding exposure to

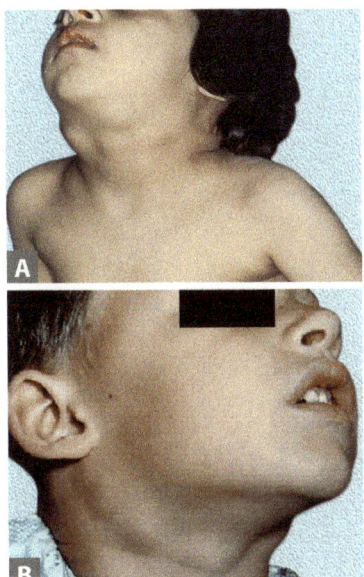

Figs 23.8A and B: Persistent generalized lymphadenopathy (PGL)

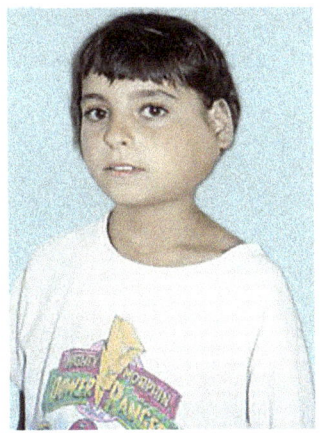

Fig. 23.9: Salivary gland enlargement

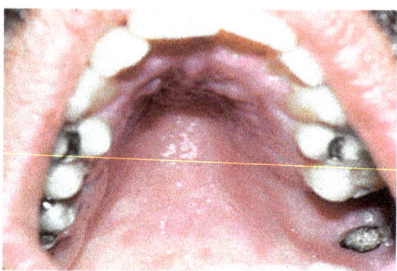

Fig. 23.10: Erythematous

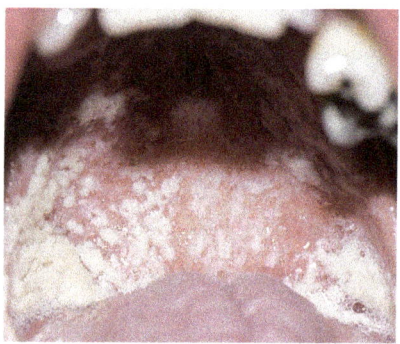

Fig. 23.11: Pseudomembranous

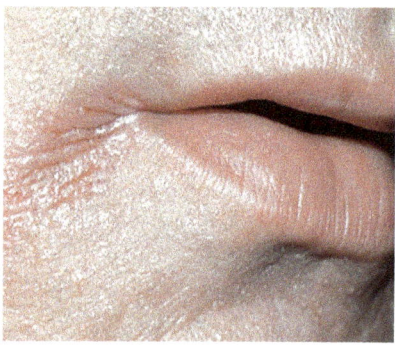

Fig. 23.12: Angular chelitis

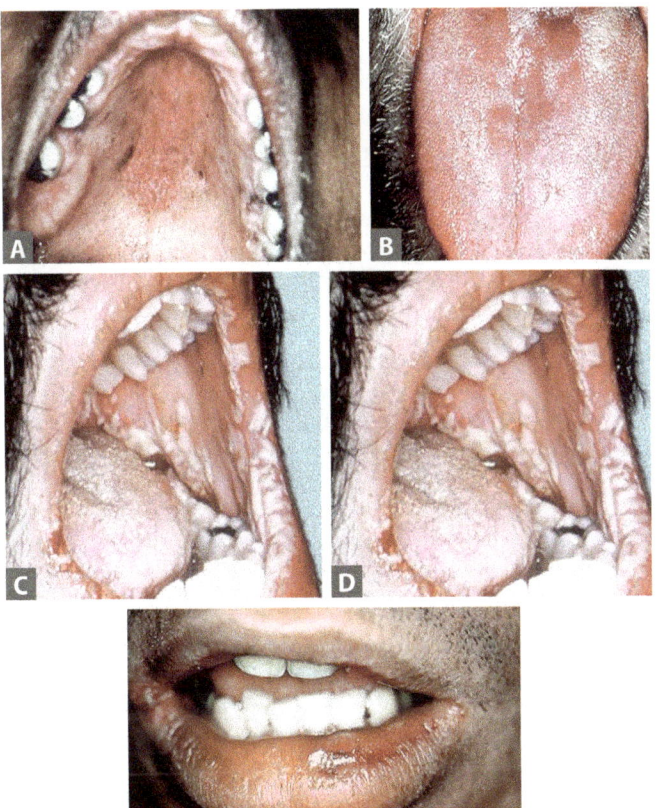

Figs 23.13A to E: Oral candidiasis

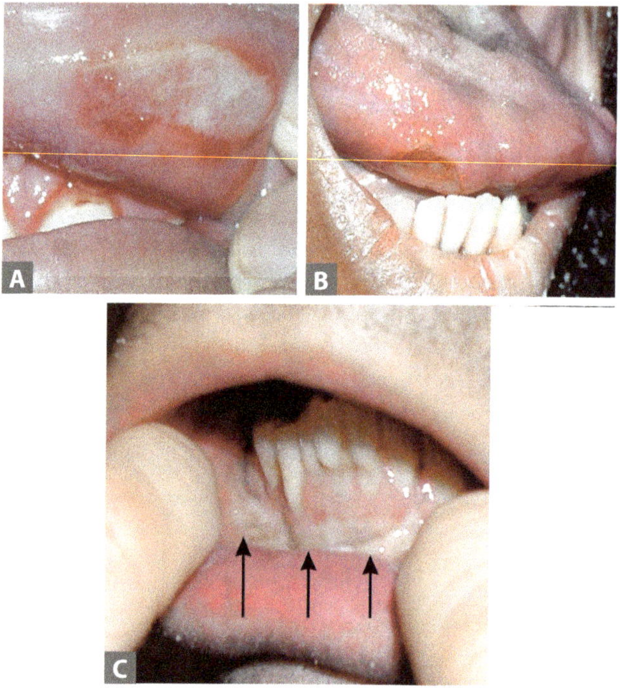

Figs 23.14A to C: Aphthous lesions: Clinical type

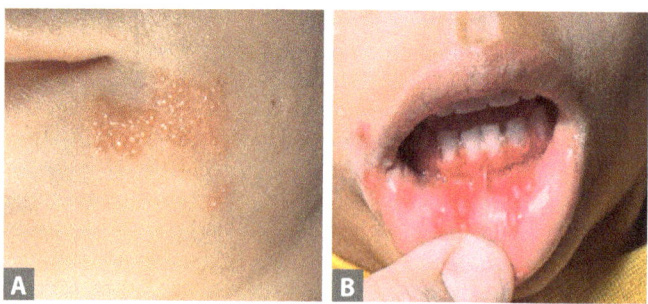

Figs 23.15A and B: Herpes simplex

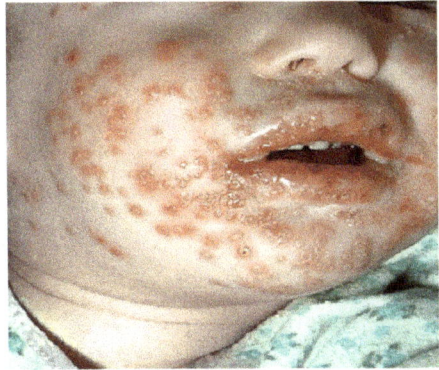

Fig. 23.16: Viral infection

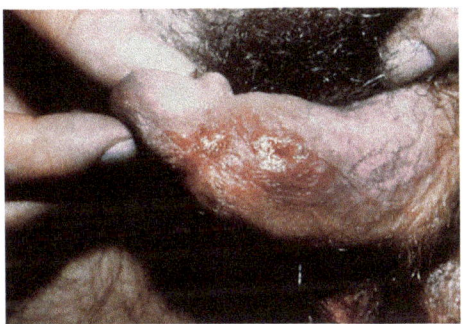

Fig. 23.17: Herpes progenitalis

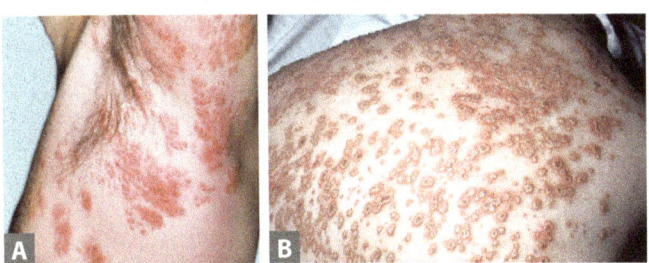

Figs 23.18A and B: Chickenpox

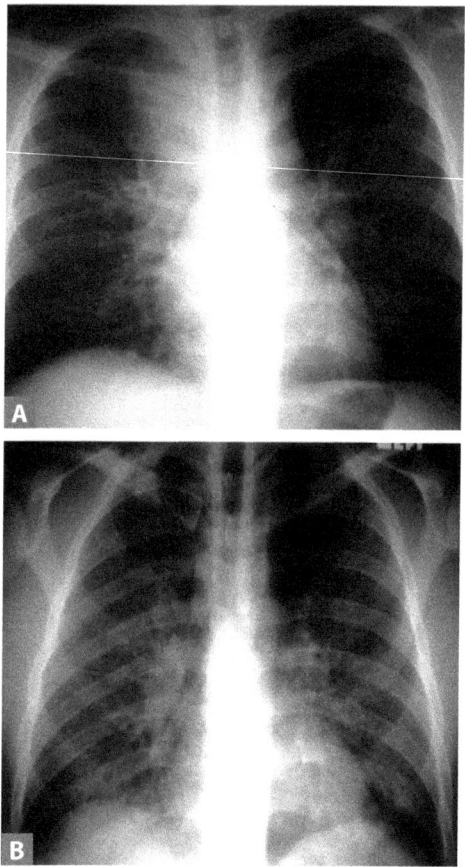

Figs 23.19A and B: X-ray picture of the TB patient along with HIV

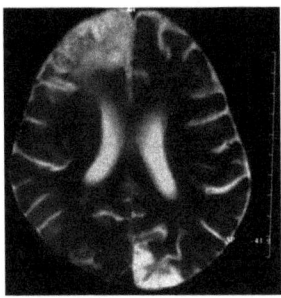

Fig. 23.20: Progressive multifocal leukoencephalopathy (PML)

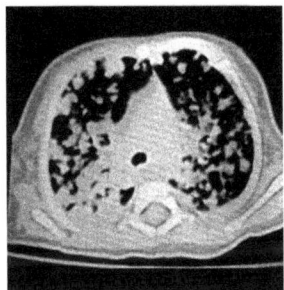

Fig. 23.21: *Pneumocystis carinii* pneumonia (PCP)

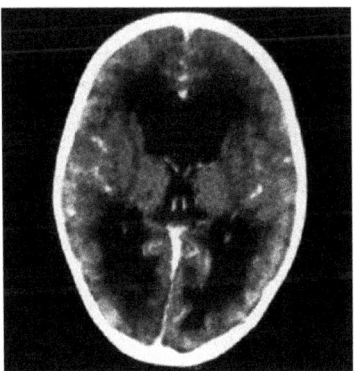

Fig. 23.22: Tuberculous meningities

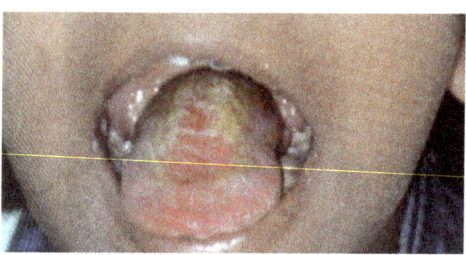

Fig. 23.23: Oral thrush

pets. It is also important to counsel patients to quit smoking, avoid alcohol and recreational drugs, reduce stress levels and obtain enough sleep and rest.

Bibliography

1. Abdalla CM, de Oliveira ZN, Sotto MN, Leite KR, Canavez FC, de Carvalho CM. Polymerase chain reaction compared to other laboratory findings and to clinical evaluation in the diagnosis of cutaneous tuberculosis and atypical mycobacteria skin infection. Int J Dermatol. 2009 Jan;48(1):27-35. doi: 10.1111/j.1365-4632.2009.03807.x.
2. AKB, ARV, et al. Future therapies for systemic sclerosis. In: Dermatology, Sexually Transmitted Diseases and Leprosy. April 2002, issue number 31.
3. Alan Menter, Baylor Psoriasis Research Institute, Dallas, TX, United States; James Signorovitch, Analysis Group, Boston, MA, United States; Parvez Mulani, Abbott Laboratories, Abbott Park, IL, United States; Shiraz Gupta, Abbott Laboratories, Abbott Park, IL, United States. Journal of the American Academy of Dermatology Volume 60, Issue 3, Supplement 1, Page AB167, March 2009 DOI: http://dx.doi.org/10.1016/j.jaad.2008.11.731 Adalimumab reduces symptoms of depression in patients with moderate to severe psoriasis.
4. Ameet R valia. Review acne vulgaris: new insights. In: Dermatology, Sexually Transmitted Diseases and Leprosy. April 2002, issue number 31.
5. Anandan V, Parveen B, Prabhavathy D, Priyavarthini V. Adams Oliver syndrome--a variant. Int J Dermatol. 2008 Dec;47(12):1260-2. doi: 10.1111/j.1365-4632.2008.03884.x.
6. Asero R, Tedeschi A, Cugno M. Treatment of refractory chronic urticaria: current and future therapeutic options. Am J Clin Dermatol. 2013 Dec;14(6):481-8. doi: 10.1007/s40257-013-0047-3.

7. Azzam OA, Leheta TM, Nagui NA, Shaarawy E, Hay RM, Hilal RF. Different therapeutic modalities for treatment of melasma. J Cosmet Dermatol. 2009 Dec;8(4):275-81. doi: 10.1111/j.1473-2165.2009.00471.x.

8. Bonifaz A, Tirado-Sánchez A, Graniel MJ, Mena C, Valencia A, Ponce-Olivera RM. The efficacy and safety of sertaconazole cream (2 %) in diaper dermatitis candidiasis. Mycopathologia. 2013 Apr;175(3-4):249-54. doi: 10.1007/s11046-013-9642-3. Epub 2013 Apr 2.

9. Chan CS, Van Voorhees AS, Lebwohl MG, Korman NJ, Young M, Bebo BF Jr, et al. Treatment of severe scalp psoriasis: from the Medical Board of the National Psoriasis Foundation. J Am Acad Dermatol. 2009 Jun;60(6):962-71. doi: 10.1016/j.jaad.2008.11.890. Epub 2009 Apr 17.

10. Choi M, Choi JW, Lee SY, Choi SY, Park HJ, Park KC, Youn SW, Huh CH. Low-dose 1064-nm Q-switched Nd:YAG laser for the treatment of melasma. J Dermatolog Treat. 2010 Jul;21(4):224-8. doi: 10.3109/09546630903401462.

11. Chun SI1, Calderhead RG. Carbon assisted Q-switched Nd:YAG laser treatment with two different sets of pulse width parameters offers a useful treatment modality for severe inflammatory acne: a case report. Photomed Laser Surg. 2011 Feb;29(2):131-5. doi: 10.1089/pho.2010.2786. Epub 2010 Dec 23.

12. Dertlioglu SB, Cicek D, Suleyman A. Increased serum apelin-12 and lipid profile in patients with and without psoriasis. Eur J Dermatol. 2013 Nov-Dec;23(6):885-6. doi:10.1684/ejd.2013.2097.

13. Duschek N, Skvara H, Kittler H, Delir G, Fink A, Pinkowicz A. Melanoma epidemiology of Austria reveals gender-related differences. Eur J Dermatol. 2013 Nov-Dec;23(6):872-8. doi: 10.1684/ejd.2013.2192.

14. Fawzy MM, Hegazy RA. "Impact of vitiligo on the health-related quality of life of 104 adult patients, using Dermatology Life Quality Index and stress score: first Egyptian report." Eur J Dermatol. 2013 Sep-Oct;23(5):733-4. doi: 10.1684/ejd.2013.2139.

15. First Indian algorithm on hyperpigmentation by Indian hyperpigmentation panel.

16. For the acne prevention. Derma Digest.
17. Galliker NA, Trüeb RM. Value of trichoscopy versus trichogram for diagnosis of female androgenetic alopecia. Int J Trichology. 2012 Jan;4(1):19-22. doi: 10.4103/0974-7753.96080.
18. Gupta S, Gargi PD. Habit reversal training for trichotillomania. Int J Trichology. 2012 Jan-Mar; 4(1): 39–41. doi: 10.4103/0974-7753.96089- PMCID: PMC3358939.
19. Held BL, Nader S, Rodriguez-Rigau LJ, Smith KD, Steinberger E. Acne and hyperandrogenism. J Am Acad Dermatol. 1984 Feb;10(2 Pt 1):223-6.
20. Hinz T, Ehler LK, Bieber T, Schmid-Wendtner MH. Complete remission of extensive cutaneous metastatic melanoma on the scalp under topical mono-immunotherapy with diphenylcyclopropenone. Eur J Dermatol. 2013 Jul-Aug; 23(4):532-3. doi: 10.1684/ejd.2013.2066.
21. Hyperpigmentation and melasma. Dermatology Updates, issue 23.
22. Kalb RE, Strober B, Weinstein G, Lebwohl M. Methotrexate and psoriasis: 2009 National Psoriasis Foundation Consensus Conference.- J Am Acad Dermatol. 2009 May;60(5):824-37. doi: 10.1016/j.jaad.2008.11.906.
23. Kim JE, Lee JH, Choi KH, Lee WS, Choi GS, Kwon OS, et al. Phototrichogram analysis of normal scalp hair characteristics with aging. Eur J Dermatol. 2013 Nov-Dec;23(6):849-56. doi: 10.1684/ejd.2013.2170.
24. Li W, Yamada I, Masumoto K, Ueda Y, Hashimoto K. Photodynamic therapy with intradermal administration of 5-aminolevulinic acid for port-wine stains. J Dermatolog Treat. 2010 Jul;21(4):232-9. doi: 10.3109/09546630903159099.
25. Oldenburg M, Kuechmeister B, Ohnemus U, Baur X, Moll I. Extrinsic skin ageing symptoms in seafarers subject to high work-related exposure to UV radiation. Eur J Dermatol. 2013 Sep-Oct;23(5):663-70. doi: 10.1684/ejd.2013.2142.
26. Olivier JX Morel, Robert M Christie. Current Trends in the Chemistry of Permanent Hair Dyeing-dx.doi.org/10.1021/cr1000145|-Chem.Rev.2011, 111,2537–2561, Xennia Technology Ltd., onroe House, Works Road, Letchworth SG6 1LN, U.K.School of Textiles & Design, Heriot-Watt University, Scottish Borders Campus, Netherdale, Galashiels TD1 3HF, Scotland, U.

27. Ono S, Miyachi Y, Arakawa A. Hair regrowth following TNF-α blockade in coexisting psoriasis vulgaris and alopecia areata. Eur J Dermatol. 2013 Jul-Aug;23(4):537. doi: 10.1684/ejd.2013.2074.
28. Pandya AG, Hynan LS, Bhore R, Riley FC, Guevara IL, Grimes P, et al. Reliability assessment and validation of the Melasma Area and Severity Index (MASI) and a new modified MASI scoring method. J Am Acad Dermatol. 2011 Jan;64(1):78-83, 83.e1-2. doi: 10.1016/j.jaad.2009.10.051. Epub 2010 Apr 15.
29. Preneau S, Dessinioti C, Nguyen JM, Katsambas A, Dreno. Predictive markers of response to isotretinoin in female acne. Eur J Dermatol. 2013 Jul-Aug;23(4):478-86. doi: B.10.1684/ejd.2013. 2033.
30. Psoriasis a Review. Skin Readers Digest, issue 3, 2013.
31. Ra'her PA, Hassan I. Human Demodex Mite: The Versatile Mite of Dermatological Importance- doi: 10.4103/0019-5154.123498 PMCID: PMC3884930- Indian J Dermatol. 2014 Jan-Feb; 59(1): 60–66.
32. Relhan V, Goel K, Bansal S, Garg VK. Management of chronic paronychia-Indian J Dermatol. 2014 Jan-Feb; 59(1): 15–20; year=2014;volume=59; issue=1;spage=15;epage=20 DOI: 10.4103/0019-5154.123482 PMID: 2447065.
33. Ring J, Kowalzick L, Christophers E, Schill WB, Schöpf E, Ständer M, et al. Calcitriol 3 microg g-1 ointment in combination with ultraviolet B phototherapy for the treatment of plaque psoriasis: results of a comparative study. Br J Dermatol. 2001 Mar; 144(3):495-9.
34. Stoevesandt J, Hamm H. Transverse nasal novelties: a critical re-evaluation of the "allergic salute". Eur J Dermatol. 2013 Jul-Aug;23(4):526-7. doi: 10.1684/ejd.2013.2067.
35. The pathogenesis of psoriasis: A conundrum yet unresolved- Anil patki, Pune.
36. Uday Khopkar, et el. Urticaria: its rare forms. In: Dermatology, Sexually Transmitted Diseases and Leprosy. April 2002, issue number 31.
37. Wheeland RG, Dhawan S. Evaluation of self-treatment of mild-to-moderate facial acne with a blue light treatment system. J Drugs Dermatol. 2011 Jun;10(6):596-602.

38. Xu AE, Zhang DM, Wei XD, Huang B, Lu LJ. Efficacy and safety of tarcrolimus cream 0.1% in the treatment of vitiligo. Int J Dermatol. 2009 Jan;48(1):86-90. doi: 10.1111/j.1365-4632.2009.03852.x.
39. Yung-gang Lu, et el. Photodynamic therapy of port-wine stains. J Dermatolog Treat. 2010;2115-19.
40. Zirbs M, Reindel U, Hermann K, Church MK, Behrendt H, Ring J, Brockow K. Reduced skin reactivity to vasoconstrictor and vasodilator substances in atopic eczema. Eur J Dermatol. 2013 Nov-Dec;23(6):812-9. doi: 10.1684/ejd.2013.2191.

Further Reading

1. Behl PN. Practice of Dermatology, Second Edition, 1972.
2. Canter A. Changes is mood during incubation of a acute febrile disease and the effects of preexposure psychologic status Psychosom Med. 1972;34:424.
3. Cipla, Essence Series, HIV and AIDS, September, 2004.
4. Coe CL, et al. Mother - infant attachment in the squirrel monkey: Adrenal response to seperation. Behav Biol. 1978;22:256.
5. Desai SC. The Indian Practitioner. 1962;15:61.
6. Dilman VM. Metabolic immunodepression which increases the risk of Cancer. Lancet. 1977;2:1207.
7. Franken Haeser M. Experimental approaches to the study of human behaviour as related to neuroendocrine functions. In: L Levi (ed). Society, Stress and Disease Oxford University Press, New York. 1971;1:22.
8. Froberg J, et al. Physiological and biochemical stress reactions induced by psychosocial stimullin. In: L Levi (ed). Society, Stress and Disease. Oxford University Press, New York. 1971;1:20.
9. Fungus diseases in India, Published by Calcutta School of Tropical Medicine, 1962.
10. Galderma. Perspective in Clinical Dermatology, 2005;1.
11. Greenfield et al. Ego, strength and length of recovery from infections mono nucleosis. J Nerv Ment Dis. 1959;128:125.
12. Holdman L et al. Human fecal flora. Variation in bacterial composition within individual and a possible effect of emotional stress. Appl Eviron Microbiol. 1976;31:359.
13. Kasals SV, et al. Changes in serum uric acid and cholestrol levels in men under going job loss. JAMA. 1968;296:7500.

14. Katcher AH, et al. Prediction of the incidence of recurrent herpes labialis and systemic illness from psychological measurements. J Dent Res. 1973;52:49.
15. Khanna N. Dermatology and Sexually Transmitted Diseases. Modern Publishers, New Delhi, 2002.
16. Kramj, et al. Cutaneous immediate hypersenitivity in man - effect of systemically administered adrenergic drugs. J Allergy Clin immunol. 1975;56:387.
17. Krishnamurthi. Aid to Dermatology. Published by Geeta Devi, Bellary. First Edition, 1967.
18. Lahiri KD. A Treatise on Tropical Skin Diseases. Thakar spink and Co, Calcutta - First Edition, 1956.
19. Lawlor, Fischer, Adelman. Manual of Allergy and Immunology Little, Brown and Company, Boston/New York/Toronto/London, 3rd Edition, 1988.
20. Lewis and Wheeler. Practical Dermatology, WB Saunders Company London, 1967.
21. LIVA. Dermatology Update. 2005;35.
22. Luborsky L. et al. A Herpes simplex virus and moods, a longitudinal study. J Psychosom Res. 1976;29:543.
23. Pasricha JS. Treatement of Skin Diseases, Arnod-Heinemann, New Delhi.
24. Pillsbury DM, Shelly WB and Kligman AM. Dermatology. WB Saunders Co Philadelphia, London, First Edition, 1957.
25. Behl PN. Practice of Dermatology, Sixth Edition. CBS Publishers, and Distributors. Delhi, 1987.
26. Behl PN. Skin Diseases. Skin Institute, Jangpura, Delhi, 1976.
27. Punshi SK. A Clinical trial with tolnaftate in dermatomycosis. Mah Med Jr. March, 1969;15(12).
28. Punshi SK. A clinical trial with trisoralen in vitiligo. Mah. Medical Journal. 1969;16:313.
29. Punshi SK. Acne vulgaris. Mah Med Jr. September. 1968;15(6).
30. Punshi SK. A Hand Book of Vitiligo and Colour Atlas. Jaypee Brothers Medical Publishers, New Delhi, 2004.
31. Punshi SK. Alopecia. Mah Medical Journal. Jan 1968;14(10).
32. Punshi SK. Clinico therapeutic evaluation of Capyna Compound in leprosy and lepra reactions prob. Jan. March 1970;9(2).

33. Punshi SK. Cutaneous tuberculosis and its management. Souvenir—X Maharashtra tuberculosis and Chest Disease Conference, Amravati, Janevari, 1972.
34. Punshi SK. et al. Leprosy in children. The Indian Practitioner. Jan. 1970;23(1).
35. Punshi SK. Lepra reactions. Punjab Medical Journal. September 1970;20(2).
36. Punshi SK. Lepra reactions—etiology and treatment. Journal of the Academy of Medical Sciences, Nagpur Annual Number, 1970.
37. Punshi SK. Leucoderma "Voice of Homeopathy" Souvenir. All India Homeo Conference, Amravati, 1974.
38. Punshi SK. Liv 52 in vitiligo probe. Oct-Dec 1970;10(1): 12-3.
39. Punshi SK. Livoderm in Different types of Ulcers, Maharashtra Medical Journal December, 1967;14(9).
40. Punshi SK. Oil Dermatitis. Journal of Academy of Medical Sciences, Nagpur. Annual Number 1976-77.
41. Punshi SK. Recent trends and advances, in pigmentary disorders. Journal of the Academy of Medical Sciences, Nagpur, 1972-73.
42. Punshi SK. Role of biogenous stimulator, placental extract. All India Seminar on Biogenous Stimulators in Modern Treatment. Calcutta, April 1976.
43. Punshi SK. Scabies Common Skin disorder India. Journal BAMS College, Mozri, 1972.
44. Punshi SK. Skin Survey - Maharashtra Medical Journal. 1969;S6(8).
45. Punshi SK. Survey for vitiligo (school survey). J Acad Med Sc. Nagpur, 1975-76.
46. Punshi SK. Toxic effects of DDS therapy in leprosy. Mah Med Jr. September 1969;16(6).
47. Punshi SK. Use of B 663 in vitiligo - proceeding. Seminar on Leucoderma, Hyderabad published council for Research Unani Medical (Ministry of Health and Family Welfare, Government of India), New Delhi-1980, March 1979.
48. Punshi SK. Use of Bakuchi extract in vitiligo. Journal of Vid Ayur Mah. April 1970; p 17.

49. Punshi SK. Veneral affection in female genitalia. Punjab Medical Journal. 1971;21(5).
50. Punshi SK. "Topical use of Bouchi - Liver extract in vitiligo. Punjab Medical Journal. Volume June 1971;(20)11:417-420.
51. Punshi SK, et al. Vitiligo probe. 1969; p. 9,18.
52. RG Valia and Ameet R Valia. Dermatology Update. Bhalani Publishing House, Mumbai, India, 1998.
53. Sacher EJ. Neuroendocrine in depressive illness. In: Topics in Psychoendocrinology. Crune and Stratton, New York. 1975; p.135.
54. Saraf V, Fernandez R, Sarangi K. Vitiligo: A monograph and Color Atlas, First Edition. Fulford India Ltd, Oxford House, Mumbai. Jan 2000.
55. Sehgal VN. A Text Book of Veneral Diseases. Vikas Publishing House Pvt Ltd, New Delhi, First Edition, 1978.
56. Sulzberger MB. Dermatology Diagnosis and Treatment. Oxford and I.B.H. Publishing House, Calcutta, First Indian Edition, 1965.
57. Totman R, et al. Cognitive dissonance, stress and virus induced common colds. J Psychosom Res. 1977; p. 21,55.
58. Trasi MS. Management of early syphilis. Maharahstra, Medical Journal. July 1970;17(4).
59. Treatment of Common Disease, Published by British Medical Association, Tevistock Square WC, 1967.
60. Udary Khopkar. An Illustrated Hand Book of Skin and STDs with an Update on HIV Infection. Bhalani Book Depot, 1999.
61. Willcox RR. Text Book of Veneral Dieases, William Heinemann Medical Book, Second Edition, 1964.
62. Yawalkar SJ, Kuchbal SD, Deshpande. Acne vulgaris. Maharashtra Med Jr. December 1969;16(9).
63. Yawalkar SJ. Bombay J 4. 55-162.
64. Yawalkar SJ. Indian Med. Gaz 1962;22:28.
65. Yawalkar SJ. Leprosy For Practitioner, Popular Prakashn Bombay, First Edition, 1967.
66. Yawalkar SJ et al. Current drug therapy of leprosy. The Indian Practitioner. Jan 1969;22(1).

Index

Page numbers followed by *f* refer to figure and *t* refer to table

A

Abdomen 361*f*
Absorption 22
Acanthosis nigricans 195, 357
Acarus scabiei 42
Acne 188*f*, 191*f*, 195
    aggravate 238
    cysts of 196*f*
    juvenile 202*f*
    nodulocystis 242*f*
    propionibacterium 187
    rosacea 198
    scars, classification of 193
    systemic therapy of 190*t*
    topical therapy of 188*t*
    vulgaris 47*f*, 186-189, 196*f*, 197*f*, 202*f*, 204*f*, 206*f*, 207*f*, 241*f*
Actinomycetoma 106
Adams Oliver syndrome 394
Adjuvant triamcinolone acetonide injections 354
Advanced antiviral therapy simplifying herpes management 137*t*, 138*t*
AIDS 443
    related complex 448
Albinism 247
Allergic contact dermatitis 169, 170, 172, 172*t*, 174
Alopecia 42, 304, 335
    areata 235, 305, 314*f*-320*f*, 328*f*
Aminolevulinic acid for port-wine stains 366
Androgenetic alopecia 195, 306, 312, 325
Androgens 186
Angioedema 383
Angular cheilitis 84*f*, 464*f*
Ankylosing spondylitis 229*t*
Antifungal drugs, classification of 104*f*
Antihistamines 162
Anti-inflammatory drugs 388
Antiretroviral drugs 455*t*
Aphthous
    lesions 466
    ulcer 379
Apocrine glands 17
Arciform 43
Arms elbows, psoriasis of 244*f*
Arthritis 226*t*

Asteatotic eczema 180
Atopic
  dermatitis 47*f*, 148, 149, 150, 153, 156*f*, 179*t*, 185
  eczema 147, 151*f*, 152*f*
Atrophy 42
Autoimmune diseases 259*f*, 375
Azithromycin 238

B

Bacterial infection 63*f*, 89*f*, 153*f*
  pitted keratolysis therapy of 70
  treatment of 72
Bakuchi plants 163*f*
Basal cell carcinoma 355
Bichrome vitiligo 266*f*
Bindi dermatitis 171*f*
Blastomycosis 107
Body heat regulation 21
Borderline lepromatus 410
Borderline tuberculoid 410
Brain mind-body axis 6*f*
Bulla 34, 35*f*
Bullous impetigo 65*f*
Bullous lesions, classification of 337*t*
Bullous pemphigoid 344, 345
Butterfly rash 332, 334*f*, 335

C

Calcipotriol 230
Calcitriol 230
Calymmatobacterium granulomatis 435
Candida albicans 69, 87
Candidal
  balanoposthitis 86
  intertrigo 81, 82, 87
  paronychia 82, 85, 87
  vulvovaginitis 86
Candidiasis 81, 82
  synopsis of 87
Capitis 102
Carbuncle 68
Carotinemia 358
Cellulitis 70
Chancre 76
Chancroid 435, 440*f*
Chickenpox 127, 132*f*, 134*f*, 135*f*, 136*f*, 467*f*
Chlamydia trachomatis 433
Chlamydial urethritis 433
Chromophytosis 80
Chronic paronychia, management of 321
Clavus 358
Cleft lips 397*f*
Clotrimazole 88, 102
Cold urticaria 386*f*
Collagen vascular diseases 331
Comedones 42, 201*f*, 202*f*, 207*f*
Congenital melanocytic nevus 362*f*
Congenital syphilis 428, 429
  stigmata of 430
Congress grass 161*f*
Contact allergy 172
Contact
  dermatitis 148, 166*f*, 168*f*, 170*f*, 171*f*, 175*f*, 182*f*
  eczema 185*f*
Corporis 102

Crawling sensation 29
C-reactive protein 222
Cruris 102
Crust 38, 38f
Cryotherapy 123, 124
Cryptosporidium 449
Cutaneous
   hyperplasias 358
   infections 64
   infestations 52
   malformations 359
   neoplasms 355
   tuberculosis 73-76, 77t
Cyst 42
Cytocrine secretion 11

D

Deep fungal infections 102-106, 113
Deformities, correction of 412
Demodex folliculorum 62, 198
Dermatitis 140, 144-146, 146f, 155, 156, 158
   herpetiformis 346, 347
Dermatological diseases 27, 28, 30, 37
Dermatology, scope of 3
Dermatomycosis 80, 88
Dermis 18
   composition of 19f
Dermoepidermal
   bullae 344
   junction 19
Diabetes mellitus 88
Diaper dermatitis 92, 180, 185
   candidiasis 92

Diaper rash, development of 93f
Discoid lesions 332
Discoid lupus erythematosus 332, 333f
Dithranol 230
Donovanosis 435
Drug
   eruptions, therapy of 294
   reactions 293
Dry eczema 157f, 159f

E

Eccrine glands 17
Ecthyma 64
Ectoderm 22
Eczema 140, 141, 141f, 142f, 144-146, 155, 158, 176f, 374
   bilateral chronic 184f
   chemical 184f
   common patterns of 147
   of leg 183f
Elephantiasis 43
Encephalitis 449
Endogenous eczemas 141
Epidermal
   appendages 13
   cell multiplication cycle 11
Epidermis
   important cells of 12
   layers of 10
Epidermodysplasia verruciformis 121
Epidermophyton 90, 93, 97
Epidermopoiesis 12

Erosion 39, 40f
Erysipelas 70
Erythema 43
    multiforme 294, 296
    nodosum 348, 370
Erythematopapular lesions 32
Erythematosquamous 43
Erythematous papules 99f
Erythematous patches 130f, 132f
Erythrasma 67f
Erythroderma 43, 349, 350
Erythrodermic psoriasis 205
Exfoliative dermatitis 43, 349, 349f
Exogenous eczemas 141

F

Face 102
    fungus infection of 107f, 108f
    hyperpigmentation of 173f, 291f
    postherpetic scar on 136f
Facial eruptions 188f
Facial erythema 332
Famciclovir 137t
Feet, psoriasis of 223, 223f, 224f, 244f
Female pattern hair loss 308f
Filariasis 439
Filiform warts 117
Fissure 39
Fixed drug eruption 294, 295, 302f
Follicular keratinization 187
Folliculitis 36, 65

Foot 102
Fordyce spots 18
Fungal infections 79, 80, 81, 86, 87, 90, 91, 93, 94, 97, 108f-109f, 111f
Furfuracea 80
Furuncle 68
Furunculosis 36

G

Genital candidiasis 86, 87
Genital herpes 128
Genital ulcer 434, 441
Genital ulcerative disease 434
Genitalia 437t
Glans penis 429f
Gonorrhea 433f
    treatment of 432
Granular layer 10
Granules 102
Granuloma 44
    inguinale 436f
Granulomatous disorders 367
Gravitation eczema 178
Groin, fungus infection of 109f
Guttate psoriasis 205, 217f

H

Haemophilus ducreyi 435
Hair
    anatomy of 14f
    and nails, disorders of 304
    and scalp evaluation 327
    changes, types of 309f
    cycle 308f
    life cycle of 14, 15f
    regeneration therapy 328

Halo nevus 260, 288*f*
Hamilton-Norwood scale of male pattern baldness 307*f*
Hanging growth innocent tumor 396*f*
Hansen's disease 407
Head louse 60*f*
   life cycle of 59*f*
Headache, complaint of 278*f*
Heat, sense of 29
Hemangioma 360*f*
Herpes
   genitalis 136
   labialis 135
   lesions, distribution of 129*f*
   progenitalis 467*f*
   simplex 134, 466*f*
   zoster 127, 130, 130*f*, 131, 132, 132*f*, 133
      complications of 133
      typical lesions of 131*f*
Hidradenitis suppurativa 292, 392*t*, 293*t*
Hirsutism 311, 376
Histoplasmosis 106
HIV 222, 443, 450*f*
   disease 446
      intermediate stage 448
      late stage 448
   infection 445, 454, 458*t*, 461
      asymptomatic 446
      immunopathogenesis of 444
      mucocutaneous manifestations of 447*t*
      stages of 446
   transmission of 444
   vaccines 453
   virus 451*f*, 452*f*
Hollow nevus 359*f*
Horny layer 10, 44
HPV 125*f*, 126*f*
Human demodex mite 62
Human hair, structure of 14, 15*f*, 310*f*
Human immunodeficiency virus 443, 448*f*
Human papilloma virus (HPV) 116
Human viruses, classification of 114
Hydroquinone compound, application of 270*f*
Hyperandrogenism 195
Hyperpigmentation 142*f*, 272, 274*f*, 278*f*, 290*f*, 298*f*, 299*f*
Hypersensitivity phenomena 367, 374, 375
Hypertrichosis 313
   causes of 313*t*
Hypertrophic scar 378*f*, 379*f*
Hypopigmented patch 269*t*

I

Ichthyosis 382, 400, 401*t*
   acquired 400
   nigra 404
   vulgaris 401-403, 404*t*
Immune system, organs of 24
Immunosuppressive
   drugs 343
   therapy 88

Impetigo 64
    contagiosa 64, 65f, 66f
Incubation period 408
Infantile
    eczema 150, 151f, 153, 156f
    seborrheic dermatitis 154f
Infection scaling 142f
Inflammatory vitiligo 290
Ingrowing toenail, treatment
    of 313
Inguinal bubo 442
Insects, common types of 61f
Insulin resistance 195
Intertriginous
    candidiasis 84f
    pustular psoriasis 238
Inverse pityriasis rosea 240f
Irritant contact dermatitis 167,
    169
Isospora 449
Itchy erythematous 384f
Itraconazole 167

K

Keloid 358, 372f
Keratinocytes 11
Keratoderma 44, 400
Keratosis 44
Ketoconazole 167
Klebsiella 65
Koebner phenomenon 45, 116

L

Lamellar ichthyosis 403t
Late congenital syphilis 430
Latent HIV infection 446
Latent syphilis 427
Legs ulcer 67f
Lepra reactions
    classification of 409t
    treatment of 410
Lepromatus leprosy 410
Leprosy 81, 407-409, 414f
    control of 422
    deformities 420f
    prevention of 421
    recent advances in 421t
    rehabilitation in 422
    tuberculoid patch of 416f
Lesions of scabies, distribution
    of 53f
Leukemia 88
Leukoderma 264f, 287f, 289f
Lice infestation 58
Lichen
    nitidus 240f
    planus 183f, 239, 242f, 245f
    simplex chronicus 142f,
        143f, 173f, 176, 177, 182f
Lichenoid 45
Linear keloid 398f
Linear vitiligo 265
Lips, swelling of 399f
Louse, common types of 60f
Ludwig classification 308f
Lupus
    erythematosus 331, 333f
    valgaris 74f, 76
Lymph node structure 24f
Lymphogranuloma venereum
    439, 441f

M

Macule 30, 30*f*
Maculo-anesthetic leprosy, patch of 411*f*
Madura foot 102-106
Male pattern baldness 318*f*
Malignant melanoma 364*f*, 365*f*
Malignant tumor 449
Maxacalcitol 230
Medical Board of National Psoriasis Foundation 219
Meibomian gland 18
Melanin pigment
   classification of 13*f*
   pathway of 13*f*
Melanocyte 11, 12
   structure of 12*f*
Melanocytic nevi 360
Melanoma 356
Melasma 274
   area and severity index 284, 284*f*
Melisma
   classification of 271, 280*t*, 282
   management of 282
   treatment of 290
Mesoderm 22
Microsporum 90, 93
Miliaria 380
Miliary tuberculosis 73
Modified MASI scoring method 284
Moisturize skin 195
Molluscum contagiosum 115, 115*f*
Mosaic warts 117
Mucocutaneous candidiasis, chronic 86
Multiple sweat gland abscesses 69
Mycetoma 102-106
   organisms of 103*t*
Mycobacterium leprae 407, 413*f*
Mycobacterium tuberculosis 73, 74
Mycoplasma 433
   urethritis 433
Mycosis 79, 80, 81, 86, 87, 90, 91, 93, 94, 97

N

Nails 102, 313, 322
   functions of 17
   psoriasis of 196*f*, 216*f*
   structure of 16, 16*f*
Napkin candidiasis 90*f*
Neoplasms, benign 357
Neurodermatitis 177
Nevus achromicus 261*f*
Niacin deficiency 352
Nodules 201*f*, 204*f*
Non-steroidal topical immunomodulator 160
Non-viral infections 375
Norwegian scabies 55
Nummular eczema 177, 178
Nutritional deficiency 351
   anemia 321*f*
Nystatin 88

O

Opportunistic infections, treatment of 460*t*
Oral and nasopharyngeal ulceration 332
Oral candidiasis 84*f*, 86, 87, 465*f*
Oral therapy 283
Oral thrush 470*f*
Oropharyngeal pemphigus vulgaris 354
Osteoarthritis 229*t*
Outer root sheath 329

P

Pain killers 302*f*
Palmoplantar keratoderma 358
Palmoplantar psoriasis 218*f*
Palms
    contact dermatitis of 182*f*
    psoriasis of 218*f*, 231*f*
Papules 32, 32*f*, 201*f*, 202*f*, 204*f*, 206*f*, 207*f*
    and nodules, shapes of 45*t*
Papulosquamous diseases 200
Paronychia
    acute 69
    chronic 82, 85, 324
Parthenium hysterophorus 161*f*
Pediculosis 52, 58, 60*f*
    capitis 58
    corporis 59
    pubis 59
Pedis 102
Pellagra 352

Pemphigus 338, 339*f*, 340, 342, 343
    foliaceus 341*f*, 342*t*
    vulgaris 342*t*
Perifolliculitis decalvans 314*f*, 319*f*
Perioral dermatitis 198
Periorbital melanosis 271, 276*f*
Periorificial tuberculosis 73
Periporitis 69
Persistent generalized lymphadenopathy 446, 463*f*
Photodermatitis 173*f*
Photosensitive
    dermatoses 297, 374
    disorders, management of 303
Photosensitivity 297
    hyperpigmentation on face and arms 300*f*
Phototrichogram analysis 311, 325
Phrynoderma 351, 353*f*
    knees 183*f*
Phytophotodermatitis 161*f*, 163*f*
Pigmentation, disorders of 246
Pigmented nevus 361*f*
Pityriasis
    alba 273*f*
    rosea 238
    versicolor 50*f*, 80
Plaque psoriasis 216*f*
Pneumocystis carinii 443, 449
    pneumonia 469*f*
Pompholyx 174-176

Port-wine stains,
    photodynamic therapy of 366
Postchemical leukoderma 267f
Post-exposure prophylaxis 459, 462f
Prickle cell layer 10
Progressive multifocal leukoencephalopathy 469f
Propionibacterium 189
Prurigo mitis 379
Pruritus 28, 380
Pseudofolliculitis 66f
Pseudomonas 65, 70
Psoralea corylifolia plants 163f
Psoralen ointment, application of 175f
Psoriasis 48f, 200, 213f-215f, 217f, 222, 227, 228, 245f
    complications of 208
    management of 236
    treatment of 226
    vulgaris 210f, 227f, 228f, 231f, 233f, 234f, 235
Psoriatic arthritis 205, 214t, 229t, 236
Psychosoma 6f
Pubic louse 60f
Purpura 335
Pustular psoriasis 205
Pustules 36, 36f, 201f, 202f, 207f
PUVA therapy 263
Pyoderma 72f
    classification of 68
Pyogenic bacteria 64

Q

Quaternary syphilis 427

R

Radiculitis 449
Rash with fever 374
Raynaud's phenomenon 332
Refractory chronic urticarial, management of 388
Rheumatoid arthritis 229t
Ringworm 111f
Rodent ulcer 355
Rosacea 198
Round nodule 377f

S

Salicylic acid 283
Salivary gland enlargement 463f
Savin hair density scale 316f
Scabies 50f, 52, 53f
    treatment of 54f, 57t
    types of 54f
Scale 37, 37f
    hair 102
    psoriasis 225f
Scarring and nonscaring alopecia 305
Scars 41, 201f
Scleroderma 331
Scratch marks 381f, 396f
Scrofuloderma 73, 76
Sebaceous
    and sweat glands, disorders of 186
    cyst 376f
    glands 18, 21

Sebopsoriasis 205
Seborrhea 195
Seborrheic dermatitis 49*f*, 148, 162, 164, 165
   scalp 159, 166*f*
Seborrheic keratosis 357, 360, 363*f*
Segmental vitiligo 260*f*
Sense organ 20
Severe scalp psoriasis, treatment of 219
Sexually transmitted diseases (STDs) 423
Skin
   and internal disease 330
   color of 246, 252*f*
   diseases 2, 3, 8*f*
   embryology of 22
   immune system 22
      components of 23*f*
   irritation, physiology of 7*f*
   lesions, shapes of 46*t*
   malignant tumor of 355
   parasitosis 4*f*
   parts of 9*f*
   physiology of 20
   storage function of 21
   structure of 9, 10*f*, 14, 16-18
   tags soft warts 378*f*
   three layers of 11*f*
   tumors 355
Soft chancre 435
Soft skin 376*f*
Sole of feet, psoriasis of 244*f*
Spiny dry chronic knee 183*f*
Spongiosis 141
Sporothrix schenckii 106
Sporotrichosis 106
Squamous cell carcinoma 355
Stasis eczema 157*f*, 178
STDs
   practical management of 439
   prevention of 424
   syndromic management of 439
   vertical transmission of 425
Stevens-Johnson syndrome 294, 296
Stretch marks, development of 368*t*
Striae marks 397*f*
Strong irritants 167
Subcutaneous nodules 367
Superficial fungal infection 110*f*, 112*f*
   classical ring of 111*f*
Superficial plantar warts 117
Sutton's disease 359*f*
Sweat apparatus, common disorders of 199
Sweat glands 17
   types of 17*f*
Swelling 142*f*
Syphilis 426, 429*f*
   acquired 426
   therapy of 428
Systemic
   antibiotics 70
   candidiasis 86
   lupus erythematosus (SLE), skin manifestations of 332
   steroids 162
   therapy 160

T

Tacalcitol 230
Tazarotene, benefits of 234
Telangiectasia 45, 335
Telogen effluvium 306
Thayer Martin medium 432
Thoracic dermatome 130*f*
Thyroid insufficiency 327
Tichophyton 98
Tinea
    barbae 93
    capitis 90, 91, 96*f*, 99*f*
    corporis 89*f*, 93
    cruris 94, 95*f*, 96*f*, 99*f*, 110*f*, 113*f*
    faciei 88*f*
    manuum 85*f*, 88*f*, 97, 98, 102
    pedis 96*f*, 97, 98, 102
    unguium 97*f*, 98, 100*f*, 101*f*
    versicolor 80, 82*f*, 83*f*, 112*f*
Toxic epidermal necrolysis 296
Trichomonas 433
Trichophyton 90, 93, 97
Trichotillomania 324
Trophic ulcer 418*f*, 419*f*
Tuberculoid 409
    leprosy 415*f*
Tuberculosis
    cutis orificiales 77
    verrucosa cutis 75*f*, 76
Tuberculous
    chancre 73
    meningitis 469*f*

U

Ulcer 40, 40*f*, 437*t*
Urethral discharge 442
Urethritis 431, 432
    non-gonococcal 433, 434, 436*f*
Urticaria 383, 384*f*

V

Vaginal discharge 442
Valcivir 138*t*
Varicella 127
    zoster virus 127
Vascular nevus 360*f*
Vellus hair 14
Verruca
    plana 116, 121
    vulgaris 116, 117
Verrucous vegetations 45
Vesicobullous
    dermatoses, chronic 374
    disorders 337
    eruptions 339*f*
Vesicular
    erupion over abdomen 132*f*
    rash 373
Viral infections 114, 153, 374, 467*f*
Viral warts, types of 116, 121-123
Vitamin A deficiency 351
Vitamin B complex 352
Vitamin C 353
Vitamin E 353
Vitamin K 353
Vitiligo 81, 247, 247f-249*f*, 250, 252, 251*f*, 255f-258*f*, 261*f*, 265*f*, 286f-288*f*, 289*f*, 291*f*, 292*f*
    patches 175*f*
    treatment of 253, 253*f*, 285
    vulgaris 254*f*

W

Warts 116, 117, 118*f*, 119*f*, 139*f*
 anogenital 125*f*
 deep palmoplantar 117
 genital 121
 hanging 139*f*
 juvenile 124
 multiple 123*f*
 nasal 120*f*
 plane 119*f*, 120*f*, 121, 124
 removal of 123
 solitary 123*f*
 varieties of 124
Wrinkles, formation of 389

X

Xerotic eczema 147
X-linked ichthyosis 402*t*, 404-406

EU GSPR Authorised Reprsentative
Logos Europe, 9 rue Nicolas Poussin
1700, La Rochelle, France
Phone: +33 (0) 6 67 93 73 78
E-mail: contact@logoseurope.eu

www.ingramcontent.com/pod-product-compliance
Ingram Content Group UK Ltd.
Pitfield, Milton Keynes, MK11 3LW, UK
UKHW021827140426
52171PUK00016B/1233